Body Structures & Functions

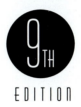

9TH EDITION

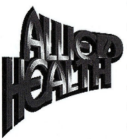

Body Structures & Functions

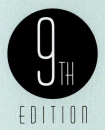

9TH EDITION

Ann Senisi Scott

Elizabeth Fong

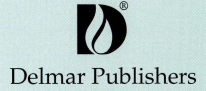

Delmar Publishers

an International Thomson Publishing company

Albany • Bonn • Boston • Cincinnati • Detroit • London • Madrid
Melbourne • Mexico City • New York • Pacific Grove • Paris • San Francisco
Singapore • Tokyo • Toronto • Washington

NOTICE TO THE READER

Delmar Staff

Publisher: Susan Simpfenderfer
Acquisitions Editor: Marlene McHugh Pratt
Developmental Editor: Helen Yackel
Team Assistant: Sandra Bruce

Art and Design Coordinator: Rich Killar
Production Manager: Linda Helfrich
Marketing Manager: Darryl L. Caron
Editorial Assistant: Sarah Holle

Cover art: courtesy of Brucie Rusch

COPYRIGHT © 1998
By Delmar Publishers
a division of International Thomson Publishing Inc.

The ITP logo is a trademark under license.

Printed in the United States of America

For more information, contact:

Delmar Publishers
3 Columbia Circle, Box 15015
Albany, New York 12212-5015

International Thomson Editores
Campos Eliseos 385, Piso 7
Col Polanco
11560 Mexico DF Mexico

International Thomson Publishing - Europe
Berkshire House 168-173
High Holborn
London, WC1V7AA
England

International Thomson Publishing GmbH
Königswinterer Strasse 418
53227 Bonn
Germany

Thomas Nelson Australia
102 Dodds Street
South Melbourne, 3205
Victoria, Australia

International Thomson Publishing Asia
221 Henderson Road
#05-10 Henderson Building
Singapore 0315

Nelson Canada
1120 Birchmount Road
Scarborough, Ontario
Canada, M1K 5G4

International Thomson Publishing - Japan
Hirakawacho Kyowa Building, 3F
2-2-1 Hirakawacho
Chiyoda-ku, Tokyo 102
Japan

1 2 3 4 5 6 7 8 9 10 XXX 03 02 01 00 99 98 97

Library of Congress Cataloging-in-Publication Data:
Scott, Ann Senisi, 1938-
      Body structures & functions. — 9th ed. / Ann Senisi Scott, Elizabeth Fong.
      p. cm.
      Rev. ed. of: Body structures & functions / Elizabeth Fong et al.
   8th ed. c1993.
      Includes bibliographical references and index.
      ISBN 0-8273-7897-1   hardcover
      ISBN 0-7668-0284-1   softcover
      1. Human physiology. 2. Human anatomy. 3. Nursing.   I. Fong,
   II. Body structures & functions.   III. Title.
   IV. Title: Body structures & functions.
   QP34.5.F66   1997
   612-dc21   97-21044
   CIP

CONTENTS

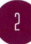

INTRODUCTION TO THE STRUCTURAL UNITS / 1

CHEMISTRY OF LIVING THINGS / 10

CELLS / 24

TISSUES AND MEMBRANES / 41

INTEGUMENTARY SYSTEM / 55

SKELETAL SYSTEM / 68

MUSCULAR SYSTEM / 92

CENTRAL NERVOUS SYSTEM / 113

THE PERIPHERAL AND AUTONOMIC NERVOUS SYSTEMS / 130

SPECIAL SENSES / 140

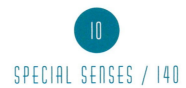

ENDOCRINE SYSTEM / 156

BLOOD / 179

HEART / 197

14

CIRCULATION AND BLOOD VESSELS / 219

15

THE LYMPHATIC SYSTEM AND IMMUNITY / 238

16

RESPIRATORY SYSTEM / 254

17

DIGESTIVE SYSTEM / 272

NUTRITION / 300

URINARY/EXCRETORY SYSTEM / 314

REPRODUCTIVE SYSTEM / 329

GENETICS AND GENETICALLY LINKED DISEASES / 356

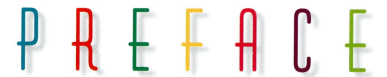

PREFACE

INTRODUCTION

The Ninth Edition of *Body Structures and Functions* has been revised to reflect the many changes that are occurring in today's health science and medical fields. The multiskilled health practitioner (MSHP) of today must know the structure and function of each body system as well as the common diseases. All diseases and disorders content is integrated within each chapter as appropriate.

The Ninth Edition has been reorganized based on customer feedback to present information in a more effective sequence. An expanded use of color and new computer-generated artwork have been added throughout to assist students in understanding each of the body systems.

Review the new "How to Study Using *Body Structures and Functions*" and "How to Use the Anatomy & Physiology CD-ROM" sections for a visual guide that will help you effectively use this learning system.

SPECIAL FEATURES

- Includes a free Anatomy and Physiology Challenge CD-ROM packaged with the text, highlighted by reference icons which appear throughout the text.

- New *Medical Highlights* give the student information on technology innovations, bioethical issues, and practical concepts.

- New *Career Profiles* provide descriptions of many health professions in today's dynamic health and medical environment.

- Reorganized chapters reflect a *more traditional organization* of anatomy and physiology, presented in an external to internal approach.

- *Key words* are listed at the beginning of each chapter, which are highlighted at the first occurrence, alerting learners to their use within the text.

- Expanded and well-organized *tables* summarize important concepts and information for ready reference.

- *End of chapter reviews* provide many critical thinking assignments, questions, and apply theory to practice exercises.

- Expanded comprehensive *glossary* of terms, with phonetic pronunciations of all entries

MAJOR CHANGES TO THE NINTH EDITION

- Chapter 2: Chemistry of Living Things—includes new information on matter and energy, isotopes, and electrolytes.

- Chapter 4: Tissues and Membranes—new tissues and membranes content.

- Chapter 5: Integumentary System—expanded with new information on burns, carcinomas, and melanoma cancers.

- Chapter 6: Skeletal System—reorganized: bone function, formation, structure, and growth, followed by bone types and disorders; additional information on arthritis, herniated disc, whiplash, and osteoporosis.

- Chapter 7: Muscular System—completely revised with additional information on muscular contractions, reorganized section of naming of skeletal muscles, and additional disorders including strain, spasm, myalgia, fibromyalgia, hernia, flatfeet, tetanus, torticollis, tennis elbow, and shin splints.

- Chapter 8: Central Nervous System—new information on brain and nerve connections, short- and long-term memory, and speech area. Completely revised information on multiple sclerosis and Alzheimer's Disease.

- Chapter 9: Peripheral and Autonomic Nervous System—new and reorganized content on functions.

- Chapter 10: Special Senses—new coverage on senses of smell and taste. Additional disorders include conjunctivitis, glaucoma, cataracts, macular degeneration, eye injuries, night and color blindness, hearing loss, Rhinitis, and deviated nasal septum.

- Chapter 11: Endocrine System—new content on hormones of pituitary gland, including vasopressin and oxytocin; new information on female hormones (estrogen and progesterone) and male hormone (testosterone); new information on pineal gland; new information on hypothyroidism and diabetes.

- Chapter 12: The Blood—clarified and revised throughout; new information on venipuncture by syringe and evacuated tube system.

- Chapter 13: The Heart—new and expanded information on circulation, heart sounds, ECGs, heart defects, and heart attacks including symptoms and prevention.

- Chapter 14: Circulation and Blood Vessels—new information on fetal circulation, pulse, peripheral vascular disease, and hypertension strokes.

- Chapter 15: Lymphatic System and Immunity—revised functions; new information on AIDS, Standard Precautions, and Personal Protective Equipment (PPE).

- Chapter 16: Respiratory System—revised functions; lung capacity and volume content; new content on hyperventilation, asthma, lung cancer, and pulmonary embolism.

- Chapter 17: Digestive System—reorganized for better sequence of information on digestive processes, new content on accessory organs (pancreas, liver, and gallbladder); new content on ingestion and digestion, gas formation, gastroesophageal reflux disease, diverticulosis, colon cancer, peptic ulcer, and hepatitis.

- Chapter 18: Nutrition—new information on fiber, cholesterol, and food labels.

- Chapter 19: Urinary and Excretory System—new content on urinary output, urinalysis, and hemodialysis.

- Chapter 20: Reproductive System—reorganized to provide a more logical sequence, new information on differentiation of reproductive system through embryonic stages, new table on hormones and functions, fertility, and contraception. New disorders include endometriosis, yeast infections, benign prostatic hypertrophy, and STDs.

Medical Highlight features include:

Career Profiles include:

SUPPLEMENTS

Student Workbook—includes activities that focus on applied academics through a variety of practical application exercises including multiple choice, fill-in-the-blank, matching, labeling, and word puzzles, basic skill problems, application of theory to practice, plus a Surf-the-Net feature.

Instructor's Manual—includes answers for all text review questions and workbook questions, as well as a comprehensive final examination.

ABOUT THE AUTHOR

Ann Senisi Scott is the author of the Ninth Edition of *Body Structures and Functions*. Ann is currently the Coordinator of Leadership Programs at Mount Mercy College, Cedar Rapids, Iowa, and was previously the Coordinator of Health Occupations and Practical Nursing at Nassau Tech Board of Cooperative Education Services, Westbury, New York. As the Health Occupations Coordinator, she worked to establish a career ladder program from health care worker to practical nurse. Before becoming the administrator of these programs, she taught Practical Nursing for over twelve years.

ACKNOWLEDGMENTS

The author of this edition wishes to thank the editors of Delmar Publishers, especially Helen Yackel, Developmental Editor who has guided and motivated me through this book. A special thanks to my husband, Wayne Scott, my personal reviewer, and my children, Vincent, Margaret, Carolyn, Daniel, Michael, and Kenneth, along with their spouses. I also want to say "thank you" to my students who made teaching a wonderful experience.

REVIEWERS

We are particularly grateful to the reviewers who continue to be a valuable resource in guiding this book as it evolves. Their insights, comments, suggestions, and attention to detail were very important in guiding the development of this textbook.

Patricia A. Stang CMA CPT
Medix School
Baltimore, MD

Sandra Shepherd
Sawyer College
Oxnard, CA

Betty White
Surrey Central High School
Dobson, NC

Tom Phelps
Poinciana High School
Kissimee, FL

Joseph Domenech MD
Blake Business School
New York, NY

Kathryn Dorsey
Huntington Junior College
Huntington, WV

Patricia Reichle RN
Simi Valley Adult School
Simi Valley, CA

Deborah Iles RN
Central Ohio J.U.S
Plain City, OH

John P. Siran MT (ASCP)
Denver Technical College
Colorado Springs, CO

Denise Abbott RN
Timpriew High School
Provo, UT

HOW TO STUDY USING
BODY STRUCTURES AND FUNCTIONS

Preview the text before attempting to study the material covered in the individual chapters. By reviewing each section of this textbook, you will better understand its organization and purpose. Reading comprehension and long-term memory levels improve dramatically when you take the time to review the text and learn how it can help you learn.

To get the most from this course, take an active role in your learning by integrating your senses to increase your retention. You may want to:

- *Visually* highlight important material.
- *Read* critically—turn headings, subheadings, and sentences into questions.
- *Recite* important material aloud in order to stimulate your auditory memory.
- *Draw* your own illustrations of anatomy or function processes and check them for accuracy.
- *Answer* (in writing or verbally) the review questions at the end of the chapter.
- *Play* the Anatomy & Physiology Challenge CD-ROM game on your own or with others, to effectively learn while having fun!

Each time you encounter a new chapter, preview it first to understand its overall structure. Review the **Objectives** presented at the beginning of each chapter to easily identify the key facts *before* you read the chapter. These objectives are also useful to review *after* you have completed a chapter. After reading a chapter, test yourself to see whether you can answer each objective. If you can't, you'll know exactly which areas to study again. The **key words** are listed at the beginning of each chapter, are highlighted in *blue* (at first usage) within the chapter and are also defined in the glossary.

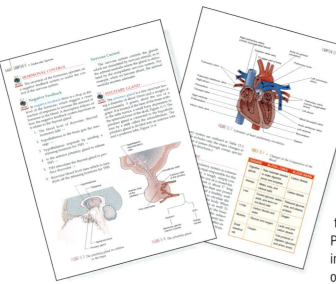

Read the **main headings**, **subheadings**, and first sentence of each paragraph—these elements serve as the outline for the whole chapter. Be careful not to overlook the **illustrations**, **photographs**, and **tables** to help you comprehend the difficult material. The **A&P Challenge Icons** highlight content that can be studied on the accompanying Anatomy & Physiology Challenge CD-ROM, a fun learning resource in a game format similar to Jeopardy™. The categories of the CD-ROM that are most appropriate for each chapter are listed on the page immediately before Chapter 1.

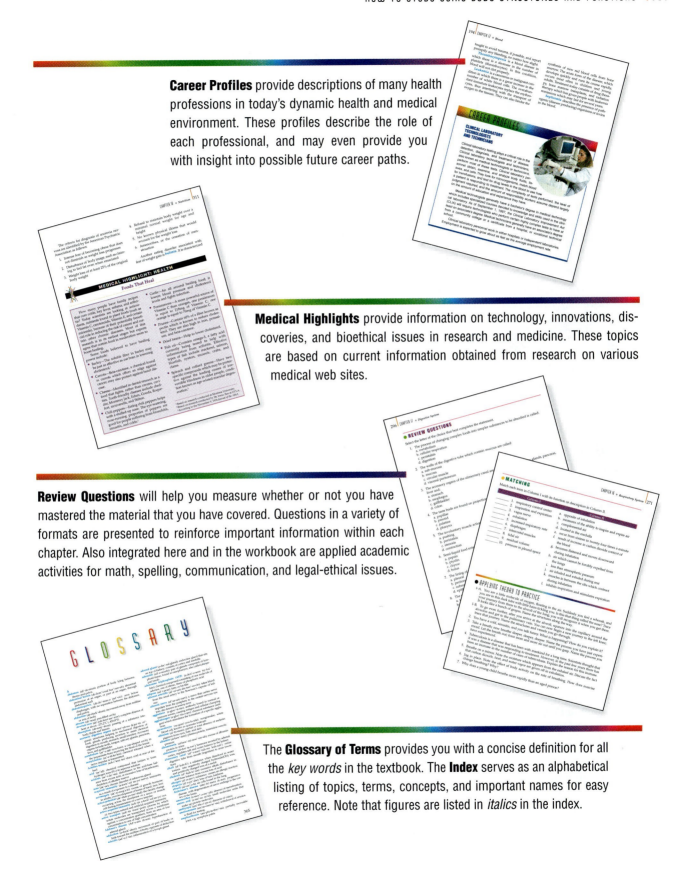

Career Profiles provide descriptions of many health professions in today's dynamic health and medical environment. These profiles describe the role of each professional, and may even provide you with insight into possible future career paths.

Medical Highlights provide information on technology, innovations, discoveries, and bioethical issues in research and medicine. These topics are based on current information obtained from research on various medical web sites.

Review Questions will help you measure whether or not you have mastered the material that you have covered. Questions in a variety of formats are presented to reinforce important information within each chapter. Also integrated here and in the workbook are applied academic activities for math, spelling, communication, and legal-ethical issues.

The **Glossary of Terms** provides you with a concise definition for all the *key words* in the textbook. The **Index** serves as an alphabetical listing of topics, terms, concepts, and important names for easy reference. Note that figures are listed in *italics* in the index.

HOW TO USE
THE A&P CHALLENGE CD-ROM

NEW ANATOMY & PHYSIOLOGY CHALLENGE

A new computer game has been added to the Ninth Edition. Delmar's Anatomy & Physiology Challenge is a great way to assess and reinforce your understanding of important anatomy & physiology principles and terminology for all major body systems. Assess your knowledge in a self-paced, non-competitive environment, or play in a team setting. Each game randomly draws from a bank of over 900 questions, so you never play the same game twice!

 The CD icon displayed throughout the text challenges students to test and reinforce their knowledge. The icon can be found next to major text topics that correspond to related coverage on the CD.

CATEGORIES

Overview of Anatomy & Physiology
Cellular Anatomy & Physiology
Biochemistry
Protective Structures and Systems
The Skeletal System
The Muscular System
The Cardiovascular System
The Blood and Lymphatic System

The Respiratory System
The Digestive System
The Renal System
The Endocrine System
The Nervous System
The Special Sense Organs
Human Reproduction

MINIMUM SYSTEM REQUIREMENTS

IBM-compatible computer
486 or higher, with CD-ROM drive

16 MB RAM
(800 x 600 x 256 colors)

OPERATING INSTRUCTIONS

1. Insert the CD into the CD-ROM drive.
2. From the Program Manager, select File → Run.
3. Type in D:\setup, where D: is the drive letter for the CD-ROM drive.
4. Follow the setup instructions from the installation procedure.

For Windows 95, most systems are set up to run a program as soon as a CD is inserted into the CD-ROM drive. In this case, the setup program runs automatically. If not, the following procedures can be used:
1. Insert the CD into the CD-ROM drive.
2. From the Start button, select Run.
3. Type in D:\setup, where D: is the drive letter of the CD-ROM drive.
4. Follow the setup instructions from the installation procedure.

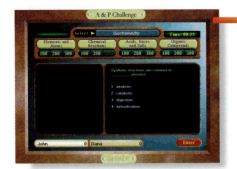

Game categories are organized into four subcategories. Select *point values* for each question; point values range in difficulty (100-easiest, 200-intermediate, 300-advanced). Play until all questions have been answered or until time runs out.

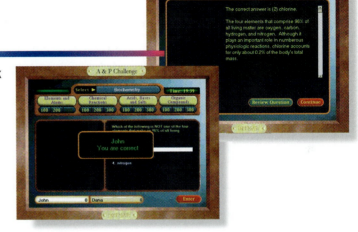

Answers are accompanied by feedback

One or two players, or teams can play the game.

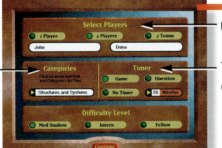

Up to 15 **categories** can be selected

The **timer** can be set for each question or for the entire game—you choose the duration.

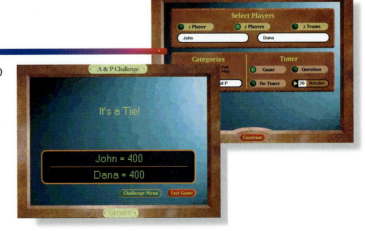

Once a game is completed, players can return to a new game, or take the **Final Challenge**.

CHAPTER CORRELATION
TO THE A&P CHALLENGE CD-ROM

For additional practice questions, refer to the following sections of the CD for each chapter.

Chapter	Challenge Sections
1. Introduction to the Structural Units	Overview of Anatomy and Physiology
2. Chemistry of Living Things	Overview of Anatomy and Physiology Biochemistry
3. Cells	Cellular Anatomy and Physiology
4. Tissues and Membranes	Overview of Anatomy and Physiology The Respiratory System The Digestive System
5. Integumentary System	Protective Structures and Systems
6. Skeletal System	The Skeletal System
7. Muscular System	The Muscular System
8. Central Nervous System	The Nervous System
9. The Peripheral and Autonomic Nervous System	The Nervous System
10. Special Senses	The Special Sense Organs
11. Endocrine System	The Endocrine System
12. Blood	The Blood and Lymphatic Systems
13. Heart	The Cardiovascular System
14. Circulation and Blood Vessels	The Cardiovascular System
15. The Lymphatic System and Immunity	The Blood and Lymphatic Systems
16. Respiratory System	The Respiratory System
17. Digestive System	The Digestive System
18. Nutrition	The Digestive System
19. Urinary/Excretory System	The Renal System
20. Reproductive System	Human Reproduction
21. Genetics and Genetically Linked Diseases	Human Reproduction

CHAPTER

1

Introduction to the Structural Units

OBJECTIVES

- Identify and discuss the different branches of anatomy
- Identify the terms referring to location, direction, planes, and sections of the body
- Identify the body cavities and the organs they contain
- Identify and discuss the life functions and related body systems
- Define the key words that relate to this chapter

KEY WORDS

abdominal cavity
abdominopelvic cavity
anabolism
anatomical position
anatomy
anterior
biology
buccal cavity
catabolism
caudal
comparative anatomy
coronal (frontal) plane
cranial
cranial cavity
cytology
deep
dermatology
developmental anatomy
distal

dorsal
dorsal cavity
embryology
endocrinology
epigastric
external
gross anatomy
histology
homeostasis
hypogastric region
inferior
internal
lateral
life function
medial
metabolism
microscopic anatomy
mid-sagittal plane
morphology
nasal cavity
neurology

oral cavity
orbital cavity
organs
organ system
pelvic cavity
planes
physiology
posterior
proximal
sagittal plane
section
spinal cavity
superficial
superior
systematic anatomy
thoracic cavity
tissues
transverse
umbilical
ventral

ANATOMY AND PHYSIOLOGY

Both anatomy and physiology are branches of a much larger science called biology. Biology is the study of all forms of life. Biology studies microscopic one-celled organisms, multicelled organisms, plants, animals, and humans.

Anatomy studies the shape and structure of an organism's body and the relationship of one body part to another. The word anatomy comes from the Greek, *ana*, meaning apart, and *temuein*, to cut; thus, the acquisition of knowledge on human anatomy comes basically from dissection. However, one cannot fully appreciate and understand anatomy without the study of its sister science, physiology. Physiology studies the function of each body part and how the functions of the various body parts coordinate to form a complete living organism.

Branches of Anatomy

Anatomy is subdivided into many branches based on the investigative techniques used, the type of knowledge sought after, or the parts of the body under study.

1. **Gross Anatomy.** Gross anatomy is the study of large and easily observable structures on an organism. This is done through dissection and visible inspection with the naked eye. In it the different body parts and regions are studied with regard to their general shape, external features, and main divisions. The study of shape is called morphology.

2. **Microscopic Anatomy.** With the invention and perfection of the microscope, the knowledge of gross anatomy can be extended down to the microscopic level. Microscopic anatomy is subdivided into two branches. One is called cytology, which is the study of the structure, function, and development of cells that make up the different body parts. For example, cytology can study the heart cells or the nerve cells comprising the brain. The other subdivision is histology, which studies the tissues and organs making up the entire body of an organism.

3. **Developmental Anatomy.** This part of anatomy studies the growth and development of an organism during its lifetime. More specifically, embryology studies the formation of an organism from the fertilized egg to birth.

4. **Comparative Anatomy.** Man is one of many animals found in the Animal Kingdom. The different body parts and organs of man can be studied with regard to similarities and differences to other animals in the Animal Kingdom.

5. **Systematic Anatomy.** Systematic anatomy is the study of the structure and function of various organs or parts making up a particular organ system. Depending upon the particular organ system under study, a specific term is applied, for example:

   a. dermatology—study of the integumentary system (skin, hair, and nails).
   b. endocrinology—study of the endocrine or hormonal system.
   c. neurology—study of the nervous system.

ANATOMIC TERMINOLOGY

In the study of anatomy and physiology, special words are used to describe the specific location of a structure or organ, or the relative position of one body part to another.

The following terms are used to describe the human body as it is standing in the anatomical position, Figure 1-1. A human being in such a position is standing erect, with face forward, arms at the side, and palms forward.

Terms Referring to Location or Position and Direction

● See Figure 1-2.

● anterior or ventral means "front" or "in front of." For example, the knees are located

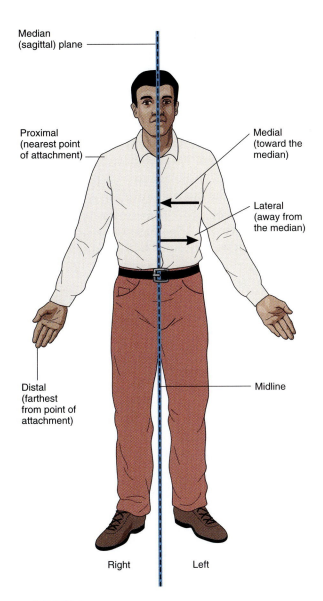

FIGURE 1-1 *Anatomical terms are used to describe body division into parts.*

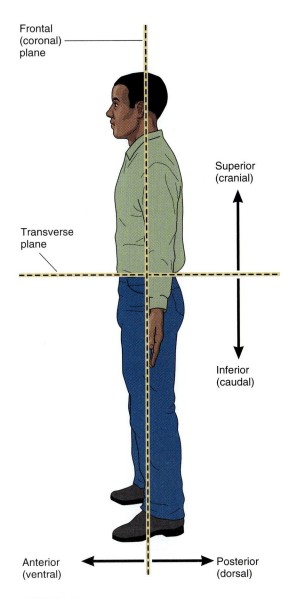

FIGURE 1-2 *Imaginary lines, or places, separate body structures.*

on the anterior surface of the human body. A ventral hernia may protrude from the front or belly of the abdomen.

- **posterior** or **dorsal** means "back" or "in back of." For example, human shoulder blades are found on the posterior surface of the body. The dorsal aspect of the foot is the back or sole of the foot.

- **cranial** and **caudal** refer to direction; cranial means the head end of the body, caudal means the tail end. For example, cranial pressure causes headache. Caudal anesthesia is injected in the lower spine.

- **superior** and **inferior**—superior means "upper" or "above another," inferior refers to "lower" or "below another." For example, the heart and lungs are situated superior to the diaphragm, while the intestines are inferior to it.

- **medial** and **lateral**—medial signifies "toward the mid-line or median plane of the body," while lateral means "away, or toward the side of the body."

- **proximal** and **distal**—proximal means "toward the point of attachment to the body, or toward the trunk of the body," distal means "away from the point of attachment or origin, or farthest from the trunk." For example, the hand is proximal to the wrist; the elbow is distal to the shoulder. Note: these two words are used primarily to describe the appendages or extremities.

- **superficial** or **external** and **deep** or **internal**—superficial implies on or near the surface of the body. For instance, a superficial wound just involves an injury to the outer skin. A deep injury involves damage to an internal organ such as the stomach. The terms external and internal are specifically used to refer to body cavities and hollow organs.

Terms Referring to Body Planes and Sections

Planes are imaginary anatomical dividing lines which are useful in separating body structures, Figure 1-2. A **section** is a cut made through the body in the direction of a certain plane.

The **sagittal plane** divides the body into right and left parts, (refer to Figures 1-1 and 1-2). If the plane started in the middle of the skull and proceeded down, bisecting the sternum and the vertebral column, the body would be divided equally into right and left halves. This would be known as the **mid-sagittal plane**.

A **coronal (frontal) plane** is a vertical cut at right angles to the sagittal plane, dividing the body into anterior and posterior portions. The term coronal comes from the coronal suture which runs perpendicular (at a right angle) to the sagittal suture. A **transverse** or cross section

is a horizontal cut that divides the body into upper and lower parts.

Terms Referring to Cavities of the Body

The organs which comprise most of the body systems are organized into four cavities: cranial, spinal, thoracic, and abdominopelvic, Figure 1-3. The cranial and spinal cavities are within a larger region known as the dorsal (posterior) cavity. The thoracic and abdominopelvic cavities are found in the ventral (anterior) cavity.

The **dorsal cavity** contains the brain and spinal cord: the brain is in the **cranial cavity** and the spinal cord is in the **spinal cavity**, see Figure 1-3. The diaphragm divides the ventral cavity into two parts: the upper thoracic and lower abdominopelvic.

The central area of the thoracic cavity is known as the mediastinum. It is between the lungs and extends from the sternum (breast bone) to the vertebrae of the back. The esophagus, bronchi, lungs, trachea, thymus gland, and heart are located in the thoracic cavity. The heart itself is contained within a smaller cavity, called the pericardial cavity.

The **thoracic cavity** is further subdivided into two pleural cavities: the left lung is in the left pleural cavity, the right lung is in the right. Each lung is covered with a thin membrane which we call the pleura.

The **abdominopelvic cavity** is really one large cavity with no separation between the abdomen and pelvis. In order to avoid confusion, this cavity is usually referred to separately—as the abdominal cavity and the pelvic cavity. The **abdominal cavity** contains the stomach, liver, gallbladder, pancreas, spleen, small intestine, appendix, and part of the large intestine. The kidneys are close to but behind the abdominal cavity.

The urinary bladder, the reproductive organs, the rectum, the remainder of the large intestine, and the appendix are in the **pelvic cavity**.

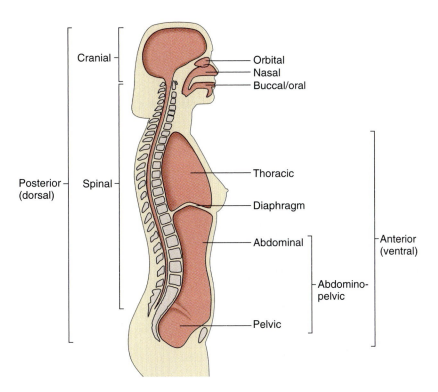

FIGURE I-3 *Cavities of the body*

 Terms Referring to Regions in the Abdominopelvic Cavity

In order to locate the abdominal and pelvic organs more easily, anatomists have subdivided the abdominopelvic cavity into nine regions, see Figure 1-4.

The nine regions are located in the upper, middle, and lower parts of the abdomen:

- *Upper*—or **epigastric** region located just below the sternum (breast bone) and the right hypochondriac and the left hypochondriac regions located below the ribs.

- *Middle*—or **umbilical** area located around the navel or umbilicus, the right lumbar region and the left lumbar region which extend from anterior to posterior. (A person will complain of back pain or lumbar sprain.)

- *Lower*—or **hypogastric region** which may also be referred to as the pubic area, the left iliac and right iliac which may also be called the left inguinal and right inguinal areas.

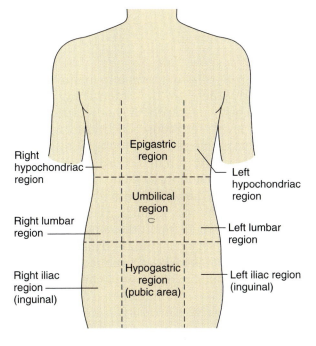

FIGURE I-4 *The nine regions of the abdominal area*

Smaller Cavities

In addition to the cranial cavity, the skull also contains several smaller cavities. The eyes, eyeball muscles, optic nerves, and lacrimal (tear) ducts are within the orbital cavity. The *nasal cavity* contains the parts that form the nose. The *oral* or *buccal* cavity encloses the teeth and tongue.

A & P CHALLENGE

LIFE FUNCTIONS

When we examine humans, plants, one-celled organisms, or multicelled organisms, we recognize that all of them have one thing in common: that of being alive.

All living organisms are capable of carrying on life functions. Life functions are a series of highly organized and related activities which help living organisms to live, grow, and maintain themselves.

These vital life functions include movement, ingestion, digestion, transport, respiration, synthesis, assimilation, growth, secretion, excretion, regulation (sensitivity) and reproduction, see Table 1-1.

A & P CHALLENGE

HUMAN DEVELOPMENT

A person is born, grows into maturity, and eventually dies. In the intervening years between birth and death, the body carries on a number of life functions which keep us alive and active. As is true of all living things, each one of us inherits a range of size, form, and a lifespan. We inherit these many characteristics through the gametes from our parents. Gametes are the sperm and egg cells.

Living depends upon the constant release of energy in every cell of the body. Powered by the energy that is released from food, the cells are able to maintain their own living condition and thus, the life of human beings.

A complex life form like a human being consists of over fifty thousand billion cells. Early in human development, certain groups of cells become highly specialized for specific functions, like movement or growth.

TABLE 1-1 • *Review of the Life Functions and Body Systems*

LIFE FUNCTIONS/ Body systems	DEFINITION
Movement / Muscle System	The ability of the whole organism—or a part of it—to move.
Ingestion / Digestive System	The process by which an organism takes in food.
Digestion / Digestive System	The breakdown of complex food molecules into simpler food molecules.
Transport / Circulatory System	The movement of necessary substances to, into, and around cells, and of cellular products and wastes out and away from cells.
Respiration / Respiratory System	The burning or oxidation of food molecules in a cell to release energy, water and carbon dioxide.
Synthesis / Digestive System	The combination of simple molecules into more complex molecules to help an organism build new tissue.
Assimilation / Digestive System	The transformation of digested food molecules into living tissue for growth and self-repair.
Growth / Skeletal System	The enlargement of an organism due to synthesis and assimilation, resulting in an increase in the number and size of its cells.
Secretion / Endocrine System	The formation and release of hormones from a cell or structure.
Excretion / Urinary System	The removal of metabolic waste products from an organism.
Regulation (sensitivity) / Nervous System	The ability of an organism to respond to its environment so as to maintain a balanced state (homeostasis).
Reproduction / Reproductive System	The ability of an organism to produce offspring with similar characteristics. This is *essential* for species survival as opposed to individual survival.

Special cells, grouped according to function, shape, size, and structure are called tissues. Tissues, in turn, form larger functional and structural units known as organs. For example, human skin is an organ made up of epithelial, connective, muscular, and nervous tissue. In much the same way, our kidneys are composed of highly specialized connective and epithelial tissue.

The organs of the human body do not operate independently. They function interdependently with one another to form a live, functioning organism. Some organs are grouped together because they are needed to perform a function. Such a grouping is called an organ system. One example is the digestive system composed of the teeth, esophagus, stomach, small intestine and large intestine. In this text you will study the various body systems and the organs which make up these systems.

BODY PROCESSES

A&P CHALLENGE

The functional activities of cells that result in growth, repair, energy release, use of food, and secretions are combined under the heading of metabolism. Metabolism consists of two processes which are opposite to each other: anabolism and catabolism. Anabolism is the building up of complex materials from simpler ones such as food and oxygen. Catabolism is the breaking down and changing of complex substances into simpler ones, with a release of energy and carbon dioxide. The sum of all the chemical reactions within a cell is, therefore, called metabolism.

The proper function and maintenance of the human body depends upon a number of activities. The body must constantly respond to changes in the environment by exchanging substances between its surroundings and its cells. Maintaining the body's cellular environment and function helps to insure regular body functions. Thus optimum cell functioning requires a stable cellular environment (within very narrow limits of acidity, nutrients, oxygen, temperature and fluid balance).

The maintenance of such (optimal) internal environmental conditions is known as homeostasis. Human survival depends on maintenance or restoration of homeostasis.

● REVIEW QUESTIONS

Select the letter of the choice that best completes the statement.

1. Anatomy is the study of:
   a. the structure of a body part
   b. the structure and function of a body part
   c. the function of a body part
   d. the formation of a body part

2. The study of the function of cells is called:
   a. anatomy
   b. physiology
   c. histology
   d. cytology

3. The anatomical position is described as:
   a. body erect, arms at the side, palms forward
   b. body supine, arms at the side, palms forward
   c. body erect, arms at the side, palms backward
   d. body supine, arms at the side, palms backward

4. A plane that divides the body into right and left parts is:
   a. transverse plane
   b. coronal plane
   c. sagittal plane
   d. frontal plane

5. If a wound occurred near the surface of the skin, it would be:
   a. deep
   b. superficial
   c. medial
   d. lateral

6. The heart is described as superior to the diaphragm because it is:
   a. in back of the diaphragm
   b. in front of the diaphragm
   c. above the diaphragm
   d. below the diaphragm

7. The brain and the spinal cavity are located in the:
   a. ventral cavity
   b. spinal cavity
   c. cranial cavity
   d. dorsal cavity

8. The epigastric region of the abdominal area is located:
   a. just above the sternum
   b. in the umbilical area
   c. just below the sternum
   d. in the pelvic area

9. The sum of the chemical reactions in a cell is known as:
   a. homeostasis
   b. metabolism
   c. anabolism
   d. catabolism

10. The formation and release of hormones from a cell or structure is called:
    a. digestion
    b. excretion
    c. synthesis
    d. secretion

● MATCHING

Match each term in Column I with its correct description in Column II.

Column I	Column II
_____ 1. catabolism	a. balanced cellular environment
_____ 2. pelvic cavity	b. constructive chemical processes which use food to build complex materials of the body
_____ 3. pericardial cavity	
_____ 4. anabolism	c. useful breakdown of food materials resulting in the release of energy
_____ 5. abdominal cavity	
_____ 6. diaphragm	d. contained within the oral cavity
_____ 7. homeostasis	e. cavity in which the reproductive organs, urinary bladder, and lower part of large intestine are located
_____ 8. tissue	
_____ 9. kidneys	f. cavity in which the stomach, liver, gallbladder, pancreas, spleen, appendix, cecum, and colon are located
_____ 10. teeth and tongue	
_____ 11. cranial cavity	g. the cavity containing the heart
_____ 12. organ system	h. a group of cells which together perform a particular job
	i. portion of the dorsal cavity containing the brain
	j. divides the ventral cavity into two regions
	k. structure located behind the abdominal cavity
	l. organs grouped together because they have a related function
	m. an activity that a living thing performs to help it live and grow

● APPLYING THEORY TO PRACTICE

1. In each of the examples below, choose the term which correctly describes the human body according to anatomical position:
   a. in the anatomical position the palms are forward or backward
   b. the liver is superior or inferior to the diaphragm
   c. the hand is proximal or distal to the elbow
   d. the sole of the foot is on the anterior or posterior part of the body
   e. cranial refers to the head or tail end of the body
   f. the coronal plane divides the body into front and back or right and left sections
   g. the arms are located on the medial or lateral side of the body
   h. the transverse plane divides the body into superior and inferior or anterior and posterior parts

2. Describe the following to a physician using the correct anatomical term:
   a. the location of an appendectomy scar
   b. a wound that is on the front of the leg
   c. the end of the spine
   d. a pain near the breast bone

3. Think about what your body does within a twenty-four hour period and name the life functions that take place.

CHAPTER

2

Chemistry of Living Things

OBJECTIVES

- Relate the importance of chemistry and biochemistry to health care
- Define matter and energy
- Explain the structure of an atom, an element and a compound
- Describe the four main groups of organic compounds: carbohydrates, fats, proteins, and nucleic acids
- Explain the difference between the DNA molecule and the RNA molecule
- Explain the difference between an acid, base, and salt
- Describe why homeostasis is necessary for good health
- Define the key words that relate to this chapter

KEY WORDS

acid
alkali
amino acid
atom
base
biochemistry
buffer
carbohydrate
chemistry
cholesterol
coenzyme
compound
deoxyribonucleic
   acid (DNA)
disaccharide
electrolytes

element
energy
enzyme
extracellular fluid
fat (triglyceride)
glycogen
hydroxide
intracellular fluid
ion
isotopes
kinetic energy
lipid
matter
molecule
monosaccharide
multicellular

neutralization
nucleic acid
organic catalyst
organic compound
pH scale
phospholipid
polysaccharide
potential energy
property
radioactive
ribonucleic acid
   (RNA)
salt
steroid
unicellular

In order for an individual to be an effective health care professional, an understanding of the normal and abnormal functioning of the human body is essential. A knowledge of basic chemistry and biochemistry is needed.

CHEMISTRY

Chemistry is the study of the structure of matter, the composition of substances, their properties, and their chemical reactions. There are many chemical reactions that occur in the human body. These reactions can range from the digestion of a piece of meat in the stomach and formation of urine in the kidneys to the manufacture of proteins in a microscopic human cell. Ultimately, the chemical reactions necessary to sustain life occur in the cells. Thus, the study of the chemical reactions of living things is called biochemistry.

MATTER AND ENERGY

Chemistry studies the nature of matter and how its atoms are put together and interact with each other. Matter is defined as anything that has weight (mass) and occupies space. Matter exists in the forms of solid, liquid, and gas. An example in our bodies of solid matter is bone; liquid matter is blood; gas is oxygen.

Matter is neither created nor destroyed, but it can change form through physical or chemical means. A physical change occurs when we chew a piece of food and it breaks up into smaller pieces. A chemical change occurs when the food is acted on by various chemicals in the body to change its composition. For example, imagine a piece of toast that becomes molecules of fat and glucose to be used by the body for energy.

Energy is defined as the ability to do work or to put matter into motion. Energy exists in our body as potential energy or kinetic energy. Potential energy is energy stored in cells waiting to be released, while kinetic energy is work resulting in motion. Lying in bed is an example of potential energy; getting out of bed is an example of kinetic energy.

ATOMS

An atom is the smallest piece of an element. Atoms are invisible to the human eye, yet they are all around us everywhere and are part of our human structure. Hydrogen is an example of an atom.

The normal atom is made up of subatomic particles: protons, neutrons and electrons. The protons have a positive (+) electric charge; the neutrons have no electric charge. The protons and the neutrons make up the nucleus of the atom (which differs from the nucleus of the cell), Figure 2-1. The electrons have a negative

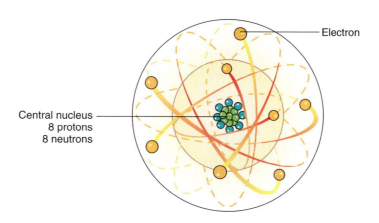

Electron

Central nucleus
8 protons
8 neutrons

FIGURE 2-1 *Structure of an atom. Eight protons and eight neutrons are tightly bound in the central nucleus, around which the eight electrons revolve.*

(–) electric charge and are arranged around the nucleus in orbital zones or electron shells. Atoms usually have more than one electron shell. The arrangement of the subatomic particles is how the atoms of one element differ from atoms of another element; the structure of the hydrogen atom is different from the structure of the oxygen atom.

The number of protons of an atom is equal to the number of electrons; atoms are electrically neutral, neither negative or positive. An atom can share or combine an electron with another atom to form a chemical bond. If one atom gives up an electron to another atom to form this bond, it will now have more protons than electrons and will have a positive charge. The atom which took the extra electron will now have more electrons than protons and have a negative charge. These charged atoms are then called ions.

Atoms of a specific element that have the same number of protons but different number of neutrons are called isotopes. All isotopes of a specific element have the same number of electrons. Certain isotopes are called radioactive isotopes because they are unstable and may decay (come apart). As they decay they give off (emit) energy in the form of radiation which can be picked up by a detector. The detector not only detects the emission from a radioactive isotope but, with the aid of a computer, can also form the image of its distribution within the body. Radioactive isotopes can be used to study structure and function of particular tissue. In addition, strong radiation from certain isotopes may destroy body tissue. This radiation is useful in the treatment of cancer and other diseases.

MEDICAL HIGHLIGHT: TECHNOLOGY

Medical Imaging

In 1950, nuclear medicine was introduced that used radionuclides (also known as radioisotopes) to scan the body. This innovative technique was hailed as a diagnostic breakthrough. It can be used to identify abnormal and normal body structures that are unable to be seen by x-ray. Since the 1970s, we have seen the development of Computerized Axial Tomography (CAT or CT scan), Positron Emission Tomography (PET scan), Sonography, and Magnetic Resonance Imaging (MRI).

CAT or CT scan combines x-ray emission with nuclear medicine in order to look inside the body. The images produced are cross-sectional, patterned much like slices of bread. By taking a series of such images a CAT scan can create a multi-dimension view of the body. The main feature of the equipment is a large "ring." The patient passes through the ring while the x-ray tube rotates 360 degrees around the patient and takes pictures. After taking many pictures, the computer has enough information to combine segments of the pictures and create views of the internal organs. These views are projected onto a television screen. Still photos are taken to record significant findings. CAT scans have all but eliminated exploratory surgery. They are most useful in evaluating brain and abdominal findings.

Positron Emission Tomography or PET scan is a procedure in which the patient is given an injection of a short lived radionuclide and then positioned in the PET scanner. The radionuclides are absorbed by active brain cells and high energy gamma rays are released as a result. A computer analyzes these rays and produces a color picture of the brain's biochemical activity. The patient must remain alert for this test. Blindfolds and earplugs may be used to reduce external stimuli to the brain. The patient is also asked questions or told to recite to see how the brain activity changes for reasoning and remembering. PET scans are most useful to diagnose the effects of stroke, some aspects of Alzheimer's disease, epilepsy, and mental illness.

Sonography or ultrasound imaging uses high frequency sound waves for diagnostic purposes. Ultrasound is completely noninvasive and uses no radiation. To date, no harmful effects on living tissue have been noted. Sound waves are sent into the body tissues by a small transducer, which also receives returning sound echoes which are deflected back as they bounce off various internal structures. (A transducer is a device that changes electrical energy into sound waves.) The returning sound waves are converted into electric signals which are fed into a computer. The computer transforms the signals into scans or graphs which are used to construct visual images of the body. This is the imaging choice for obstetrics to visualize the fetal embryo and placenta. It is useful to examine the pelvic and abdominal areas. The Doppler method is a variation of sonography in which returning sound waves are transformed into audible sounds which can be detected by earphones. Doppler method measures blood flow by moving the transducer along the path of a blood vessel. Data can be

obtained concerning the velocity of flow in the area over which the transducer moves.

Magnetic Resonance Imaging or MRI uses a magnetic field along with radio frequency waves to produce cross-section images of the body. The patient is inserted into a chamber that is built within a huge magnet. The magnetic field causes the atomic ions in the tissue to line up in a parallel fashion. Radio waves are sent into the patient and the lined up ions pick up this energy and change their orientation. When the radio waves are turned off, the ions revert back to the lined up fashion produced by the magnetic field. These changes in the energy field are sensed and translated by a computer into a visual image. MRI is a good diagnostic tool for degenerative disease such as multiple sclerosis. Caution must be used, however, since strong magnetic fields may damage pacemakers and metal protheses such as hips and knees. Patients must remove all hair clips, jewelry, and watches when receiving an MRI.

Health care workers must be aware of the anxiety people feel when they see the huge CAT scan and MRI machines. Patient education is critical. Explain to the patient that they may hear loud noises which are common during the test. No one can be in the room with them during the test but a technician will always be in voice contact with the patient.

ELEMENTS

Atoms which are alike combine to form the next stage of matter which is an **element**. An element is a substance which can neither be created nor destroyed by ordinary means. Elements can exist in more than one phase in our bodies. Our bones are solid and contain the element calcium. The air we take into our lungs contains the element oxygen which is a gas. Our cells are bathed in fluids which contain the elements of hydrogen and oxygen. When these two elements unite they form water.

There are ninety-two elements found naturally in our world; additional elements have

been man-made by scientists. Each of the elements is represented by a chemical symbol or an abbreviation. Table 2-1 shows a sampling of elements and their chemical symbols.

COMPOUNDS

Various elements can combine together, in a definite proportion by weight, to form **compounds**. A compound has different characteristics or properties from the elements that make them up. For example, the compound water (H_2O) is made of two parts of hydrogen and one part of oxygen. Separately hydrogen

TABLE 2-1 • *Some Sample Elements and their Symbols*

ELEMENT	SYMBOL
Calcium	Ca
Carbon	C
Chlorine	Cl
Hydrogen	H
Iodine	I
Iron	Fe
Magnesium	Mg
Nitrogen	N
Oxygen	O
Phosphorus	P
Potassium	K
Sodium	NA
Zinc	Zn

and oxygen are gaseous elements, but when combined together to form water, the resulting compound is a liquid. Common table salt is a compound made from the two elements sodium (Na) and chlorine (Cl), and it is chemically called sodium chloride (NaCl). Separately, sodium is a metallic element. It is light, silver-white, and shiny when freshly cut, but rapidly becomes dull and gray when exposed to air. Chlorine, on the other hand, is an irritating, greenish-yellow poisonous gas with a very suffocating odor. However, the chemical combination of both sodium and chlorine results in sodium chloride, which is a crystalline powder that can be dissolved in water.

Just as elements are represented by symbols, compounds are represented by something called a formula. A formula shows the types of elements present and the proportion of each element present by weight. Some common formulas are H_2O (water), NaCl (common table salt), HCl (hydrogen chloride or hydrochloric acid), $NaHCO_3$ (sodium bicarbonate or baking powder), NaOH (sodium hydroxide or lye), $C_6H_{12}O_6$ (glucose or grape sugar), $C_{12}H_{22}O_{11}$ (sucrose or common table sugar), CO_2 (carbon dioxide), and CO (carbon monoxide).

A living organism, whether it is a **unicellular** (one-celled) microbe or a **multicellular** animal or plant, can be compared to a chemical factory. Most living organisms will take the twenty essential elements and change them into needed compounds for the maintenance of the organism. In many living organisms, the elements carbon, hydrogen, and oxygen are united to form **organic compounds** (compounds found in living things containing the element carbon). One group of organic compounds manufactured are carbohydrates, such as sugars and starches.

Molecules

The smallest unit of a compound that still has the properties of the compound and has the capability to lead its own stable and independent existence is called a **molecule**. For example, the common compound water can be broken down into smaller and smaller droplets. Finally, when the absolutely smallest unit is reached, one has a molecule of water, H_2O.

A & P
CHALLENGE

IONS AND ELECTROLYTES

In addition to combining to form elements, atoms can share or combine their electrons with other atoms to form chemical bonds. If one atom gives up an electron to another atom to form a bond, it will have more protons than electrons and will have a positive (+) charge. The atom that took the extra electron will now have more electrons than protons and have a negative (-) charge. Such a positively or negatively charged particle is called an **ion**. The attraction between the opposite charges produces an ionic bond.

When compounds are in solution and they act as if they have broken into individual pieces (ions), the elements of the compound are **electrolytes**. For example, a salt solution consists of sodium (Na^+) ions with a positive charge and chlorine (Cl^-) ions with a negative charge.

In the cells and tissue fluids of the body, ions make it possible for materials to be altered, broken down, and recombined to form new substances or compounds. Electrolytes are responsible for the acidity or alkalinity of solutions and can conduct an electrical charge.

The ability to record electric charges within the tissue are invaluable for diagnostic tools such as an electrocardiogram, which measures the electrical conduction of the heart.

TYPES OF COMPOUNDS

The various elements can combine to form a great number of compounds. All known compounds, whether natural or synthetic, can be classified into two groups: inorganic compounds and organic compounds.

Inorganic Compounds

Inorganic compounds are made of molecules that do not contain the element carbon (C). A few exceptions are carbon dioxide (CO_2) and calcium carbonate ($CaCO_3$). Water is an inorganic compound and makes up between fifty-five to sixty-five % of body weight. Water is the most important inorganic compound to living organisms.

Organic Compounds

Organic compounds are compounds found in living things and the products they make. These compounds always contain the element carbon combined with hydrogen and other elements. Carbon has the ability to combine with other carbons and other elements to form a large number of organic compounds. There are more than a million known organic compounds. Their molecules are comparatively large and very complex. By comparison, inorganic molecules are much smaller. There are four main groups of organic compounds: carbohydrates, lipids, proteins, and nucleic acids.

CARBOHYDRATES

All carbohydrates are compounds composed of the elements carbon (C), hydrogen (H), and oxygen (O). These compounds have twice as many hydrogen as oxygen and carbon atoms. Carbohydrates are divided into three groups. They are the monosaccharides, disaccharides, and polysaccharides.

Monosaccharides

Monosaccharides (from the Greek words *mono*, meaning one, and *sakcharon*, meaning sugar) are sugars that cannot be broken down any further. Hence, they are also called single or simple sugars. The types of monosaccharide sugars are glucose, fructose, galactose, ribose, and deoxyribose.

Glucose is a very important sugar. It is the main source of energy in cells. Glucose, sometimes referred to as blood sugar, is carried by the bloodstream to individual cells, and is stored in the form of glycogen in the liver and muscle cells. Glucose combines with oxygen in a chemical reaction called oxidation that produces energy.

Fructose is the sweetest of the monosaccharides and is found in fruit and honey. Deoxyribose sugar is found in deoxyribonucleic acid (DNA) and ribose sugar is found in ribonucleic acid (RNA).

Disaccharides

A disaccharide is known as a double sugar because it is formed from two monosaccharide molecules by a chemical reaction called dehydration synthesis. Dehydration synthesis involves the synthesis of a large molecule from small ones by the loss of a molecule of water. Table 2-2 illustrates the process of dehydration synthesis.

TABLE 2-2 • *The Monosaccharide Composition of Sucrose, Maltose, and Lactose*

MONOSACCHARIDE + MONOSACCHARIDE - H₂O (DEHYDRATION SYNTHESIS)	FORMS	DISACCHARIDE
Glucose + Fructose - H_2O	⟶	Sucrose
Glucose + Glucose - H_2O	⟶	Maltose
Glucose + Galactose - H_2O	⟶	Lactose

The opposite reaction to dehydration synthesis is hydrolysis. In this reaction, a large molecule is broken down into smaller molecules by the addition of water. Examples of disaccharides are sucrose (table sugar), maltose (malt sugar), and lactose (milk sugar).

Disaccharides must be broken down by the process of digestion to monosaccharides to be absorbed and used by the body.

Polysaccharides

A large number of carbohydrates found in or made by living organisms and microbes are polysaccharides. Polysaccharides are large, complex molecules made up of hundreds to thousands of glucose molecules bonded together in one long chainlike molecule. Examples of polysaccharides are starch, cellulose, and glycogen. Under the proper conditions, polysaccharides can be broken down into disaccharides and then finally into monosaccharides. Starch is a polysaccharide found in grain products and root vegetables such as potatoes. Cellulose is the main structural component of plant tissue.

LIPIDS

Lipids are molecules containing the elements carbon, hydrogen, and oxygen. Lipids are different from carbohydrates because there is proportionately much less oxygen in relation to hydrogen. Examples of lipids are fats, phospholipids and steroids.

Characteristics of Lipids

Everywhere you look today you see the words "no fat," and yet lipids or fats are essential to health. Lipids are an important source of stored energy. They make up the essential steroid hormones and help to insulate our bodies. It is when the intake of lipids in the form of fat becomes excessive that a health problem may occur.

Fats are made up of glycerol and fatty acids. Fats also may be known as triglycerides.

This type of lipid is the most abundant in the body.

Phospholipids are lipids which contain carbon, hydrogen, oxygen and phosphorus. This type of lipid may be found in the cell membranes, the brain and the nervous tissue.

Steroids are the lipids which contain cholesterol. Cholesterol is essential in the structure of the semi-permeable membrane of the cell. It is necessary in the manufacture of Vitamin D and in the production of male and female hormones. Cholesterol is needed to make the adrenal hormone cortisol. However, in certain people, cholesterol can accumulate in the arteries, becoming a problem. The most common food sources of cholesterol are meat, eggs and cheese. Yet, even without these food sources, the liver will still manufacture cholesterol.

PROTEINS

Proteins are organic compounds containing the elements carbon, hydrogen, oxygen, and nitrogen and, most times, phosphorus and sulfur. Proteins are among the most diverse and essential organic compounds found in all living organisms. Proteins are found in every part of a living cell. Proteins are also an important part of the outer protein coat of all viruses. Proteins also serve as binding and structural components of all living things. For example, large amounts of protein are found in fingernails, hair, cartilage, ligaments, tendons, and muscle.

The small molecular units that make up the very large protein molecules are called amino acids. There are twenty-two different amino acids that can be combined in any number and sequence to make up the various kinds of proteins.

Table 2-3 gives a list of the nine essential amino acids. Essential amino acids must be ingested because they cannot be made by the body.

Large protein molecules are constructed from any number and sequence of these amino acids. The number of amino acids in any given protein molecule can number from 300 to several thousand. Therefore, the structure of proteins is quite complicated.

TABLE 2-3 • *The Nine Essential Amino Acids*

ESSENTIAL AMINO ACIDS	SYMBOL
Histidine	His
Isoleucine	Ileu
Leucine	Leu
Lysine	Lys
Methionine	Met
Phenylalanine	Phe
Threonine	Trp
Tryptophan	Try
Valine	Val

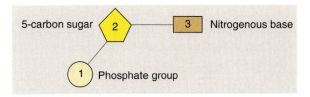

FIGURE 2-2 *Structure of a typical nucleotide*

ENZYMES

Enzymes are specialized protein molecules that are found in all living cells. They help to finely control the various chemical reactions occurring in a cell, so each reaction occurs at just the right moment and at the right speed. Enzymes help provide energy for the cell, assist in the making of new cell parts, and control almost every process in a cell. Because enzymes are capable of such activity, they are known as **organic catalysts**. An enzyme or organic catalyst affects the rate or speed of a chemical reaction without itself being changed. Enzymes can also be used over and over again. An enzyme molecule is highly specific in its action. Enzymes are made up of all protein or part protein (apoenzyme) attached to a nonprotein part (**coenzyme**).

The name of an enzyme usually ends in *-ase*.

NUCLEIC ACIDS

Nucleic acids are very important organic compounds containing the elements carbon, oxygen, hydrogen, nitrogen, and phosphorus. There are two major types of nucleic acids: one is **deoxyribonucleic acid** (**DNA**) and the other is **ribonucleic acid** (**RNA**).

Structure of Nucleic Acids

Nucleic acids are the largest known organic molecules. They are very high molecular-weight polymers made from thousands of smaller, repeating subunits called nucleotides. A nucleotide is a very complex molecule. It is composed of three different molecular groups. Figure 2-2 shows a typical nucleotide. Group 1 is a phosphate or phosphoric acid group, H_3PO_4, while group 2 represents a five-carbon sugar. Depending upon the nucleotide, the sugar could be either a ribose or a deoxyribose sugar. Finally, group 3 represents a nitrogenous base. There are two groups of nitrogenous bases: one is the purines and the other is the pyrimidines. The purines are either adenine (A) or guanine (G), while the pyrimidines are cytosine (C) and thymine (T).

DNA Structure and Function

DNA is involved in the process of heredity. The nucleus of every human cell contains forty-six (twenty-three pairs of) chromosomes, which is a long coiled molecule of DNA. The chromosomes contain about 100,000 genes. This genetic information tells a cell what structure it will possess and what function it will have. The DNA molecule passes on this genetic information from one generation to the next.

DNA is a double-stranded molecule referred to as a double helix. This structure resembles a twisted ladder. The sides of the ladder are formed by alternating bands of a sugar (deoxyribose) unit and a phosphate unit. The rungs of the ladder are formed by the nitrogenous bases which always pair in specific ways: thymine (T) pairs with adenine (A), and cytosine (C) pairs with guanine (G), Figure 2-3.

RNA Structure and Function

The RNA nucleotide consists of a phosphate group, the ribose sugar, and any one of

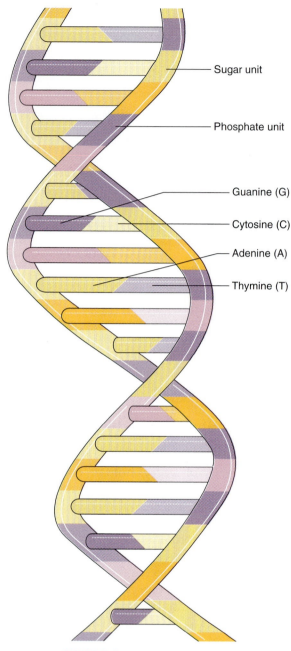

Sugar unit

Phosphate unit

Guanine (G)

Cytosine (C)

Adenine (A)

Thymine (T)

FIGURE 2-3 *Schematic of DNA*

Messenger RNA carries the instructions for protein synthesis from the DNA molecule located in the nucleus of a cell into the cytoplasm. The m-RNA molecule carries the code for protein synthesis from the DNA in the nucleus to the ribosomes in the cytoplasm. The transfer RNA molecule picks up amino acid molecules in the cytoplasm and transfers them to the ribosomes where they are put together to form proteins. The ribosomal RNA helps in the attachment of the m-RNA to the ribosome. Table 2-4 shows the basic differences between the DNA molecule and the RNA molecule.

ACIDS, BASES, AND SALTS

Before ending the discussion of basic chemistry and biochemistry, a brief discussion of acids, bases, salts, and pH is essential.

Many inorganic and organic compounds found in living organisms are ones that we use in our daily lives. They can be classified into one of three groups: acids, bases, and salts. We are familiar with the sour taste of citrus fruits (grapefruits, lemons, and limes) and vinegar. The sour taste is due to the presence of compounds called acids. What characteristics do acids have to set them apart from the bases and salts?

Acids

An **acid** is a substance that, when dissolved in water, will **ionize** into positively charged hydronium ions (H_3O^+) or hydrogen ions (H^+) and negatively charged ions of some other element. (Basically, an acid is a substance that yields hydronium ions (H_3O^+) in solution.) For example, hydrogen chloride (HCl) in pure form is a gas. But when bubbled into water, it becomes hydrochloric acid. How does this happen? Simply. In a water solution, hydrogen chloride ionizes into one hydronium ion and one negatively charged chloride ion.

$$HCl + H_2O \longrightarrow H_3O^+ + Cl^-$$

Hydrogen chloride in solution $\longrightarrow$ Hydronium ion + Chloride ion

the following nitrogenous bases: adenine, cytosine, guanine, and uracil instead of thymine. The RNA molecule is a single-stranded molecule, while the DNA molecule is a double-stranded molecule.

There are three different types of RNA in a cell: the messenger RNA (m-RNA), the transfer RNA (t-RNA), and the ribosomal RNA (r-RNA).

TABLE 2-4 • *Differences Between the DNA and RNA Molecules*

TYPE OF NUCLEIC ACID	TYPE OF SUGAR PRESENT	TYPES OF BASES PRESENT	PHOSPHATE GROUP	LOCATION	NUMBER OF STRANDS PRESENT
DNA	Deoxyribose	A, T, G, C	Same as RNA	Cell nucleus, chromosomes	2
RNA	Ribose	A, U, G, C	Same as DNA	Cytoplasm, nucleoli, ribosomes	1

TABLE 2-5 • *Names, Formulas, Locations or Uses of Some Common Acids*

NAME OF ACID	FORMULA	WHERE FOUND OR USAGE
Acetic acid	CH_3COOH	Found in vinegar
Boric acid	H_3BO_3	Weak eyewash
Carbonic acid	H_2CO_3	Found in carbonated beverages
Hydrochloric acid	HCl	Found in stomach
Nitric acid	HNO_3	Industrial oxidizing acid
Sulfuric acid	H_2SO_4	Found in batteries and industrial mineral acid

It is the presence of the hydronium ions that gives hydrochloric acid its acidity and sour taste. (However, one should *not* taste any substance to identify it as an acid. There are other more reliable and safer methods for the identification of an acid.) A substance can be tested for its acidity through the use of specially-treated paper called litmus paper. In the presence of an acid, blue litmus paper turns red. Table 2-5 gives the name of some common acids, their formulas, and where they are found or how they are used.

Bases

A **base** or **alkali** is a substance that, when dissolved in water, ionizes into negatively charged **hydroxide** (OH^-) ions and positively charged ions of a metal. For example, sodium hydroxide (NaOH) ionizes into one sodium ion (Na^+) and one hydroxide ion (OH^-). The reaction can be shown as follows:

$$NaOH \longrightarrow Na^+ + OH^-$$

Sodium hydroxide ⟶ Sodium + Hydroxide
in solution   ion   ion

Bases have a bitter taste and feel slippery between the fingers. They turn red litmus paper blue. Table 2-6 gives the names of some common bases, their formulas, and location or use.

Neutralization and Salts

When an acid and a base are combined, they form a salt and water. This type of reaction is called a **neutralization**, or exchange reaction. In a neutralization reaction, hydrogen

TABLE 2-6 • *Names, Formulas, Locations or Uses of Some Common Bases*

NAME OF BASE	FORMULA	WHERE FOUND OR USAGE
Ammonium hydroxide	NH_4OH	Household liquid cleaners
Magnesium hydroxide	$Mg(OH)_2$	Milk of magnesia
Potassium hydroxide	KOH	Caustic potash
Sodium hydroxide	$NaOH$	Lye

ions (H^+) from the acid and hydroxide ions (OH^-) from the base join to form water. At the same time, the negative ions of the acid combine with the positive ions of the base to form a compound called a salt. For example, hydrochloric acid and sodium hydroxide combine to form sodium chloride and water. The hydrogen ions from the acid unite with the hydroxide ions from the base to form water. The sodium ions (Na^+) combine with the chloride ions (Cl^-) to form sodium chloride ($NaCl$). When the water evaporates, solid salt remains. The neutralization reaction is written as shown in Figure 2-4.

THE pH SCALE

pH is a measure of the acidity or alkalinity (basicity) of a solution. Special pH meters determine the hydrogen or hydroxide ion concentration of a solution on a scale called the pH scale. The pH scale, which is used to measure the acidity or alkalinity of a solution, ranges from 0 to 14. A pH of 7 indicates that a particular solution has the same number of hydrogen ions as hydroxide ions. This is a neutral pH, and distilled water is neutral with a pH value of 7.0. Any pH value between zero and 6.9 indicates an acidic solution. The lower the pH number, the stronger the acid or higher hydrogen ion concentration. Any pH value between 7.1 and 14.0 means a solution is basic or alkaline. Thus, the greater the number above 7.0, the stronger the base or greater hydroxide ion concentration. Figure 2-5 shows the pH values of some common acids, bases, and human body fluids. It also shows the color changes that occur on a pH strip.

Homeostasis

As shown in Figure 2-5, living cells and the fluids they produce are usually neither strongly acidic nor strongly alkaline. These fluids, in fact, are nearly neutral. For instance, human tears have a pH of 7.3 and human blood has a pH range of 7.35 to 7.45.

In order for living cells to function optimally, their biochemical reactions must maintain homeostasis. In humans and other living organisms, the maintenance of a balanced pH is achieved through a compound called a buffer. Sodium bicarbonate ($NaHCO_3$) acts as a buffer in many living organisms. Buffers help

Hydrochloric Acid	+	Sodium Hydroxide	→	Sodium Chloride (Salt)	+	Water
HCL	+	NaOH	→	NaCl	+	H_20

FIGURE 2-4 *The neutralization reaction or exchange reaction*

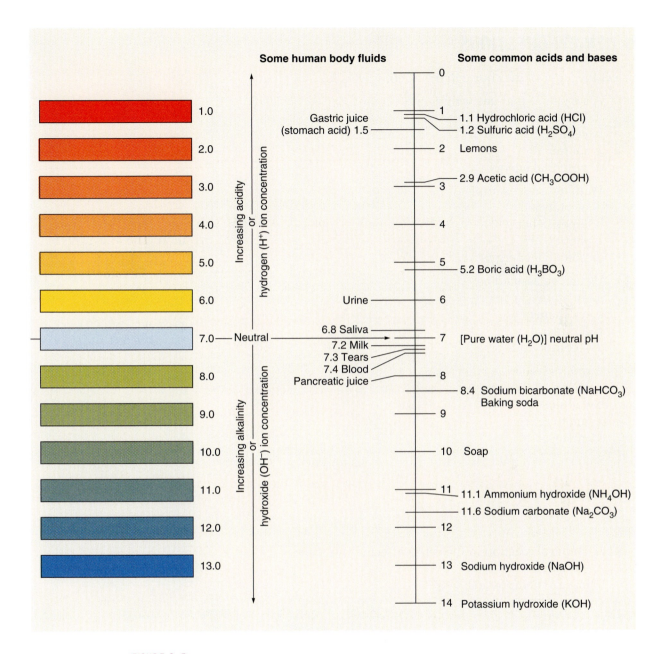

FIGURE 2-5 *pH values of some common acids, bases, and human body fluids*

a living organism to maintain a constant pH value which contributes to the homeostasis or balanced state within all living things.

It is important that the fluid within the cell (**intracellular fluid**) and the fluid surrounding the cell (**extracellular fluid**) maintain the proper chemical balance in order for the cell to func-tion. A state of homeostasis is required for the body to function at an optimum level of health. If a control system like the acid-base or elec-trolyte balance is not maintained, cells and tis-sue will become damaged. A moderate dys-function causes illness; a severe dysfunction causes death.

● REVIEW QUESTIONS

Select the letter of the choice that best completes the statement.

1. A substance that has weight and occupies space is called:
   a. kinetic energy
   b. catalyst
   c. matter
   d. potential energy

2. Walking is an example of:
   a. a catalyst
   b. kinetic energy
   c. matter
   d. potential energy

3. Water is classified as:
   a. an atom
   b. an element
   c. a mineral
   d. a compound

4. A monosaccharide sugar is:
   a. sucrose
   b. cellulose
   c. maltose
   d. glucose

5. Sugar stored in the liver and muscle cells for energy is called:
   a. glucose
   b. glycogen
   c. fructose
   d. ribose

6. A chemical reaction in the cell is affected by:
   a. enzymes
   b. organic compounds
   c. nucleic acids
   d. energy

7. The strongest acid is found in the stomach. It is:
   a. sulfuric
   b. acetic
   c. hydrochloric
   d. nitric

8. A compound with a pH of 8.4 is alkaline and it is:
   a. milk of magnesia
   b. baking soda
   c. ammonia
   d. lye

9. When proper amounts of an acid and base are combined, the products formed are a salt and:
   a. gas
   b. water
   c. another base
   d. another acid

10. The name given to the atomic particle that is found outside the nucleus of an atom is:
    a. proton
    b. neutron
    c. electron
    d. ion

● MATCHING

Match each term in Column I with its correct description in Column II.

Column I	Column II
_____ 1. glucose	a. fluid within the cell
_____ 2. electrolyte	b. double sugar
_____ 3. intracellular	c. triglycerides
_____ 4. disaccharides	d. chromosomes
_____ 5. HCL	e. conducts an electrical charge in a solution
_____ 6. steroid	f. blood sugar
_____ 7. energy	g. positively or negatively charged particle of an atom
_____ 8. ion	h. ability to do work
_____ 9. DNA	i. cholesterol
_____ 10. fats	j. found in the stomach

● APPLYING THEORY TO PRACTICE

1. Read the label on a loaf of bread and state why the bread can be advertised as "no cholesterol."

2. Compare the fat content in one slice of pizza, a fast food quarter pound hamburger, a serving of ice cream, and a serving of yogurt.

3. Should DNA identification be required at birth? Have a panel discussion on the "ethics" of DNA testing as part of a pre-employment physical.

CHAPTER

3

Cells

OBJECTIVES

- Identify the structure of a typical cell
- Define the function of each component of a typical cell
- Relate the function of cells to the function of the body
- Describe the processes that will transport materials in and out of a cell
- Describe what a tumor is and define cancer
- Define the key words that relate to this chapter

KEY WORDS

active transport
adenosine triphos-
    phate (ATP)
anaphase
benign cancer
cell
cell membrane
centriole
centrosome
chromatid
chromatin
chromosome
cytoskeleton
cytoplasm
diffusion
endoplasmic reticu-
    lum (smooth and
    rough)
equilibrium
filtration

Golgi apparatus
hypertonic
    solution
hypotonic solution
interphase
isotonic solution
lysosome
malignant
meiosis
metaphase
metastases
mitochondria
mitosis
neoplasm
nuclear membrane
nucleolus
nucleoplasm
nucleus
organelle

osmosis
osmotic pressure
perioxisome
phagocytosis
phase
pinocytic vesicle
pinocytosis
prophase
protein synthesis
replication
ribosome
selective permeable
    membrane
solutes
somatic cell
telophase
tumor
vacuole
wart (papilloma)

When a field of grass is seen from a distance it looks just like a solid green carpet. Closer observation, however, shows that it is not a solid mass but is made up of countless separate blades of grass. So it is with the body of a plant or animal; it seems to be a single entity, but when any portion is examined under a microscope it is found to be made up of many small, discrete parts. These tiny parts, or units, are called **cells**. (*Note:* These units were first discovered in the 1600s by Robert Hook. When examining a piece of cork under a crude microscope, the units reminded him of a monk's room, which was called a cell). All living things, whether plant or animal, unicellular or multicellular, large or small, are composed of cells. A cell is microscopic in size. *The cell is the basic unit of structure and function of all living things.*

Since cells are microscopic, a special unit of measurement is employed to determine their size. This is the micrometer (μm), or micron (μ). It is used to describe both the size of cells and their cellular components, Table 3-1.

To better understand the structure of a cell, let us compare a living entity—such as a human being—to a house. The many individual cells of this living organism are comparable to the many rooms of a house. Just as each room is bounded by four walls, floor and ceiling, a cell is bounded by a specialized cell membrane with many openings. Cells, like rooms, come in a variety of shapes and sizes. Every kind of room or cell has its own unique function. A house can be made up of a single room or many. In much the same fashion, a living thing can be made up of only one cell (unicellular), or many cells (multicellular).

TABLE 3-1 • *Units of Length in the Metric System*

1 meter = 39.37 inches
1 centimeter (cm) = 1/100 or 0.01 meters
1 millimeter (mm) = 1/1000 or 0.001 meters
1 micrometer (μm) or micron (μ) = 1/1,000,000 or 0.000001
1 nanometer (nm) = 1/1,000,000,000 or 0.000000001 meters
1 angstrom (Å) = 1/10,000,000,000 or 0.0000000001 meters

"Basic" and "typical" are terms used to identify structures common to most living cells.

CELL MEMBRANE

Every cell is surrounded by a cell membrane. It is sometimes called a plasma membrane. The **cell membrane** separates the cell's cytoplasm from its external environment and from the neighboring cells. It also regulates the passage or transport of certain molecules into and out of the cell, while preventing the passage of others. This is why the cell membrane is often called a "selective semi-permeable membrane." The cell membrane is made of protein and lipid (fatty substance) molecules arranged in a double layer. This arrangement is rather like a sandwich: the lipid molecules are the filling, and the two layers of protein molecules are the slices of bread.

NUCLEUS

The **nucleus** is the most important organelle within the cell. It has two vital functions: to control the activities of the cell and to facilitate cell division. This spherical organelle is usually located in or near the center of the cell. Various dyes or stains, like iodine, can be used to make the nucleus stand out. The nucleus stains vividly because it contains DNA and protein. Both readily absorb stains. Surrounding the nucleus is a membrane called the nuclear membrane.

The DNA and protein are arranged in a loose and diffuse state called **chromatin**. When the cell is ready to divide, the chromatin condenses to form short, rodlike structures called **chromosomes**. There is a specific number of chromosomes in the nucleus for each species. The number of chromosomes for the human being is 46, or 23 pairs.

When a cell reaches a certain size, it may divide to form two new cells. When this occurs, the nucleus divides first by a process called **mitosis**. During this process, the nuclear material is distributed to each of the two new nuclei. This is followed by division of the cytoplasm into two approximately equal parts through the formation of a new membrane between the two nuclei. It is only during the process of nuclear division that the chromosomes can be seen.

Chromosomes are important because they store the hereditary material—deoxyribonucleic acid (DNA)—which is passed on from one generation of cells to the next.

Nuclear Membrane

The nuclear membrane, or nuclear envelope, is a double-layered membrane that has openings at regular intervals. Through these pores materials can pass from either the nucleus to the cytoplasm or from the cytoplasm to the nucleus. The outer layer of the nuclear membrane is continuous with the endoplasmic reticulum of the cytoplasm and may have small round projections on it called ribosomes. (A discussion of the ribosomes and endoplasmic reticulum follows shortly.)

Nucleoplasm

The nucleoplasm is a clear, semi-fluid medium that fills the spaces around the chromatin and the nucleoli.

Nucleolus and the Ribosomes

Within the nucleus are one or more nucleoli. Each nucleolus is a small, round body, Figure 3-1. It contains ribosomes made up of ribonucleic acid and protein. The ribosomes can pass from the nucleus through the nuclear pores into the cytoplasm. There the ribosomes aid in protein synthesis. They may exist freely in the cytoplasm, be in clusters called polyribosomes, or be attached to the walls of the endoplasmic reticulum.

CYTOPLASM

The cytoplasm is a sticky semi-fluid material found between the nucleus and the cell membrane. Chemical analysis of the cytoplasm shows that it consists of proteins, lipids, carbohydrates, minerals, salts, and water (70%-90%). Each of these substances other than water varies greatly from one cell to the next and from one organism to the next. The cytoplasm is the background for all the chemical reactions which take place in a cell, such as protein synthesis and cellular respiration. Molecules are transported about the cell by the circular motion of the cytoplasm. Embedded in the cytoplasm are organelles, or cell structures that help a cell to function. Table 3-2, page 28, summarizes the organelles and their functions.

Centrosome and Centrioles

The centrioles are two cylindrical organelles found near the nucleus in a tiny round body called the centrosome. The centrioles are perpendicular to each other. Figure 3-1 shows two centrioles near the nucleus. During mitosis, or cell division, the two centrioles separate from each other. In the process of separation, thin cytoplasmic spindle fibers form between the two centrioles. This structure is called a spindle-fiber apparatus. The spindle fibers attach themselves to individual chromosomes to help in the even and equal distribution of these chromosomes to two daughter cells.

Endoplasmic Reticulum

Crisscrossing the cellular cytoplasm is a fine network of tubular structures called the endoplasmic reticulum (reticulum means "network"). Some of this endoplasmic reticulum connects the nuclear membrane to the cell membrane. Thus it serves as a channel for the transport of materials in and out of the nucleus. Sometimes the endoplasmic reticulum will accumulate large masses of proteins and act as a storage area.

There are two types of endoplasmic reticulum: rough endoplasmic reticulum and smooth endoplasmic reticulum. Rough endoplasmic reticulum has ribosomes studding the outer membrane. The ribosomes are the sites for protein synthesis in the cell. The smooth endoplas-

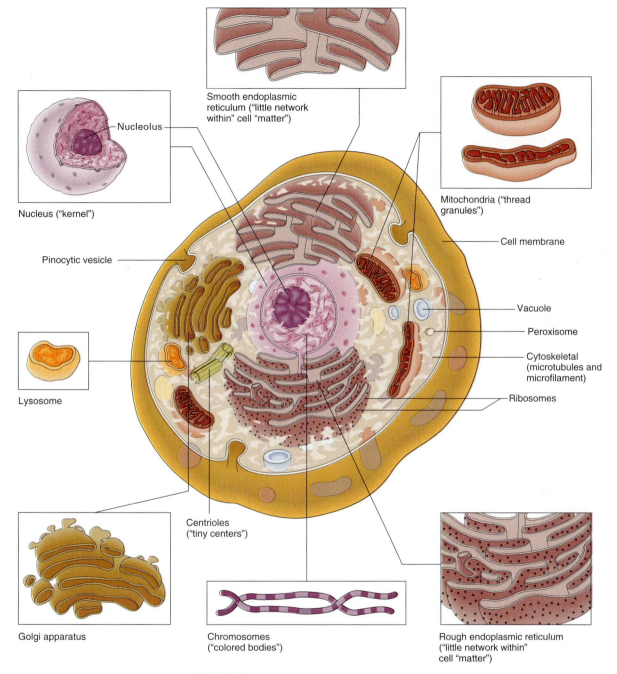

Smooth endoplasmic reticulum ("little network within" cell "matter")

Nucleolus

Nucleus ("kernel")

Pinocytic vesicle

Lysosome

Golgi apparatus

Centrioles ("tiny centers")

Chromosomes ("colored bodies")

Mitochondria ("thread granules")

Cell membrane

Vacuole

Peroxisome

Cytoskeletal (microtubules and microfilament)

Ribosomes

Rough endoplasmic reticulum ("little network within" cell "matter")

FIGURE 3-1 *Structure of a typical animal cell*

mic reticulum has a role in cholesterol synthesis, fat metabolism, and detoxification of drugs.

Mitochondria

A&P CHALLENGE

Most of the cell's energy comes from spherical or rod-shaped organelles called **mitochondria** (singular, mitochondrion; *mito*

means thread, *chondrion* means granule). These mitochondria vary in shape and number. There can be as few as a single one in each cell or as many as a thousand or more. Cells that need the most energy have the greatest number of mitochondria. Because they supply the cell's energy mitochondria are also known as the "powerhouses" of the cell.

TABLE 3-2 ● *Summary Table of Cell Organelles*

ORGANELLE	FUNCTION
Cell membrane	Regulates transport of substances into and out of the cell.
Cytoplasm	Provides an organized watery environment in which life functions take place by the activities of the organelles contained in the cytoplasm.
Nucleus	Serves as the "brain" for the control of the cell's metabolic activities and cell division.
Nuclear membrane	Regulates transport of substances into and out of the nucleus.
Nucleoplasm	A clear, semifluid medium that fills the spaces around the chromatin and the nucleoli.
Nucleolus	Functions as a reservoir for RNA.
Ribosomes	Serve as sites for protein synthesis.
Endoplasmic reticulum	Provides passages through which transport of substances occurs in cytoplasm.
Mitochondria	Serve as sites of cellular respiration and energy production; stores ATP.
Golgi apparatus	Manufactures carbohydrates and packages secretions for discharge from the cell.
Lysosomes	Serve as centers for cellular digestion.
Peroxisome	Enzymes oxidize cell substances.
Centrosome and centrioles	Contains two centrioles that are functional during animal cell division.
Cytoskeleton	Forms internal framework.

The mitochondria have a double-membraned structure which contains enzymes. These enzymes help to break down carbohydrates, fats and protein molecules into energy to be stored in the cell as **adenosine triphosphate**, otherwise known as **ATP**. All living cells need ATP for their activities.

Golgi Apparatus

The **Golgi apparatus** is also called Golgi bodies or the Golgi complex. It is an arrangement of layers of membranes resembling a "stack of pancakes." Scientists believe that this organelle synthesizes carbohydrates and combines them with protein molecules as they pass through the Golgi apparatus. In this way the Golgi apparatus stores and packages secretions for discharge from the cell. These organelles are abundant in the cells of gastric glands, salivary glands and pancreatic glands.

Lysosomes

Lysosomes are oval or spherical bodies found in the cellular cytoplasm. They contain powerful digestive enzymes that digest protein molecules. The lysosome thus helps to digest old, wornout cells, bacteria and foreign matter. If a lysosome should rupture, as sometimes happens, the lysosome will start digesting the cell's proteins, causing it to die. For this reason lysosomes are also known as "suicide bags."

Perioxisomes

Membranous sacs which contain oxidase enzymes are called **perioxisomes**. These enzymes help to digest fats and detoxify harmful substances.

Cytoskeleton

Cytoskeleton is the internal framework of the cell which is made up of microtubules, intermediate filaments, and microfilaments. The filaments provide support for the cells and the microtubules are thought to aid in movement of substances through cytoplasm.

Pinocytic Vesicles

Large molecules like protein and lipids, which cannot pass through the cell membrane, will enter a cell by way of the pinocytic vesicles. The **pinocytic vesicles** form by having the cell membrane fold inward to form a pocket. The edges of the pocket then close and pinch away from the cell membrane, forming a bubble or **vacuole** in the cytoplasm. This process by which a cell forms pinocytic vesicles to take in large molecules is called pinocytosis or "cell drinking."

CELL DIVISION

Both the growth and the maintenance of all the cells in the human body are achieved through cell division. Some human body cells (**somatic cells**) live only a short time, while others are subjected to continual "wear and tear" and are destroyed. The process of cell division or mitosis will produce new cells. All cells do not reproduce at the same rate. Blood-forming cells of the bone marrow, the cells of the skin, and the cells of the intestinal tract reproduce continuously. Muscle cells only reproduce every few years; however, muscle tissue may be enlarged with exercise. Neurons or nerve cells do not reproduce.

Mitosis

Cell division or mitosis is divided into two distinct processes: the first stage is the division of the nucleus, and the second stage is the division of the cytoplasm.

Mitosis essentially is an orderly series of steps by which the DNA in the nucleus of a cell is precisely and equally distributed to two daughter nuclei. The process of cell division of the sex cell or gamete is called **meiosis**. During meiosis, the ovum from the female and the spermatozoa from the male *reduce* their respective chromosomes to 23 or one-half the normal amount. When fertilization (the union of the ovum and sperm) occurs, the two cells combine to form a simple cell called the zygote, which will then have the full set of 46 chromosomes, 23 from each parent, Figure 3-2.

Mitosis in a Typical Animal Cell

Mitosis is a smoothly continuing process. However, for ease and convenience of study,

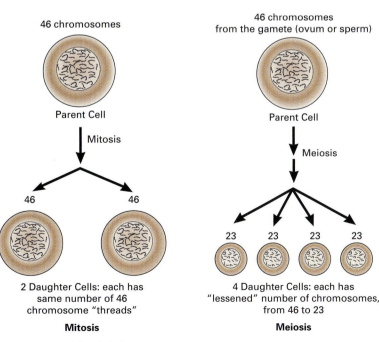

FIGURE 3-2 *The processes of meiosis and mitosis*

five stages or **phases** have been identified by the cell biologist. These five phases are discussed subsequently with accompanying diagrams, Figure 3-3. The normal human somatic cell contains 46 chromosomes in the nucleus, which is equal to 23 pairs of chromosomes. This particular chromosome number (46) is called the diploid number of chromosomes. The illustration of a cell in interphase that follows is a representative animal cell with a diploid number of 46 chromosomes. This cell will help to

illustrate the process of mitosis. (Refer to Figure 3-3 for the following, Phases 1-5.)

Phase 1—Interphase (Resting Stage). In the interphase or "resting" stage, an animal cell undergoes *all* metabolic cellular activities to help in the maintenance of cell homeostasis. The term "resting" *only* refers to the fact that the cell is not undergoing the visible steps of mitosis yet. Interphase occurs between nuclear divisions. During early interphase, an

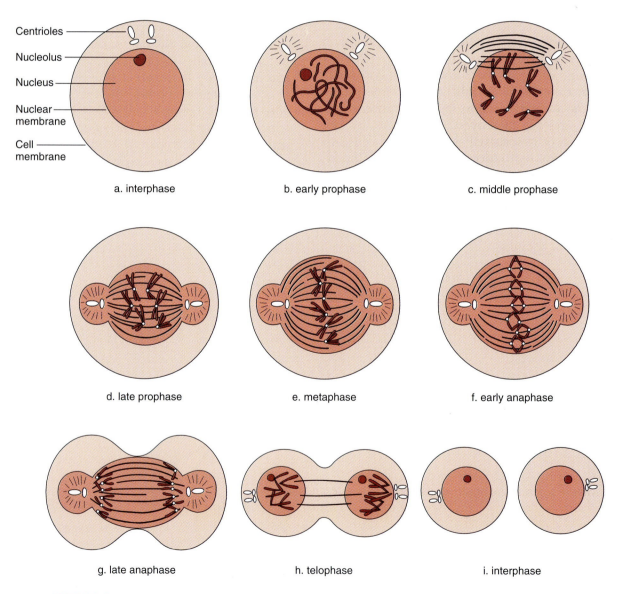

Centrioles
Nucleolus
Nucleus
Nuclear membrane
Cell membrane

a. interphase b. early prophase c. middle prophase

d. late prophase e. metaphase f. early anaphase

g. late anaphase h. telophase i. interphase

FIGURE 3-3 *The five phases of mitosis: interphase, prophase, metaphase, anaphase, and telophase*

exact duplicate of each nuclear chromosome is made. This process is called **replication**. Replication is the duplication of the molecules of DNA within a chromosome.

At the start of mitosis, each chromosome has already replicated. Each strand of the replicated chromosome is called a **chromatid**. The two chromatid strands are joined together by a small structure called the centromere. During interphase, two centrioles located near the periphery of the nucleus are quite visible. The two centrioles are found in an area called the centrosome. They also replicate during interphase in preparation for the next cell division.

Phase 2—Prophase. During prophase, the two pairs of centrioles start to separate towards the opposite ends or poles of the cell. As the two pairs of centrioles migrate, an array of cytoplasmic microtubules forms between them.

There are changes in the nucleus as well. The nuclear membrane starts to dissolve and the nucleolus disappears. The DNA in the chromosomes becomes more highly coiled or condensed and forms very deeply-staining, rod-like structures.

 Phase 3—Metaphase. During metaphase, the nuclear membrane has dissolved completely. The chromatid pairs arrange themselves in a single file, one chromatid pair per spindle fiber between the two centrioles. The area that the chromatid pairs line up along is called the equatorial plate.

 Phase 4—Anaphase. During anaphase, the chromatid pairs separate and are pulled by the shortening spindle fibers towards the centrioles. The two chromatids of each replicated chromosome are now fully separated.

Phase 5—Telophase. During telophase, the chromosomes migrate to the opposite poles of the cell. There they start to uncoil or decondense to become loosely arranged chromatin granules. The nuclear membrane and the nucleolus reappear to help reestablish the nucleus as a definite organelle again.

When cytoplasmic division is finished, two new daughter cells are formed.

PROTEIN SYNTHESIS

Cells produce proteins which are essential to life such as albumin or globulin through a process called **protein synthesis**. Within each cell is the DNA which determines the kinds of proteins that are produced. The blueprint for each individual kind of protein is contained within a specific gene which resides in the DNA chain.

 ## MOVEMENT OF MATERIALS ACROSS CELL MEMBRANES

The cell membrane controls passage of substances into and out of the cell. This is important because a cell must be able to acquire materials from its surrounding medium, after which it either secretes synthesized substances or excretes wastes. The physical processes which control the passage of materials through the cell membrane are: diffusion, osmosis, filtration, active transport, phagocytosis, and pinocytosis. Diffusion, osmosis, and filtration are passive processes, which means they do not need energy in order to function. Active transport, phagocytosis, and pinocytosis are active processes which do require an energy source.

Diffusion

Diffusion is a physical process whereby molecules of gases, liquids, or solid particles spread or scatter themselves evenly through a medium. When solid particles are dissolved within a fluid, they are known as **solutes**. Diffusion also applies to a slightly different process, where solutes and water pass across a membrane to distribute themselves evenly throughout the two fluids, which remain separated by the membrane. Generally, *molecules move from an area where they are greatly concentrated to an area where they are less concentrated.* The molecules will, eventually, distribute themselves evenly within the space available; when this happens, the molecules are said to be in a state of **equilibrium**, Figure 3-4.

The three common states of matter are gases, liquids, and solids. Molecules will diffuse

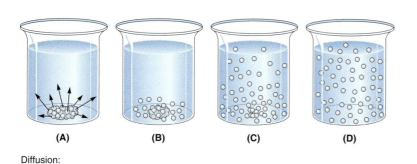

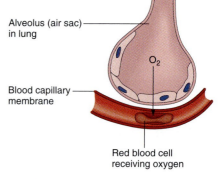

Diffusion:

(A) A small lump of sugar is placed into a beaker of water, its molecules dissolve and begin to diffuse outward. **(B&C)** The sugar molecules continue to diffuse through the water from an area of greater concentration to an area of lesser concentration. **(D)** Over a long period of time, the sugar molecules are evenly distributed throughout the water, reaching a state of equilibrium.

Example of diffusion in the human body: Oxygen diffuses from an alveolus in a lung where it is in greater concentration, across the blood capillary membrane, into a red blood cell where it is in lesser concentration.

FIGURE 3-4 *The process of diffusion. The sugar molecules eventually reach a state of equilibrium.*

more quickly in gases and more slowly in solids. Diffusion occurs due to the heat energy of molecules. As a result of this, molecules are always in constant motion, except at absolute zero (-273°C). In all cases, the movement of molecules increases with an increase in temperature.

A few familiar examples of the rates of diffusion may be helpful. For instance, if one thoroughly saturates a wad of cotton with ammonia and places it in a far corner of a room, the entire room will soon smell of ammonia. Air currents quickly carry the ammonia fumes throughout the room. Another test for diffusion is to place a pair of dye crystals on the bottom of a water-filled beaker. Eventually, they will uniformly permeate and color the water. This diffusion process will take quite a while, especially if no one stirs, shakes or heats the beaker. In still another test, a dye crystal placed on an ice cube moves even more slowly through the ice. Diffusion of the dye can be accelerated by melting the ice.

The diffusion rate of molecules in the various media (gas, liquid, and solid) depends upon the distances between each molecule and how freely they can move. In a gas, molecules can move more freely and quickly; within a liquid, molecules are more tightly held together. In a solid substance, molecular movement is highly restricted and thus very slow.

Diffusion plays a vital role in permitting molecules to enter and leave a cell. Oxygen diffuses from the bloodstream, where it dwells in greater concentration. From the bloodstream, the oxygen enters the fluid surrounding a cell, then into the cell itself, where it is far less concentrated. In this manner, the flow of blood through the lungs and bloodstream provides a continuous supply of oxygen to the cells. Once oxygen has entered a cell, it is utilized in metabolic activities.

Osmosis

Osmosis is the diffusion of water or any other *solvent* molecule through a selective permeable membrane (like the cell membrane). A **selective permeable membrane** is any membrane through which some solutes can diffuse, but others cannot.

Sausage casing is a selective permeable membrane which can be used to substitute for a cell membrane. A solution of salt, sucrose (table sugar), and gelatin is placed into the sausage casing. This mixture is then suspended into a beaker filled with distilled water, Figure 3-5. The sausage casing is permeable to

Initial stage

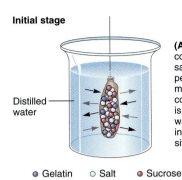

Distilled
water

(A) Initially, the sausage casing contains a solution of gelatin, salt and sucrose. The casing is permeable to water and salt molecules only. Since the concentration of water molecules is greater outside the casing, water molecules will diffuse into the casing. The opposite situation exists for the salt.

10-12 hours later

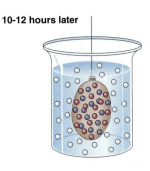

(B) The sausage casing swells due to the net movement of water molecules inward. However, the volume of distilled water in the beaker remains constant.

● Gelatin   ○ Salt   ● Sucrose

FIGURE 3-5 *Osmosis: the diffusion of water through a selective permeable membrane (A sausage casing is an example of a selective permeable membrane.)*

water and salt, but not to gelatin and sucrose. Thus only the water and salt molecules can pass through the casing. Eventually more salt molecules will move out because we began with a greater concentration of these molecules inside. At the same time, more water molecules move into the casing, since there were more outside when we began.

The volume of water increases inside the casing, causing it to expand because of the entry of water molecules. When the number of water molecules entering the casing are equal to the number exiting, an equilibrium has been achieved: the casing will expand no further.

The pressure exerted by the water molecules within the casing at equilibrium is called the **osmotic pressure**.

Osmosis is the movement of water molecules across a semi-permeable membrane from an area of higher concentration of a solution to an area of lower concentration of a solution. The key word is *solute*, the amount of concentration of a dissolved substance.

In the human body this is well illustrated by a red blood cell in blood plasma, Figure 3-6. If a red blood cell is put into blood plasma, which has the same number of sodium particles as a red blood cell, the osmotic pressure of the red blood cell and that of the plasma are the same representing an **isotonic solution**.

If a red blood cell is put into freshwater, which has less sodium particles than the red blood cell, water will rush into the red blood cell. The freshwater represents a **hypotonic solution**.

Hypertonic solution

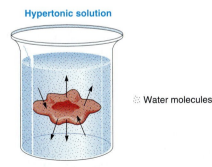

Hypotonic solution

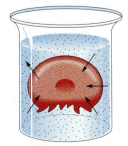

Water molecules

Isotonic solution

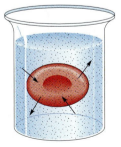

Hypertonic solution (seawater)
a red blood cell will shrink and wrinkle up because water molecules are moving out of the cell.

Hypotonic solution (freshwater)
a red blood cell will swell and burst because water molecules are moving into the cell.

Isotonic solution (human blood serum)
a red blood cell remains unchanged, because the movement of water molecules into and out of the cell are the same.

FIGURE 3-6 *Movement of water molecules in solutions of different osmotic pressure*

If a red blood cell is put into sea water, which has more sodium particles than the red blood cell, water will leave the red blood cell to dilute the sea water. The sea water represents a **hypertonic solution**.

The health care worker needs to know about which type of solutions are used in health care. When a physician orders intravenous fluids, the patient's condition will determine what type of solution is ordered. Most intravenous fluids are isotonic solutions. Hypertonic solution is used for patient with edema; hypotonic for patients with dehydration.

Filtration

Filtration is the movement of solutes and water across a semi-permeable membrane. This results from some mechanical force, such as blood pressure or gravity. The solutes and water move from an area of higher pressure to an area of lower pressure. The size of the membrane pores determines which molecules are to be filtered. Thus filtration allows for the separation of large and small molecules. Such filtration takes place in the kidneys. The process allows larger protein molecules to remain within the body and smaller molecules to be excreted as waste, Figure 3-7.

Active Transport

Active transport is a process whereby molecules move across the cell membrane from an area of lower concentration against a concentration gradient, to an area of higher concentration. This process requires the high energy chemical compound ATP (adenosine triphosphate). The ATP is supplied by cell metabolism.

How does active transport work? One theory suggests that a molecule is picked up from the outside of the cell membrane and brought inside by a carrier molecule. Both molecule and carrier are bound together, forming a temporary carrier-molecule complex. This carrier-molecule complex shuttles across the cell mem-

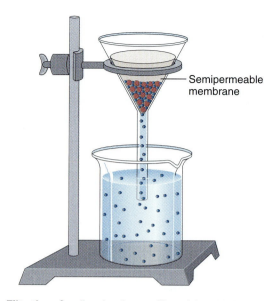

Filtration: Small molecules are filtered through the semipermeable membrane, while the large molecules remain in the funnel.

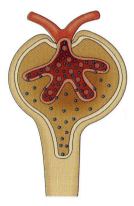

Example of filtration in the human body: Glomerulus of kidney, large particles like red blood cells and proteins remain in the blood, and small molecules like urea and water are excreted as a metabolic excretory product—urine.

FIGURE 3-7   *Example of filtration: a passive transport process*

brane; the molecule is released at the inner surface of the membrane, from where it enters the cytoplasm. At this point, the carrier acquires energy at the inner surface of the cell membrane. Then it returns to the outer surface of the cell membrane to pick up another molecule for transport. Accordingly, the carrier can also convey molecules in the opposite direction, from the inside to the outside, Figure 3-8.

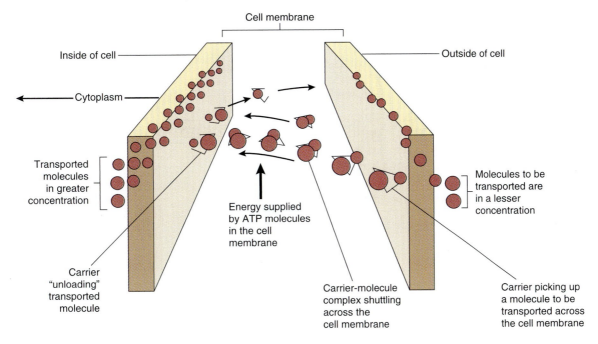

Cell membrane

Inside of cell

Cytoplasm

Outside of cell

Transported
molecules
in greater
concentration

Molecules to be
transported are
in a lesser
concentration

Energy supplied
by ATP molecules
in the cell
membrane

Carrier
"unloading"
transported
molecule

Carrier-molecule
complex shuttling
across the
cell membrane

Carrier picking up
a molecule to be
transported across
the cell membrane

FIGURE 3-8   *The active transport of molecules from an area of lesser concentration to an area of greater concentration, according to one theoretical model*

Phagocytosis

Phagocytosis, or "cell eating," is quite similar to pinocytosis, with an important difference: in pinocytosis, the substances engulfed by the cell membrane are in solution; however, in phagocytosis, the substances engulfed are within particles. Human white blood cells undergo phagocytosis. The particulate substance will be engulfed by an enfolding of the cell membrane to form a vacuole enclosing the material. When the material is completely enclosed within the vacuole, digestive enzymes pour into the vacuole from the cytoplasm to destroy the entrapped substance.

Pinocytosis

As stated earlier, **pinocytosis** or "cell drinking" involves the formation of pinocytic vesicles which engulf large molecules in solution. The cell then ingests the nutrient for its own use.

SPECIALIZATION

There are many kinds of cells of different shapes and sizes. Most of them have the characteristics shown in Figure 3-1, which is a generalized diagram of a basic cell. Some of the more specialized types, such as nerve cells and red blood cells, look very different, Figure 3-9.

Human beings are composed entirely of cells and the nonliving substances which cells build up around themselves. The interaction of the various parts of the cell within the cellular structure constitutes the life of the cell. These interactions result in the life activities, life processes, or life functions that were discussed in Chapter 1. However, in complex organisms, groups of cells become specialists in a particular function. Nerve cells, for example, have become specialized in response; red blood cells, in oxygen transport.

Specialized cells may lose the ability to perform some of the other functions, such as reproduction (cell division). Normally, when nerve cells are destroyed or damaged, others

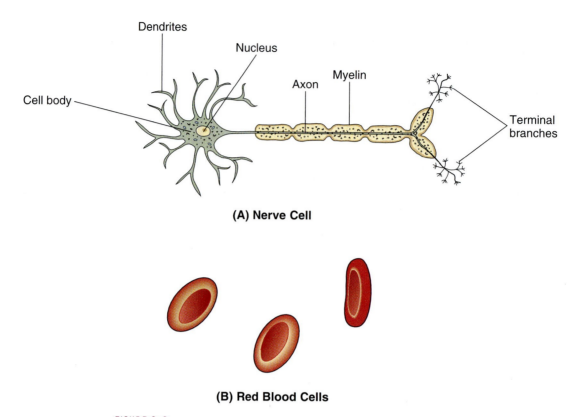

(A) Nerve Cell

(B) Red Blood Cells

FIGURE 3-9 *Specialized cells: nerve cells and red blood cells*

cannot be formed to replace them. Heart muscle cells no longer divide when they reach maturity. If a person has a heart attack there is a loss of heart muscle cells which are replaced by scar tissue. The heart then loses some of its ability to contract. Specialization also has resulted in an interdependence among cells—certain cells depend on other kinds of cells to aid them in carrying on the total life activities of the organism. In humans, this specialization and interdependence extends to the organs.

DISORDERS OF CELL STRUCTURE

Tumor

A **tumor** results when cell division does not occur in the usual pattern. If the pattern is interrupted by an abnormal and uncontrolled growth of cells, the result is a tumor. Tumors are also known as **neoplasms**. Tumors can be divided into two groups: benign or malignant.

A **benign** tumor is when cells are confined to the local area. Benign tumors are given other names depending on their type or location (e.g., **wart** or **papilloma** is a type of tumor of the epithelial tissue). Most benign tumors can be surgically removed.

A **malignant** tumor or **cancer** is when cells move rapidly from one place to another. This process is called **metastases**. These tumors will cause death. In some cases if the cancer is detected early, it may be treated, and the person may recover. It is important for health care workers to know the early signs of cancer. Some of the early signs are weight loss, general feeling of poor health, abnormal bleeding,

MEDICAL HIGHLIGHT: TECHNOLOGY AND ETHICS

Genetic Engineering

Genetic engineering is the ability to snip, rearrange, edit or program DNA. The United States Genome Project aims to identify and map the location of the more than 100,000 genes that reside on the DNA of an individual. Scientists hope to ultimately identify the genes responsible for certain disease and treat the disease with gene therapy. Studies of genes may also reveal individuals predisposed to physical and psychological problems. Is this an invasion of an individual's privacy? Could it cause healthy individuals to be discriminated against just because of their genes?

One example of genetic engineering is a new cancer vaccine. In the labs of UCLA in 1996, Habib Fakhrai, a cancer scientist, along with other researchers, developed a cancer vaccine which is successful in treating brain cancer in laboratory rats. This vaccine was obtained from genetically engineered cells. Upon approval from the Food and Drug Administration, this vaccine will be tested on humans with a particular type of brain cancer.

Cancers of the brain, breast, lung, colon, and prostate all secrete a substance called Transforming Growth Factor-Beta (TGF-B). TGF-B suppresses the body's immune system and protects the cancer from the body's normal defenses. Using rats with brain cancer, scientists removed the cancer cells and purified the DNA. They then altered some of the genes on that DNA to make a protein that blocks the secretion of TGF-B. This anti TGF-B vaccine was given to rats with brain cancer and the cancers were destroyed by the rat's immune system.

This wonderful breakthrough technology has a price. It is the question of who will govern experimentation and genetic engineering. The American and International Communities realize that humans should dictate the growth of technology rather than technology dictating the futures of humans. However, checks and balances must be developed and implemented to ensure that the studies and experiments pass strict ethical criteria.

---

wounds slow to heal, or some type of abnormal function.

Diagnostic tests can detect the early stages of cancer. Some of these tests are x-ray, mammogram, sonagram or biopsy. These tests can be conducted on an out-patient basis. If you are working in a medical office, get the procedures from your local testing center. Give the patient this information before any testing begins.

Treatment of cancer depends on the type of tumor and where it is located. Cancers may also be classified according to stages. Each stage reflects the size of the cancer and how much invasion has occurred. Treatment for cancer includes surgery, radiation, and use of drugs called antineoplastics. Other types of treatment include immunotherapy and laser treatment. Disadvantages of cancer treatment include toxic side effects from drugs and tissue damage caused by radiation. Scientists today are working to develop cancer treatments which are specific to the tumor to help eliminate the side effects of treatment.

● REVIEW QUESTIONS

Select the letter of the choice that best completes the statement.

1. Structures found in cytoplasm to help cells function are called:
   a. nucleolus
   b. organelles
   c. ribosomes
   d. vacuoles

2. Regulating transport of substances in and out of the cell is the:
   a. cell membrane
   b. nuclear membrane
   c. cytoplasm
   d. nucleus

3. A structure that digests worn out cells and bacteria is called:
   a. perioxisome
   b. ribosome
   c. lysosome
   d. mitochondria

4. The function of Golgi apparatus of the cell is:
   a. protein synthesis
   b. destroying bacteria
   c. digesting fats
   d. storing and packaging secretions

5. The internal framework of the cell is called:
   a. mitochondria
   b. cytoskeleton
   c. endoplasmic reticulum
   d. ribosomes

● COMPLETION

Fill in the blank with the correct word.

1. The powerhouse of the cell stores _____ and is called _____.

2. The rough endoplasmic reticulum is studded with _____ which serve as a site for _____ synthesis.

3. The perioxisomes contain _____ enzymes which help digest _____.

4. During the _____ stage of mitosis, the two pairs of centrioles start to move toward _____ end of the cell.

5. The _____ for each individual's kind of protein is contained within a specific _____ in the _____ chain.

● MATCHING

Match each term in Column I with its correct description in Column II.

Column I	Column II
_____ 1. solute	a. cells confined to local area
_____ 2. isotonic solution	b. has a higher concentration of Na than red blood cell
_____ 3. diffusion	c. needs ATP for energy
_____ 4. phagocytosis	d. malignant tumor
_____ 5. osmosis	e. solid particles dissolved within a fluid
_____ 6. benign	f. cell reproduction
_____ 7. hypertonic solution	g. molecules move from higher concentration to lower
_____ 8. cancer	
_____ 9. mitosis	h. has same concentration of Na as the red blood cell
_____ 10. active transport	i. engulfs bacteria
	j. diffusion of water molecules

● APPLYING THEORY TO PRACTICE

1. The cell is a miniature of how the body works. Name the cellular structure responsible for each: digestion, respiration, energy, circulation, and the reproductive process.

2. Describe how the cell takes in nutrients and name at least three products that the cell manufactures.

3. Explain to the patient, admitted with a heart attack, what happens to the cells of the heart muscle when someone has a heart attack and what the difference is between the scar tissue and the heart tissue.

4 You are working in an emergency care center. A person comes in dehydrated and the doctor orders a hypertonic solution. Explain why this solution is used instead of an isotonic solution.

5. You are asked to participate in an ethics discussion of the question "Should couples be required to undergo genetic screening before they are issued a marriage license?" State your opinion (yes/no) and list at least three positive arguments for this. Also, give three arguments for the negatives to this requirement.

● LABELING

Study the following diagram of a typical cell. Enter the names of the structures after the properly numbered callouts, as listed below.

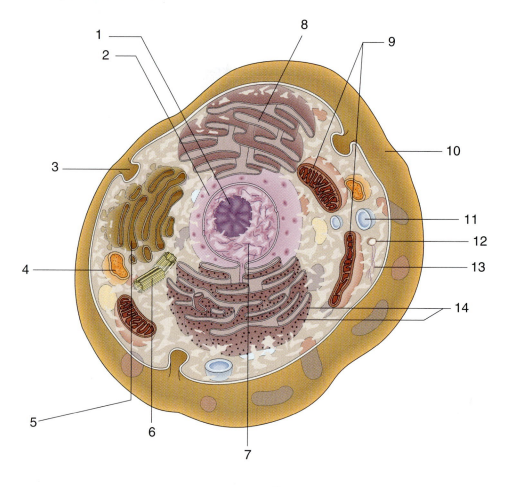

1 _____   8 _____

2 _____   9 _____

3 _____   10 _____

4 _____   11 _____

5 _____   12 _____

6 _____   13 _____

7 _____   14 _____

C H A P T E R

4

Tissues and Membranes

OBJECTIVES

- List the four main types of tissues
- Define the function and location of tissues
- Define the function and location of membranes
- Define an organ and organ system
- Relate various organs to their respective systems
- Describe the processes involved in the two types of tissue repair
- Describe the process of granulation
- Define the key words that relate to this chapter

KEY WORDS

adipose
aponeuroses
areolar
bactericidal
calcify
cardiac
cartilage
cicatrix
clean wound
collagen
connective tissue
epithelial
elastin
fasciae

graft
granulation
hyaline
ligament
membrane
mucosa
mucous membrane
muscle tissue
nervous tissue
organ system
osseous
parietal membrane
pericardial
    membrane

peritoneal membrane
pleural
    membrane
primary repair
scab
secondary repair
serous fluid
serous membrane
skeletal
sutures
synovial membrane
tissue
tendon
visceral membrane

TISSUES

Multicellular organisms are composed of many different types of cells. Although they are not randomly arranged, each of these cells performs a special function. These millions of cells are grouped according to their similarity in shape, size, structure, intercellular materials and function. Cells so grouped are called tissues. There are four main types of tissue. (1) epithelial, which protects the body by covering internal and external surfaces. The cells of the epithelial tissue also produce secretions such as digestive juices. The epithelial tissue is named according to its structure. (2) connective, which supports and connects organs and tissue. (3) muscle, which contains cell material which has the ability to contract and move the body. (4) nervous, which contains cells that react to stimuli and conduct an impulse.

Specialization of cells can be seen in a study of the epithelial cells which make up epithelial tissue. Epithelial cells that cover the body's external and internal surfaces have a typical shape, either columnar, cubical, or platelike. This variation is necessary so the epithelial cells can fit together smoothly in order to line and protect the bodily surface. Muscle cells making up muscle tissue are long and spindle-like so they can contract.

Some tissues are comprised of both living cells and various nonliving substances which the cells build up around themselves. The variations, functions, and locations of each type are described in Table 4-1.

MEMBRANES

A membrane is formed by putting two thin layers of tissue together. The cells in the membrane may secrete a fluid. Membranes are classified as epithelial or connective.

Epithelial Membranes

Epithelial membranes are classified as mucous or serous depending on the type of secretions which are produced, Figure 4-1.

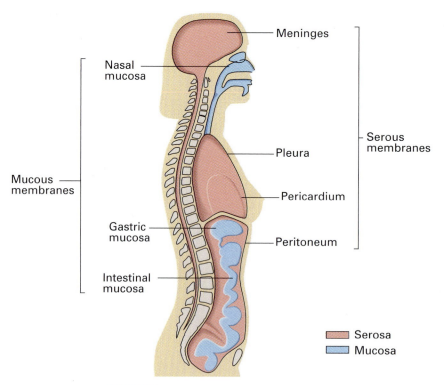

FIGURE 4-1 *Mucous and serous membranes*

Labels: Meninges, Nasal mucosa, Pleura, Pericardium, Peritoneum, Mucous membranes, Serous membranes, Gastric mucosa, Intestinal mucosa

Legend: Serosa, Mucosa

TABLE 4-1 • *Different Kinds of Human Tissue*

TYPE OF TISSUE	FUNCTION	CHARACTERISTICS AND LOCATION	MORPHOLOGY
I. EPITHELIAL	Cells form a continuous layer covering internal and external body surfaces, provide protection, produce secretions (digestive juices, hormones, perspiration), and regulate the passage of materials across themselves. **A. Covering and lining tissue** These cells can be stratified (layered), ciliated, or keratinized.	**1. Squamous epithelial cells** These are flat, irregularly-shaped cells. They line the heart, blood and lymphatic vessels, body cavities, and alveoli (air sacs) of lungs. The outer layer of the skin is composed of stratified and keratinized squamous epithelial cells. The stratified squamous epithelial cells on the outer skin layer protect the body against microbial invasion.	
		2. Cuboidal epithelial cells These are the cube-shaped cells that line the kidney tubules, and which cover the ovaries and secretory parts of certain glands.	
		3. Columnar epithelial cells Elongated, with the nucleus generally near the bottom and often ciliated on the outer surface. They line the ducts, digestive tract (especially the intestinal and stomach lining), parts of the respiratory tract, and glands.	

TABLE 4-1 • *Different Kinds of Human Tissue (Continued)*

TYPE OF TISSUE	FUNCTION	CHARACTERISTICS AND LOCATION	MORPHOLOGY
I. EPITHELIAL (continued)	**B. Glandular or secretory tissue** These cells are specialized to secrete materials like digestive juices, hormones, milk, perspiration, and wax. They are columnar or cuboidal shaped.	**Endocrine gland cells** These cells form ductless glands which secrete their substances (hormones) directly into the bloodstream. For instance, the thyroid gland secretes thyroxin, while adrenal glands secrete adrenaline. **Exocrine gland cells** These cells secrete their substances into ducts. The mammary glands, sweat glands, and salivary glands are examples.	Duct (where secretions leave) Secretory cells Exocrine (duct) gland cell e.g. sweat and mammary glands
II. CONNECTIVE		Cells whose intercellular secretions (matrix) support and connect the organs and tissues of the body.	Cytoplasm Collagen fibers Nucleus Vacuole (for fat storage)
	A. Adipose tissue This tissue stores lipid (fat), acts as filler tissue, cushions, supports, and insulates the body.	A type of loose, connective tissue composed of sac-like adipose cells; they are specialized for the storage of fat. Adipose cells are found throughout the body: in the subcutaneous skin layer, around the kidneys, within padding around joints, and in the marrow of long bones.	
	B. Areolar (loose) connective This tissue surrounds various organs and supports both nerve cells and blood vessels which transport nutrient materials (to cells) and wastes (away from cells). Areolar tissue also (temporarily) stores glucose, salts, and water.	It is composed of a large, semifluid matrix, with many different types of cells and fibers embedded in it. These include fibroblasts (fibrocytes), plasma cells, macrophages, mast cells, and various white blood cells. The fibers are bundles of strong, flexible white fibrous protein called collagen, and elastic single fibers of elastin. It is found in the epidermis of the skin and in the subcutaneous layer with adipose cells.	Mast cell Reticular fibers Collagen fibers Fibroblast cell Plasma cell Elastic fiber Matrix Macrophage cell

TABLE 4-1 • *Different Kinds of Human Tissue (Continued)*

TYPE OF TISSUE	FUNCTION	CHARACTERISTICS AND LOCATION	MORPHOLOGY
II. CONNECTIVE (continued)	**C. Dense fibrous** This tissue forms ligaments, tendons and aponeuroses. **Ligaments** are strong, flexible bands (or cords) which hold bones firmly together at the joints. **Tendons** are white, glistening bands attaching skeletal muscles to the bones. **Aponeuroses** are flat, wide bands of tissue holding one muscle to another or to the periosteum (bone covering). **Fasciae** are fibrous connective tissue sheets that wrap around muscle bundles to hold them in place.	Dense fibrous tissue is also called white fibrous tissue, since it is made from closely packed white collagen fibers. Fibrous tissue is flexible, but not elastic. This tissue has a poor blood supply and heals slowly.	Fibroblast cell — Closely packed collagen fibers
	D. Supportive **1. Bone (osseous) tissue—** Comprises the skeleton of the body, which supports and protects underlying soft tissue parts and organs, and also serves as attachments for skeletal muscles.	Connective tissue whose intercellular matrix is *calcified* by the deposition of mineral salts (like calcium carbonate and calcium phosphate). Calcification of bone imparts great strength. The entire skeleton is composed of bone tissue.	Bone lacunae — Bone cell — Cytoplasm — Nucleus
	2. Cartilage— Provides firm but flexible support for the embryonic skeleton and part of the adult skeleton. **a. Hyaline—** Forms the skeleton of the embryo.	Hyaline cartilage is found upon articular bone surfaces, and also at the nose tip, bronchi and bronchial tubes. Ribs are joined to the sternum (breastbone) by the costal cartilage. It is also found in the larynx and the rings in the trachea.	Cells (chondrocytes) — Matrix — Lacuna (space enclosing cells)
	b. Fibrocartilage— A strong, flexible, supportive substance, found between bones and wherever great strength (and a degree of rigidity) is needed.	Fibrocartilage is located within intervertebral discs and pubic symphysis between the pubic bones.	Chondrocytes — Dense white fibers

TABLE 4-1 • *Different Kinds of Human Tissue (Continued)*

TYPE OF TISSUE	FUNCTION	CHARACTERISTICS AND LOCATION	MORPHOLOGY
II. CONNECTIVE (continued)	**D. Supportive (continued)** **c. Elastic cartilage—** The intercellular matrix is embedded with a network of elastic fibers and is firm but flexible.	Elastic cartilage is located inside the auditory ear tube, external ear, epiglottis, and larynx.	Elastic fibers / Chondrocyte / Nucleus
	E. Vascular (liquid blood tissue) **1. Blood—** Transports nutrient and oxygen molecules to cells, and metabolic wastes away from cells (can be considered as a liquid tissue). Contains cells that function in the body's defense and in blood clotting.	Blood is composed of two major parts: a liquid called plasma, and a solid cellular portion known as blood cells (or corpuscles). The plasma suspends corpuscles, of which there are two major types: red blood cells (erythrocytes) and white blood cells (leukocytes). A third cellular component (really a cell fragment) is called platelets (thrombocytes). Blood circulates within the blood vessels (arteries, veins, and capillaries) and through the heart.	Lymphocyte / Basophil / Thrombocytes (platelets) / Monocyte / Eosinophil / Erythrocytes / Neutrophil
	2. Lymph— Transports tissue fluid, proteins, fats and other materials from the tissues to the circulatory system. This occurs through a series of tubes called the lymphatic vessels.	Lymph is a fluid made up of water, glucose, protein, fats, and salt. The cellular components are lymphocytes and granulocytes. They flow in tubes called lymphatic vessels, which closely parallel the veins and bathe the tissue spaces between cells.	Lymph capillary / Red blood cells / White blood cell / Lymph / Cells / Blood capillary

TABLE 4-1 ● *Different Kinds of Human Tissue (Continued)*

TYPE OF TISSUE	FUNCTION	CHARACTERISTICS AND LOCATION	MORPHOLOGY
III. MUSCLE	**A. Cardiac** These cells help the heart contract in order to pump blood through and out of the heart.	Cardiac muscle is a striated (having a cross-banding pattern), involuntary (not under conscious control) muscle. It makes up the walls of the heart.	Centrally located nucleus; Striations; Branching of cell; Intercalated disc
	B. Skeletal (striated voluntary) These muscles are attached to the movable parts of the skeleton. They are capable of rapid, powerful contractions and long states of partially sustained contractions, allowing for voluntary movement.	Skeletal muscle is: striated (having transverse bands that run down the length of muscle fiber); voluntary, because the muscle is under conscious control; and *skeletal*, since these muscles are attached to the skeleton (bones, tendons and other muscles).	Myofibrils; Nucleus
	C. Smooth (nonstriated involuntary) These provide for involuntary movement. Examples include the movement of materials along the digestive tract, controlling the diameter of blood vessels and the pupil of the eyes.	Smooth muscle is nonstriated because it lacks the striations (bands) of skeletal muscles; its movement is involuntary. It makes up the walls of the digestive, genito-urinary, respiratory tracts, blood vessels, and lymphatic vessels.	Cells separated from each other; Nucleus; Spindle-shaped cell
IV. NERVE	**Neurons (nerve cells)** These cells have the ability to react to stimuli. **1. Irritability—** Ability of nerve tissue to respond to environmental changes. **2. Conductivity—** Ability to carry a nerve impulse (message).	Nerve tissue is composed of *neurons* (nerve cells). Neurons have branches through which various parts of the body are connected and their activities coordinated. They are found in the brain, spinal cord, and nerves.	Nucleus; Myelin; Axon; Terminal branches; Dendrites; Cell body

Mucous membranes. They line surfaces and spaces that lead to the outside of the body; they line the respiratory, digestive, reproductive and urinary systems. The mucous membrane produces a substance called mucous which lubricates and protects the lining. For example, the mucous in the digestive tract protects the lining of the stomach and small intestines from the digestive juices. The term mucosa is used for a specific mucous membrane, namely:

- **respiratory mucosa**, which lines the respiratory passages

- **gastric mucosa**, which lines the stomach

- **intestinal mucosa**, which lines the small and large intestines.

Serous membrane. This is a double-walled membrane which produces a watery fluid and lines closed body cavities. The fluid produced is called **serous fluid**. The outer part of the membrane which lines the cavity is known as the **parietal** serous membrane and the part which covers the organs within is known as the **visceral** serous membrane. The fluid produced allows the organs within to move freely and prevents friction. The name serosa is given to the specific serous membranes, all beginning with the letter "p." The serous membranes are:

- **pleural membrane**, which lines the thoracic or chest cavity and protects the lungs; the fluid is called pleural fluid

- **pericardial membrane**, which lines the heart cavity and protects the heart; the fluid is called pericardial fluid

- **peritoneal membrane**, which lines the abdominal cavity and protects the abdominal organs; the fluid is called peritoneal fluid.

Cutaneous membrane, or skin. This is a specialized type of epithelial membrane which will be discussed in Chapter 5.

Connective Membranes

Connective membranes are made of two layers of connective tissue. In this classification is the **synovial membrane** which lines joint cavities. Synovial membranes secrete synovial fluid which prevents friction inside the joint cavity.

ORGANS AND SYSTEMS

An organ is a structure made up of several tissues grouped together to perform a single function. For instance, the stomach is an organ composed of highly specialized vascular, connective, epithelial, muscular, and nerve tissues. All of these tissues function together so as to enable the stomach to undergo digestion and absorption.

The skin which covers our bodies is no mere simple tissue, but a complex organ composed of connective, epithelial, muscular and nervous tissue. These tissues enable the skin to protect the body and remove its wastes (water and inorganic salts), making us sensitive to our environment.

The various organs of the human body do not function separately. Instead, they coordinate their activities to form a complete, functional organism. A group of organs which act together to perform a specific, related function is called an **organ system**, see Figure 4-2.

The digestive system has the special function of processing solid food into liquid for absorption into the bloodstream. This organ system includes the mouth, salivary glands, esophagus, stomach, small intestine, liver, pancreas, gallbladder, and large intestine. The circulatory system transports materials to and from cells. It is comprised of the heart, arteries, veins, capillaries, lymphatic vessels, and spleen.

Each of the ten organ systems is highly specialized to perform a specific function; together they coordinate their functions to form a whole, live, functioning organism.

The systems of the body are the skeletal, muscular, digestive, respiratory, circulatory,

LEVEL   EXAMPLES

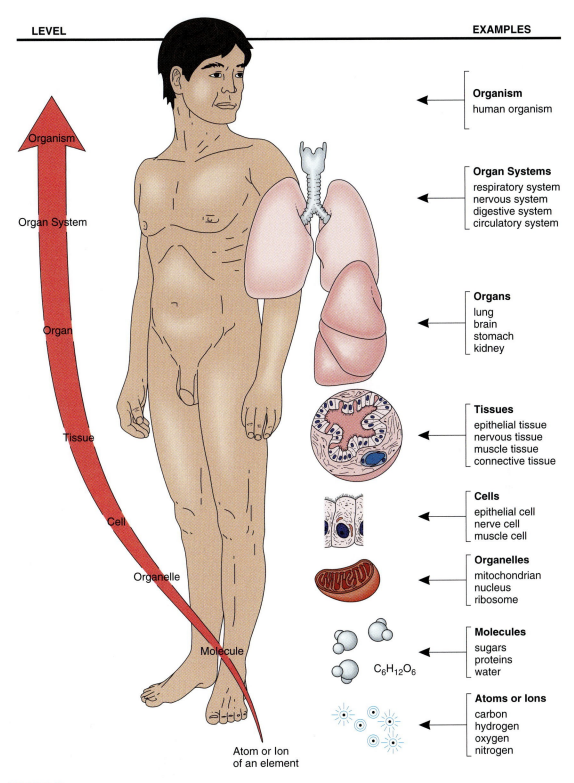

Organism
human organism

Organ Systems
respiratory system
nervous system
digestive system
circulatory system

Organs
lung
brain
stomach
kidney

Tissues
epithelial tissue
nervous tissue
muscle tissue
connective tissue

Cells
epithelial cell
nerve cell
muscle cell

Organelles
mitochondrian
nucleus
ribosome

Molecules
sugars
proteins
water

$C_6H_{12}O_6$

Atoms or Ions
carbon
hydrogen
oxygen
nitrogen

Organism

Organ System

Organ

Tissue

Cell

Organelle

Molecule

Atom or Ion
of an element

FIGURE 4-2 *The various organs of the human body function together. The formation of the human organism progresses from different levels of complexity.*

TABLE 4-2 ● *The Ten Body Systems*

SYSTEM	SYSTEM FUNCTIONS	ORGANS
Skeletal	Gives shape to body; protects delicate parts of body; provides space for attaching muscles; is instrumental in forming blood; stores minerals.	Skull, Spinal Column, Ribs and Sternum, Shoulder Girdle, Upper and Lower Extremities, Pelvic Girdle.
Muscular	Determines posture; produces body heat; provides for movement.	Striated Voluntary Muscles — Skeleletal Striated Involuntary — Cardiac Smooth — Non-striated
Digestive	Prepares food for absorption and use by body cells through modification of chemical and physical states.	Mouth (salivary glands, teeth, tongue), Pharynx, Esophagus, Stomach, Intestines, Liver, Gallbladder, Pancreas.
Respiratory	Acquires oxygen; rids body of carbon dioxide.	Nose, Pharynx, Larynx, Trachea, Bronchi, Lungs.
Circulatory	Carries oxygen and nourishment to cells of body; carries waste from cells; body defense.	Heart, Arteries, Veins, Capillaries, Lymphatic Vessels, Lymph Nodes, Spleen.
Excretory	Removes waste products of metabolism from body.	Skin, Lungs, Kidneys, Bladder, Ureters, Urethra.
Nervous	Communicates; controls body activity; coordinates body activity.	Brain, Nerves, Spinal Cord, Ganglia.
Endocrine	Manufactures hormones to regulate organ activity.	Glands (ductless): Pituitary, Thyroid, Parathyroid, Pancreas, Adrenal, Gonads (ovaries, testes).
Reproductive	Reproduces human beings.	*Male* *Female* Testes Ovaries Scrotum Fallopian tubes Epididymis Uterus Vas deferens Vagina Seminal vesicles Bartholin glands Ejaculatory duct External genitals (vulva) Prostate gland Breasts (mammary Cowper's gland glands) Penis Urethra
Integumentary	Helps regulate body temperature, establishes a barrier between the body and environment; eliminates waste; synthesizes Vitamin D; contains receptors for temperature, pressure, and pain.	Epidermis, Dermis, Sweat Glands, Oil Glands.

reproductive, excretory, endocrine, nervous, and integumentary systems. The functions and organs of each system are shown in Table 4-2.

DEGREE OF TISSUE REPAIR

Repair of damaged tissues occurs continually under the everyday activities of living.

Depending on the type and location of injury, some tissue is quickly repaired. Muscle tissue heals slowly and bone tissue repairs are slow because broken bone ends must be kept aligned and immobilized until the repair is done. Heart muscle tissue does not repair itself, and nerve cell bodies destroyed by infection or injury do *not* grow back.

PROCESS OF EPITHELIAL TISSUE REPAIR

There are two types of epithelial tissue repair. One is called **primary repair** and the other one is called **secondary repair**.

Primary Repair

Primary repair takes place in "clean" wounds. A **clean wound** is a cut or incision on the skin where infection is not present. In a simple skin injury, the deep layer of stratified squamous epithelium divides. The new stratified squamous epithelial cells "push" themselves upward toward the surface of the skin. The damage or wound is quickly and completely restored to normal. However, if the damage is over a larger area, then the underlying connective tissue cells and fibroblasts are also involved.

Primary Repair Over A Larger Skin Area

If a larger area of skin is damaged, fluid will escape from the broken capillaries. This capillary fluid dries and seals the wound, and the typical **scab** forms. Epithelial cells multiply at the edges of the scab and continue to grow over the damaged area until it is covered. If even a much larger or deeper area of skin is destroyed, skin **grafts** are needed to help in wound healing.

Primary Repair of Deeper Tissues

When there is damage to deeper tissues, the edges of the wound must be brought (sewn) together with **sutures**. For example, in operative incisions or wounds, there is a tremendous amount of serous fluid that leaks out onto the wound. This helps to form a coagulation (clot) that seals the wound. The coagulum contains tissue fragments and white blood cells. In twenty-four to thirty-six hours, the epithelial cells lining the capillaries (endothelium) and fibroblasts of connective tissue are rapidly regenerating. The newly formed cells remain along the edges of the wound. On the third day, new vascular tissue starts to form. These multiply across the wound along with connective tissue formation.

On the fourth or fifth day, fibroblast cells start to be very active. They will help to make new collagen fibers. In addition, capillaries grow and "reach" across the wound, holding the edges firmly together. Towards the end of the healing process, the collagenous fibers shorten, and scar tissue is reduced to a minimum.

Secondary Repair

A process called **granulation** occurs in a large open wound with small or large tissue loss. The granulation process will form new vertically upstanding blood vessels. These new blood vessels are surrounded by young connective tissue and wandering cells of different types. Granulation causes the surface area to have a pebbly texture. Fibroblasts will be quite active in their production of new collagenous fibers. With all this activity going on, the large open wound eventually heals up. It also should be mentioned that as granulation occurs, a fluid is secreted. This fluid has very strong bactericidal (bacterial destruction) properties. This is important to help reduce the risk of infection during wound healing.

As in any type of tissue repair, there is always some amount of scar tissue that will be formed. The amount of scar (cicatrix) tissue formed depends upon the extent of tissue damage. Much careful attention must be given to patients whose body or body parts are undergoing massive tissue repair (these include burn victims). These areas *must* be kept in alignment and immobile at the beginning. However, later on active movement should be encouraged so as new tissue forms, pulling from scar tissue will not occur. It is the role of the health care professional to help prevent or minimize excessive scar tissue formation that can lead to disfigurement.

A health care professional should also be mindful that proper nutrition plays an important part in the healing act. Newly growing tissues require lots of protein for repair, thus the need for protein-rich foods is important.

Vitamins also play an essential role in wound repair. They help the patient develop resistance to and help prevent infections. Table 4-3 gives a listing of some vitamins that are needed in tissue repair.

TABLE 4-3 ● *Vitamins Favorable to Tissue Repair*

VITAMIN	FUNCTION
Vitamin A	Repairs epithelial tissue, especially the epithelial cells lining the respiratory tract.
Vitamin B (Thiamine, nicotinic acid, and riboflavin)	Helps to promote the general well-being of the individual. Specifically helps to promote appetite, metabolism, vigor, and pain relief in some cases.
Vitamin C	Helps in the normal production of and maintenance of collagen fibers and other connective tissue substances.
Vitamin D	Needed for the normal absorption of calcium from the intestine. Possibly helps in the repair of bone fractures.
Vitamin K	Helps in the process of blood coagulation.
Vitamin E	Helps healing of tissues by acting as an antioxidant protector. It prevents important molecules and structures in the cell from reacting with oxygen. (When delicate components of living protoplasm are attacked by oxygen, they are literally "burnt.")

● REVIEW QUESTIONS

Select the letter of the choice that best completes the statement.

1. Cells that are alike in size, shape and function are called:
   a. elements
   b. tissues
   c. organs
   d. systems

2. The type of tissue found on the outer layer of skin is called:
   a. squamous epithelial
   b. stratified epithelial
   c. ciliated epithelial
   d. columnar epithelial

3. Collagen is a strong flexible protein found mainly in:
   a. adipose tissue
   b. cartilage tissue
   c. loose connective tissue
   d. bone tissue

4. Connective tissue structures that hold bones firmly together at joints are called:
   a. fascia
   b. tendons
   c. aponeuroses
   d. ligaments

5. The membrane that covers linings to the outside of the body is:
   a. cutaneous
   b. serous
   c. mucous
   d. synovial

6. The membrane that covers the lungs is called:
   a. parietal pleura
   b. visceral pleura
   c. parietal pericardial
   d. visceral pericardial

7. An inflammation of the lining of the abdominal cavity is called:
   a. pleurisy
   b. pericarditis
   c. peritonitis
   d. gastritis

8. The system that provides for movement of the body is the:
   a. skeletal
   b. nervous
   c. muscle
   d. circulatory

9. The type of repair that takes place in a clean wound is called:
   a. primary repair
   b. granulation
   c. secondary repair
   d. secretion of bactericidal fluid

10. The vitamin necessary to help as an antioxidant is:
    a. A
    b. D
    c. K
    d. E

● COMPLETION

Complete the following statements:

1. The tissue that has the ability to react to stimuli is _____.

2. The gastric mucosa is the mucous membrane lining of the _____ _____.

3. The secretion that prevents the bones in a joint from rubbing together is _____ _____.

4. The lining that protects the lung is the _____ membrane.

5. In secondary tissue repair when there is a large open wound the process of tissue repair is called _____.

● APPLYING THEORY TO PRACTICE

1. Feel your skin. What type of tissue is it? Is this tissue the same as the lining in your mouth?

2. Explain how mucous affects the air we breathe or the food we eat.

3. Name each organ system involved when you eat a slice of pizza.

4. You have fallen and scraped your knees. What type of healing will take place? Describe the process involved in the repair.

5. If you had a friend with severe injuries, describe the lunch you would prepare for this person. The menu should include the vitamins necessary for tissue repair and to help with pain relief.

CHAPTER

5

Integumentary System

KEY WORDS

acne vulgaris
albinism
alopecia
arrector pili muscle
athlete's foot
avascular
boils
basal cell carcinoma
corn
cortex
dermis
dermatitis
eczema
epidermis
first degree burn
genital herpes
hair follicle
herpes
impetigo
Integumentary system
keratin
malignant melanoma
matrix
medulla
melanin
melanoma
papilla
psoriasis
ringworm
root
rule of nines
sebaceous gland
sebum
second degree burn
shaft
shingles (herpes zoster)
skin cancer
squamous cell carcinoma
stratum corneum
stratum germinativum
sudoriferous gland
third degree burn
urticaria (hives)

The skin is our protective covering and is called the integument or **integumentary system** or cutaneous membrane. It is tough, pliable, and multi-functional.

FUNCTIONS OF THE SKIN

The skin has seven functions.

1. Skin is a covering for the underlying, deeper tissues, protecting them from dehydration, injury, and germ invasion.

2. The skin also helps regulate body temperature by controlling the amount of heat loss. Evaporation of water from the skin, in the form of perspiration, helps rid the body of excess heat. Only a very small amount of waste is eliminated through the skin.

3. Skin helps to manufacture Vitamin D. The ultraviolet light on the skin is necessary for the first stages of Vitamin D formation.

4. The skin is the site of many nerve endings, Figure 5-1. A square inch of skin contains about 72 feet of nerves and hundreds of receptors.

5. The skin has tissues for the temporary storage of fat, glucose, water, and salts like sodium chloride. Most of these substances are later absorbed by the blood and transported to other parts of the body.

6. The skin is designed to screen out any harmful ultraviolet radiation contained in sunlight.

7. The skin has special properties which absorb certain drugs and other chemical substances. We can apply drugs for local application, as in the case of treating rashes; or we can apply medications which can be absorbed through the skin and have a general effect in the body. An example of this is Nitro-Bid paste, which is used to help dilate blood vessels in the treatment of angina pectoris (chest pain).

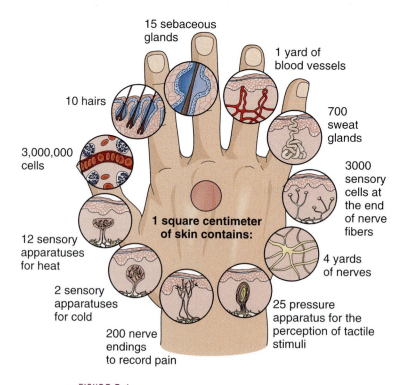

15 sebaceous glands

1 yard of blood vessels

10 hairs

700 sweat glands

3,000,000 cells

3000 sensory cells at the end of nerve fibers

1 square centimeter of skin contains:

12 sensory apparatuses for heat

4 yards of nerves

2 sensory apparatuses for cold

25 pressure apparatus for the perception of tactile stimuli

200 nerve endings to record pain

FIGURE 5-1 *The skin is well supplied with nerves.*

STRUCTURE OF THE SKIN

The skin consists of two basic layers:

1. the **epidermis** or outermost covering which is made of epithelial cells with no blood vessels present (**avascular**), and

2. the **dermis** or true skin which is made up of connective tissue and is vascular.

Epidermis

The two most functionally important cellular layers of the epidermis are the **stratum corneum** and the **stratum germinativum**. The cytoplasm of the cells making up the stratum corneum is replaced by a hard, nonliving protein substance called **keratin**. This keratin layer acts as a waterproof covering. Cells making up the stratum corneum are flattened and scale-like. They flake off from the constant friction of clothing, rubbing, and washing. For this reason the stratum corneum is sometimes called the horny layer. As the cells of the horny layer are flaked off, they are replaced by new cells from the lower stratum germinativum.

The stratum corneum forms the body's first line of defense against invading bacteria. Because it is slightly acidic, many kinds of organisms which come in contact with the stratum corneum are destroyed. The thickness of the horny layer varies in different parts of the body. It is thickest on the palms of the hands and on the soles of the feet due to constant friction. Sometimes the thickening develops outwardly in a concentrated area forming a callus. If the thickening grows inward, a **corn** may form.

The stratum germinativum is a very important epidermal layer. The replacement of cells in the epidermis depends upon the division of cells in this layer. As new germinativum cells form, they push their way upward towards the epidermis. Eventually they become keratinized like the other epidermal cells within the horny layer.

Skin pigmentation is found in germinativum cells called **melanocytes**. Melanocytes contain a skin pigment called **melanin**. Melanin can be black, brown, or have a yellow tint, depending upon racial origin. The amount of melanin (and other skin pigments like carotene and hemoglobin) in the melanocytes determines the various shades of human skin color. Caucasians have a reduced amount of melanin in their melanocytes. If there are patches of melanin present, the skin is said to be freckled. In the elderly melanin also collects in spots. These are said to be aging spots. Other races, on the other hand, possess a higher amount of melanin. Absence of pigments (other than hemoglobin) causes **albinism**. The skin of an albino has a pinkish tint. Basic skin coloring is inherited from our parents.

Environment is another factor which can modify skin coloring. For example, exposure to sunlight may result in a temporary increase in melanin within the melanocytes. This is the darkened, or tanned effect with which we are all familiar. Tanning is produced by the ultraviolet (UV) rays of sunlight. It should be noted that prolonged exposure to sunlight is unwise because it may lead to the development of skin cancers.

As seen in Figure 5-2, the lower edge of the stratum germinativum is thrown into ridges. These ridges are known as the **papillae** of the skin. The papillae actually arise from the dermal layer of the skin and push into the stratum germinativum of the epidermis. In the skin of the fingers, soles of the feet, and the palms of the hands, these papillae are quite pronounced. So much so, in fact, that they raise the skin into permanent ridges. These ridges are so arranged that they provide maximum resistance to slipping when grasping and holding objects. Thus they are also referred to as friction ridges. The ridges on the inner surfaces of the fingers create individual and characteristic fingerprint patterns used in identification. Newborn infants are also footprinted for means of identity.

Dermis

The dermis, or corium, is the thicker, inner layer of the skin. It contains matted masses of connective tissue, collagen tissue bands, elastic fibers (through which pass numerous blood

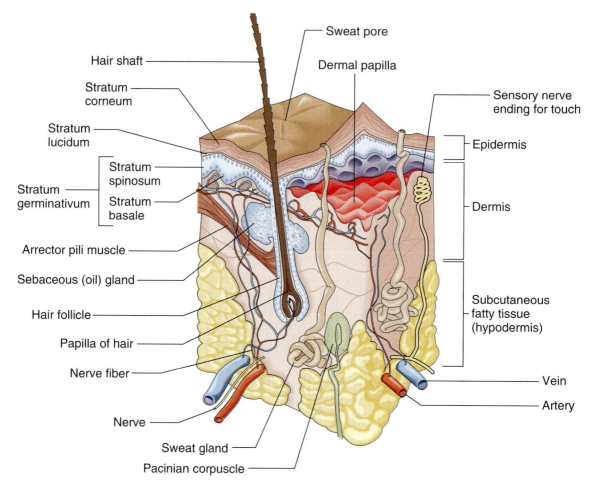

Sweat pore

Hair shaft

Dermal papilla

Stratum corneum

Sensory nerve ending for touch

Stratum lucidum

Epidermis

Stratum spinosum

Stratum germinativum

Stratum basale

Dermis

Arrector pili muscle

Sebaceous (oil) gland

Hair follicle

Subcutaneous fatty tissue (hypodermis)

Papilla of hair

Nerve fiber

Vein

Artery

Nerve

Sweat gland

Pacinian corpuscle

FIGURE 5-2   *A cross-section of the skin*

vessels), nerve endings, muscles, hair follicles, oil and sweat glands, and fat cells. The thickness of the dermis varies over different parts of the body. It is, for instance, thicker over the soles of the feet and the palms of the hand. The skin covering the shoulders and back is thinner than that over the palms, but thicker than the skin over the abdomen and thorax.

There are many nerve receptors of different types in the dermal layer. The sensory nerves end in nerve receptors which are sensitive to heat, cold, touch, pain and pressure. The nerve endings vary in where they are located. The receptors for touch are closer to the epidermis and you can feel someone touch you. However, the pressure receptors are deeper in the dermal layer. This explains why you can sit for a long period before you feel uncomfortable. There

are also nerve endings to sense pain located under the epidermis and around the hair follicles. These pain receptors are especially numerous on the lower arm, breast, and forehead.

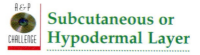

Subcutaneous or Hypodermal Layer

This layer lies under the dermis and sometimes is called superficial fascia. It is not a true part of the integumentary system. It is made up of loose connective tissue and contains about one-half of the body's stored fat. The hypodermis layer attaches the integumentary system to the surface muscles underneath. Injections frequently given in this area are called hypodermic, or subcutaneous.

APPENDAGES OF THE SKIN

The appendages of the skin include the hair, nails, the sudoriferous (sweat) glands, and the sebaceous (oil) glands and their ducts.

Hair

Hairs are distributed over most of the surface area of the body. They are missing from the palms of hands, soles of feet, the glans penis, and the inner surfaces of the vaginal labia.

The length, thickness, type, and color of hair varies with the different body parts and different races. The hairs of the eyelids, for example, are extremely short, while hair from the scalp can grow to a considerable length. Facial and pubic hair are quite thick. The hair of Asian people is straight; that of Africans is very curly.

A hair is composed of root shaft, the outer cuticle layer, the cortex, and the inner medulla. The cuticle consists of a single layer of flat, scalelike, keratinized cells that overlap each other. The cortex is comprised of elongated, keratinized, nonliving cells. Hair pigment is located in the cortex, or in the medulla if one is present. In dark hair the cortex contains pigment granules; as one ages, pigment granules are replaced with air, which looks gray or white.

The root is the part of the hair that is implanted in the skin. The shaft is that part which projects from the skin surface. The root is embedded in an inpocketing of the epidermis called the hair follicle. Toward the lower end of the hair follicle is a tuft of tissue called the papilla, which extends upward into the hair root. The papilla contains capillaries which nourish the hair follicle cells. This is important because the division of cells in the hair follicle gives rise to a new hair. There is a genetic predisposition in some males to a condition known as alopecia or baldness, which is a permanent hair loss. The normal hair is replaced by a very short hair which is transparent and for practical purposes invisible.

Attached to each hair follicle on the side toward which it slopes is a smooth muscle called the arrector pili muscle. When the pili muscle is stimulated, as by a sudden chill, it contracts and causes the skin to pucker around the hair. It may be called "goosebumps" or "gooseflesh." When this occurs, a small amount of oil is produced, due to pressure on the sebaceous glands.

Nails

The nails are hard structures covering the dorsal surfaces of the last phalanges of the fingers and toes. They are slightly convex on their upper surfaces and concave on their lower surfaces. A nail is formed in the nail bed or matrix, Figure 5-3. Here the epidermal cells first appear as elongated cells. These then fuse together to form hard, keratinized plates. As long as a nail bed remains intact, a nail will always be formed. Occasionally, a nail is lost due to an injury or disease. However, if the nail bed is not damaged, a new nail will be produced.

Sweat Glands

While actual excretion is a minor function of the skin, certain wastes dissolved in perspiration are removed. Perspiration is 99% water with only small quantities of salt and organic materials (waste products). Sweat, or sudoriferous glands are distributed over the entire skin surface. They are present in large numbers under the arms, on the palms of the hands, soles of the feet, and forehead.

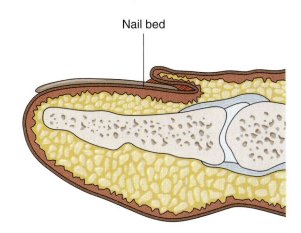

Nail bed

FIGURE 5-3 *Diagram of the fingernail bed*

Sweat glands are tubular, with a coiled base and a tube-like duct which extends to form a pore in the skin, see Figure 5-2. Perspiration is excreted through the pores. Under the control of the nervous system, these glands may be activated by several factors including heat, pain, fever, and nervousness.

The amount of water lost through the skin is almost 500 milliliters a day. However, this varies according to the type of exercise and the environmental temperature. In profuse sweating a great deal of water may be lost; it is vital to replace the loss of water as soon as possible.

Ceruminous or wax glands are modifications of the sweat (sudoriferous) glands. These are found in the ear canals and produce "ear wax."

Sebaceous Glands

The skin is protected by a thick, oily substance known as **sebum** secreted by the **sebaceous glands**. Sebum lubricates the skin, keeping it soft and pliable.

THE INTEGUMENT AND ITS RELATIONSHIP TO MICROORGANISMS

An intact skin surface is the best way the body can defend itself against pathogens, (disease producing) toxins and water loss. If skin is especially dry, use lotions or creams to prevent the skin from cracking.

Most of the surface of the skin is not a favorable place for microbial growth because it is too dry. Microbes live only on moist skin areas where they adhere to and grow on the surfaces of dead cells that compose the outer epidermal layer. The type of microbes found are of the Staphylococcus or Corynebacterium bacterial species type. The other types are *fungi** and *yeasts**.

Most skin bacteria are associated with the hair follicles or sweat glands where nutrients

are present and the moisture content is high. "Underarm perspiration odor" is caused by the interaction of bacteria on perspiration. This odor can be minimized or prevented either by decreasing perspiration with antiperspirants or killing the bacteria with deodorant soaps. Each hair follicle is associated with a sebaceous gland that secretes sebum. This lubricant fluid contains amino acids, lactic acid, lipids, salts, and urea. These are substances that can support microbial growth.

A health care worker must know that the number one way to prevent the spread of disease is by hand washing. The amount of time you spend washing depends on the amount of contamination. The least amount of time is ten to thirty seconds. If you are in contact with infectious material, the time should be from two to four minutes. If you are in contact with blood or any body secretions, you must first wash your hands, apply gloves before exposure, remove the gloves, and wash your hands again.

REPRESENTATIVE DISORDERS OF THE SKIN

Acne vulgaris is a common and chronic disorder of the sebaceous glands. The sebaceous glands secrete excessive oil, or sebum, which is deposited at the openings of the glands. Eventually this oily deposit becomes hard, or keratinized, plugging up the opening. This prevents the escape of the oily secretions, and the area becomes filled with leukocytes. The leukocytes cause the accumulation of pus. Acne occurs most often during adolescence and is marked by blackheads, cysts, pimples, and scarring.

Athlete's foot is a contagious fungal infection. The fungus infects the superficial skin layer and leads to skin eruptions. These eruptions are characterized by the formation of small blisters between the fingers and most often the toes. Accompanied by cracking and

---

* Fungi are low forms of microscopic plant life lacking chlorophyll; may be filamentous (mold) or unicellular (yeast).

* Yeast is a microscopic, single-celled member of the fungi division.

scaling, this condition is usually contracted in public baths or showers. Treatment involves thorough cleansing and drying of the affected area. In addition, special antifungal agents are administered and antifungal powders are applied liberally.

Dermatitis is an inflammation of the skin which may be non-specific. For example, some people may use a particular soap and develop contact dermatitis; they get a rash. Another cause may be emotional; stress may cause a person's skin to become covered with blotches.

Eczema is an acute, or chronic, noncontagious inflammatory skin disease. The skin becomes dry, red, itchy, and scaly. Various factors can lead to eczema. The most common type is atopic eczema, an allergic reaction that usually occurs in the first year of life. Eczema caused by ingested drugs is known as dermatitis medicamentosa. That caused by sunlight or artificial ultraviolet radiation is called dermatitis actinica. Treatment consists of removal or avoidance of the causative agent, as well as application of topical medications containing hydrocortisone. The medication, however, only helps to alleviate the symptoms.

Impetigo is an acute, inflammatory and contagious skin disease seen in babies and young children. It is caused by the staphylococcus or streptococcus organism. This disorder is characterized by the appearance of vesicles which rupture and develop distinct yellow crusts.

Psoriasis is a chronic inflammatory skin disease characterized by the development of dry reddish patches which are covered with silvery-white scales. It affects the skin surface over the elbows, knees, shins, scalp, and lower back, Figure 5-4. The cause is unknown; onsets may be triggered by stress, trauma, or infection.

Ringworm is a highly contagious fungal infection marked by raised, itchy, circular patches with crusts. It may occur upon the skin, scalp, and underneath the nails. Ringworm can be effectively treated with a drug called griseofulvin.

Urticaria or **hives** is a skin condition recognized by the appearance of intensely itching wheals or welts. These welts have an elevated

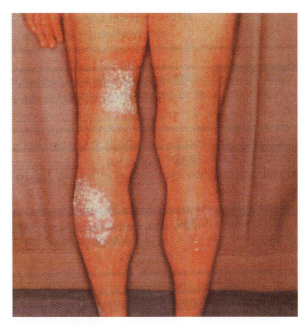

FIGURE 5-4 *Skin affected by psoriasis (photograph courtesy of Armed Forces Institute of Pathology, negative 74-16673)*

usually white, center with a surrounding pink area. They appear in clusters distributed over the entire body surface. The welts last about a day or two. Urticaria is generally a response to an allergen, such as an ingested drug or foods like citrus fruits, chocolate, fish, eggs, shellfish, strawberries, and tomatoes. Complete avoidance and elimination of the causative factor(s) alleviate the problem.

Boils, or carbuncles, are painful. A boil is a bacterial infection of the hair follicles or sebaceous glands usually caused by the staphylococcus organism. If the boil becomes more extensive and is deeply embedded, it is called a carbuncle. Treatment requires antibiotics and excision and drainage of the affected area.

Shingles (herpes zoster) is a skin eruption thought to be due to a virus infection of the nerve endings. It is commonly seen on the chest or abdomen, accompanied by severe pain known as herpetic neuralgia. The condition is especially serious in elderly or debilitated persons. Treatment consists of medication for pain and itching and protecting the area, Figure 5-5.

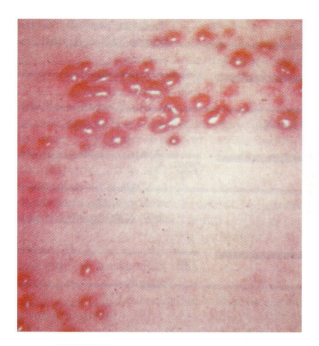

FIGURE 5-5 *Shingles is a skin eruption.*

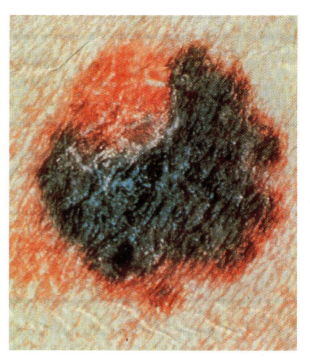

FIGURE 5-6 *Melanoma (courtesy of the American Academy of Dermatology)*

Herpes is a viral infection that is usually seen as a fever blister or cold sore. This virus may be spread through oral contact or through the respiratory route.

Genital Herpes is another form of the virus which may appear as a blister in the genital area. This virus is usually spread through sexual contact. In any type of herpes infection there are periods of remission and exacerbation (outbreak). Treatment is with acyclovir. A problem may arise when a woman becomes pregnant. If the woman has symptoms when the delivery date arrives, the baby may become infected when passing through the vaginal route for delivery. The physician must be told of a herpes condition in order to prevent infection of the newborn.

SKIN CANCER

Skin Cancer has been associated with exposure to ultraviolet light and scientists are cautioning people to limit their exposure to direct sunlight. Skin cancer is the most common type of cancer in people.

Basal cell carcinoma is the most common and least malignant type of skin cancer and it usually occurs on the face. The abnormal cells start in the epidermis and extend to the dermis or subcutaneous layer. This cancer may be treated by surgical removal or radiation. Full recovery occurs in 99% of the cases.

Squamous cell carcinoma arises from the epidermis and occurs most often on the scalp and lower lip. This type grows rapidly and metastasizes to the lymph nodes. This cancer may be treated by surgical removal or radiation. Chances for recovery are good if found early.

Malignant melanoma occurs in pigmented cells of the skin called melanocytes. The cancer cells metastasize to other areas quickly. This type of tumor may appear as a brown or black irregular patch which occurs suddenly, Figure 5-6. A color or size change in a pre-existing wart or mole may also indicate melanoma. Treatment is surgical removal of the melanoma and the surrounding area and chemotherapy.

BURNS

Burns occur as the result of radiation from the sun (sunburn), a heat lamp, or contact with boiling water, steam, fire, chemicals, or electricity. It is important to remind people that some medication causes increased sensitivity to sunlight. When the skin is burned, dehydration and infection may occur—either condition can be life threatening. The "rule of nines" measures the percent of the body burned: the body is divided into eleven areas and each area accounts for 9% of the total body surface. For example, the entire arm is 9% while the perineal area accounts for 1%.

Burns are usually referred to as first, second, or third degree, depending on the skin layers affected and the symptoms, Figure 5-7.

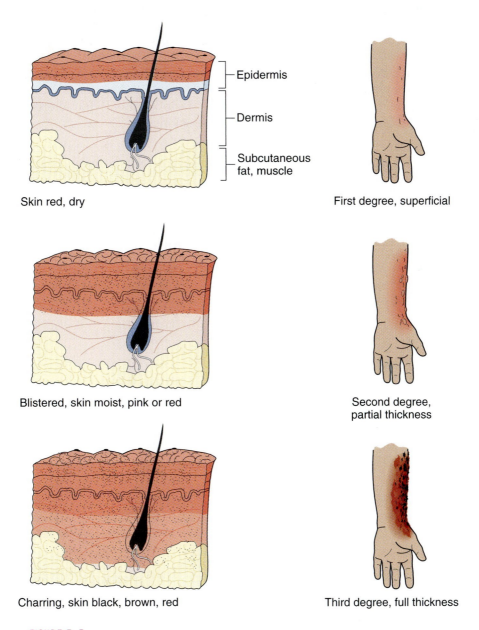

Skin red, dry

Epidermis

Dermis

Subcutaneous fat, muscle

First degree, superficial

Blistered, skin moist, pink or red

Second degree, partial thickness

Charring, skin black, brown, red

Third degree, full thickness

FIGURE 5-7 *Burns are usually referred to as first, second, or third degree burns.*

First degree burns involve only the epidermis. Symptoms are redness, swelling, and pain. Treatment consists of the application of cold water. Healing usually occurs within one week.

Second degree burns may involve the epidermis and dermis. Symptoms include pain, swelling, redness, and blistering. The skin may also be exposed to infection. Treatment may include pain medication and dry sterile dressings applied to open skin areas. Healing generally occurs within two weeks.

Third degree burns involve complete destruction of the epidermis, dermis, and subcutaneous layers. Symptoms include loss of skin, and eschar (blackened skin), yet there may be no pain. This may be a life threatening situation, depending on the amount of skin damaged, and fluid and blood plasma lost. The person requires immediate hospitalization. Treatment consists of prevention of infection, contracture, and fluid replacement. Skin grafting is done as soon as possible.

SKIN LESIONS

The health care professional should be familiar with the different types of skin disorders or lesions. This can indicate to the health professional the presence of a specific type of internal disease or disorder in the patient they are caring for. Sometimes the skin lesions indicate only an outer skin disorder. Table 5-1 and Figure 5-8 describe the different types of skin lesions, their characteristics, and their dimensions.

TABLE 5-1 ● *Different Types of Skin Lesions, Their Characteristics, Sizes, and Examples of Each*

TYPE OF SKIN LESION	CHARACTERISTICS	SIZE	EXAMPLE(S)
Bulla (blister)	Fluid-filled area	Greater than 5 mm across	A large blister
Macule	A round, flat area usually distinguished from its surrounding skin by its change in color	Smaller than 1 cm	• Freckle • Petechia
Nodule	Elevated solid area, deeper and firmer than a papule	Greater than 5 mm across	Wart
Papule	Elevated solid area	5 mm or less across	Elevated nevus
Pustule	Discrete, pus-filled raised area	Varying size	Acne
Ulcer	A deep loss of skin surface that may extend into the dermis that can bleed periodically and scar	Varies in size	Venous stasis ulcer
Tumor	Solid abnormal mass of cells that may extend deep through cutaneous tissue	Larger than 1-2 cm	• Benign (harmless) epidermal tumor • Basal cell carcinoma (rarely metastasizing)
Vesicle	Fluid-filled raised area	5 mm or less across	• Chickenpox • Herpes simplex
Wheal	Itchy, temporarily elevated area with an irregular shape formed as a result of localized skin edema	Varies in size	• Hives • Insect bites

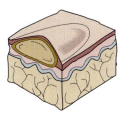

Bulla:
Same as a vesicle only greater than 0.5 cm
Example:
Contact dermatitis, large second-degree burns, bulbous impetigo, pemphigus

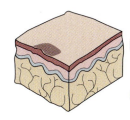

Macule:
Localized changes in skin color of less than 1 cm in diameter
Example:
Freckle

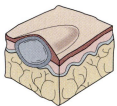

Nodules:
Solid and elevated; however, they extend deeper than papules into the dermis or subcutaneous tissues, 0.5-2 cm
Example:
Lipoma, erythema, nodosum, cyst

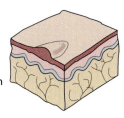

Papule:
Solid, elevated lesion less than 0.5 cm in diameter
Example:
Warts, elevated nevi

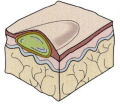

Pustule:
Vesicles or bullae that become filled with pus, usually described as less than 0.5 cm in diameter
Example:
Acne, impetigo, furuncles, carbuncles, folliculitis

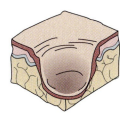

Ulcer:
A depressed lesion of the epidermis and upper papillary layer of the dermis
Example:
Stage 2 pressure ulcer

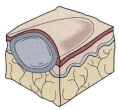

Tumor:
The same as a nodule only greater than 2 cm

Example:
Carcinoma (such as advanced breast carcinoma); **not** basal cell or squamous cell of the skin

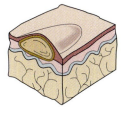

Vesicle:
Accumulation of fluid between the upper layers of the skin; elevated mass containing serous fluid; less than 0.5 cm
Example:
Herpes simplex, herpes zoster, chickenpox

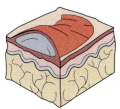

Wheal:
Localized edema in the epidermis causing irregular elevation that may be red or pale
Example:
Insect bite or a hive

FIGURE 5-8 *Different types of skin lesions*

● REVIEW QUESTIONS

Select the letter of the choice that best completes the statement.

1. The outmost layer of the skin is the:
   a. epidermis
   b. dermis
   c. hypodermis

2. The substance that serves best to keep our skin smooth and protected is:
   a. melanin
   b. keratin
   c. cortex

3. Nerve receptors are found in the:
   a. epidermis
   b. dermis
   c. hypodermis

4. Hair contains keratinized cells which are found in the:
   a. cuticle layer
   b. cortex
   c. medulla

5. The glands that secrete 99% water, small amounts of salt, and organic matter are called:
   a. endocrine glands
   b. sudoriferous glands
   c. sebaceous glands

● COMPLETION

Complete the following statements.

1. Hypodermic injections may be given in the _____ layer.

2. A common and chronic disorder that occurs in the teen years is called _____ _____.

3. Inflammation of the skin is called _____.

4. Urticaria or hives is usually a reaction to an _____.

5. A chronic inflammatory disease characterized by silvery patches is known as _____.

6. A cold sore or fever blister is known as _____.

7. Painful viral infections of the nerve endings are called _____.

8. The most common type of cancer is _____ _____.

9. A skin cancer that occurs as a large brown or black patch is _____ _____.

10. To determine the percent of the body burned, a health care worker may use a formula called the _____ _____ _____.

● APPLYING THEORY TO PRACTICE

1. If you get a cut on your skin, what may be the result?

2. Explain why you tan in the sun.

3. The skin helps to regulate body temperature by evaporation of water from the skin. Why do you feel uncomfortable on a hot, humid day?

4. A person is brought to the emergency room with third degree burns but is not complaining of pain. How is this possible?

5. The cosmetic industry sells many products that remove or prevent wrinkles. If this is true, why do people who use these creams still wrinkle as they age?

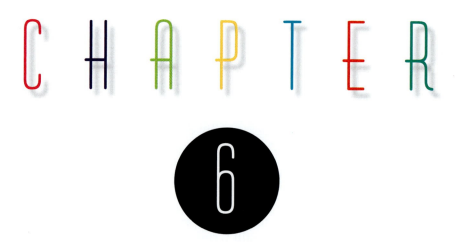

CHAPTER

6

Skeletal System

OBJECTIVES

- List the main function of the skeletal system
- Explain the formation of bone
- Name and locate the bones of the skeleton
- Name and define the main types of joint movement
- Identify common bone and joint disorders
- Define the key words that relate to this chapter

KEY WORDS

abduction
adduction
amphiarthroses
appendicular skeleton
arthritis
articular cartilage
atlas
axial skeleton
axis
ball-and-socket joint
bursa
bursitis
calcaneus
carpal
cervical vertebrae
circumduction
clavicle
coccyx
diaphysis
diarthroses
dislocation
endosteum
epiphysis
ethmoid
extension
femur
fibula
flexion
fontanel
fracture

frontal
gliding joint
gout
humerus
hinge joint
inferior concha
joint
kyphosis
lacrimal
lordosis
lumbar vertebrae
mandible
maxilla
medullary canal
metacarpal
metatarsal
nasal
occipital
ossification
osteoarthritis
osteoblast
osteoclast
osteocyte
osteomyelitis
osteoporosis
osteosarcoma
palatine
parietal
patella
periosteum

phalanges
pivot joint
pronation
radius
rheumatoid arthritis
rickets
rotation
sacrum
scapulae
scoliosis
skeletal system
slipped (herniated) disc
sphenoid
spongy bone
sprain
supination
suture
synarthroses
synovial membrane
synovial cavity
synovial fluid
tarsal
temporal
thoracic vertebrae
tibia
true ribs
vomer
whiplash injury
zygomatic

If you have ever visited a beach, you may have seen a jellyfish floating lightly near the surface. The organs of the jellyfish are buoyed up by the water. But, if a wave should chance to deposit the jellyfish upon the beach, it would collapse into a disorganized mass of tissue. This is because the jellyfish does not possess a supportive framework or skeleton. Fortunately, we humans do not suffer such a fate because we have a solid, bony skeleton to support body structures.

The **skeletal system** comprises the bony framework of the body. It is composed of 206 individual bones in the adult; some bones are hinged while others are fused to one another.

FUNCTIONS

The skeletal system has five specific functions:

1. *Supports* body structures and provides shape to the body.

2. *Protects* the soft and delicate internal organs. For example, the cranium protects the brain, the inner ear, and parts of the eye. The ribs and breastbone protect the heart and lungs; the vertebral column encases and protects the spinal cord.

3. *Movement* and *anchorage* of muscles. Muscles which are attached to the skeleton are called skeletal muscles. Upon contraction, these muscles exert a pull upon a bone and so move it. In this manner, bones play a vital part in body movement, serving as passively operated levers.

4. *Mineral storage.* Bones are a storage depot for minerals like calcium and phosphorus. In case of inadequate nutrition, the body is able to draw upon these reserves. For example, if the blood calcium dips below normal, the bone releases the necessary amount of stored calcium into the bloodstream. When calcium levels exceed normal, calcium release from the skeletal system is inhibited. In this way the skeletal system helps to maintain blood calcium homeostasis.

5. *Hemopoiesis.* The red marrow of the bone is the site of blood cell formation. Red marrow is found in long bones, sternum and ilia.

STRUCTURE AND FORMATION OF BONE

Bones are composed of microscopic cells called **osteocytes** (from the Greek word *osteon*, meaning bone). An osteocyte is a mature bone cell. Bone is made up of 35% organic material, 65% inorganic mineral salts, and water.

The organic part derives from a protein called bone collagen, a fibrous material. Between these collagenous fibers is a jelly-like material. The organic substances of bone give it a certain degree of flexibility. The inorganic portion of bone is made from mineral salts like calcium phosphate, calcium carbonate, calcium fluoride, magnesium phosphate, sodium oxide, and sodium chloride. These minerals give bone its hardness and durability.

A bony skeleton can be compared to steel-reinforced concrete. The collagenous fibers may be compared to flexible steel supports, and mineral salts to concrete. When pressure is applied to a bone, the flexible, organic material prevents bone damage, while the mineral elements resist crushing under pressure.

BONE FORMATION

The embryonic skeleton is initially composed of collagenous protein fibers secreted by the osteoblasts (primitive embryonic cells). Later on, during embryonic development, cartilage is deposited between the fibers. At this stage, the embryo's skeleton consists of collagenous protein fibers and hyaline (clear) cartilage. During the eighth week of embryonic development, **ossification** begins. That is, mineral matter starts to replace previously formed cartilage, creating bone. Infant bones are very soft and pliable because of incomplete ossification at birth. A familiar example is the soft spot on a baby's head, the **fontanel**. The bone has not yet been formed there, although it will become hardened later. Ossification due to

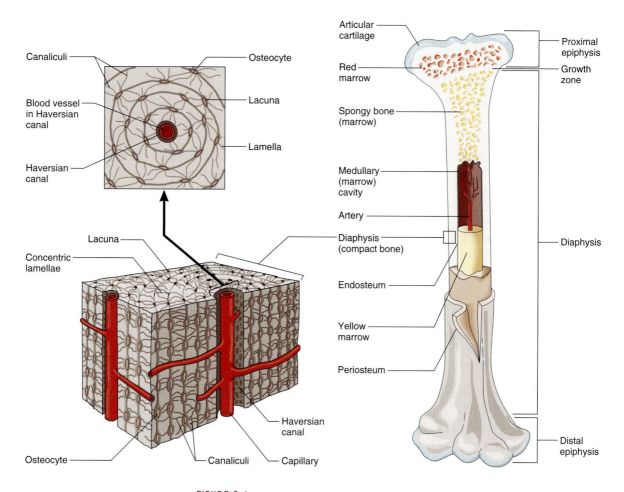

FIGURE 6-1 *Structure of a typical long bone*

mineral deposits continues through childhood. As bones ossify, they become hard and more capable of bearing weight.

STRUCTURE OF LONG BONE

A typical long bone contains a shaft, or **diaphysis**. This is a hollow cylinder of hard, compact bone. It is what makes a long bone strong and hard yet light enough for movement. At the ends (extremes) of the diaphysis are the **epiphyses**, Figure 6-1.

In the center of the shaft is the broad **medullary canal**. This is filled with yellow bone marrow, mostly made of fat cells. The marrow also contains many blood vessels and some cells which form white blood cells, called leukocytes. The yellow marrow functions as a fat storage center. The marrow canal is lined and the cavity kept intact by the **endosteum**.

The medullary canal is surrounded by compact or hard bone. Haversian canals branch into the compact bone. They carry blood vessels which nourish the osteocytes, or bone cells. Where less strength is needed in the bone, some of the hard bone is dissolved away leaving **spongy bone**.

The ends of the long bones contain the red marrow where some red blood cells called erythrocytes and some white blood cells are made. The outside of the bone is covered with the **periosteum**, a tough fibrous tissue which contains blood vessels, lymph vessels, and nerves. The periosteum is necessary for bone growth, repair, and nutrition.

Covering the epiphysis is a thin layer of cartilage known as the articular cartilage. This cartilage acts as a shock absorber between two bones that meet to form a joint.

GROWTH

Bones grow in length and ossify from the center of the diaphysis toward the epiphyseal extremities. Using a long bone by way of example, it will grow lengthwise in an area called the growth zone. Ossification occurs here, causing the bone to lengthen; this causes the epiphyses to grow away from the middle of the diaphysis. It is a sensible growth process, since it does not interfere with the articulation between two bones.

A bone increases its circumference by the addition of more bone to the outer surface of the diaphysis by osteoblasts. Osteoblasts are bone cells that deposit the new bone. As girth increases bone material is being dissolved from the central part of the diaphysis. This forms an internal cavity called the marrow cavity, or medullary canal. The medullary canal gets larger as the diameter of the bone increases.

The dissolution of bone from the medullary canal results from the action of cells called osteoclasts. Osteoclasts are very large bone cells which secrete enzymes. These enzymes digest the bony material, splitting the bone minerals, calcium, and phosphorus and enabling them to be absorbed by the surrounding fluid. The medullary canal eventually fills with yellow marrow and cells that will produce white blood cells.

The length of a bone shaft continues to grow until all the epiphyseal cartilage is ossified. At this point, bone growth stops. This fact is helpful in determining further growth in a child. First, an x-ray of the child's wrists is taken. If some epiphyseal cartilage remains, there will be further growth. If there is no epiphyseal cartilage left, the child has reached his or her full stature (height).

The average growth in females continues to about eighteen years; in males to approximately twenty or twenty-one years. However, new bone growth can occur in a broken bone at any time. Bone cells near the site of a fracture become active, secreting large amounts of new bone within a relatively short time. Bone healing proceeds efficiently depending on age and health of the individual.

BONE TYPES

Bones are classified as one of four types on the basis of their form, Figure 6-2. *Long* bones

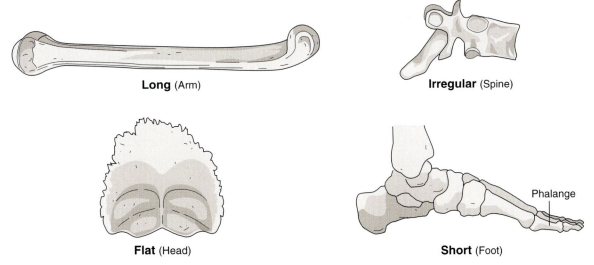

Long (Arm)

Irregular (Spine)

Flat (Head)

Short (Foot)

Phalange

FIGURE 6-2 *Bone shapes*

are found in both upper and lower arms and legs. The bones of the skull are examples of *flat* bones, as are the ribs. *Irregular* bones are represented by bones of the spinal column. The wrist and ankle bones are examples of *short* bones, which appear cube-like in shape.

The bones in the hand are short, making flexible movement possible. The same is true of the irregular bones of the spinal column. The thigh bone is a long bone needed for support of the strong leg muscles and the weight of the body. The degree of movement at a joint is determined by bone shape and joint structure.

PARTS OF THE SKELETAL SYSTEM

The skeletal system is comprised of two main parts: the axial skeleton and the appendicular skeleton. The **axial skeleton** consists of the skull, spinal column, ribs, sternum (breastbone), and hyoid bone. The hyoid bone is a U-shaped bone in the neck, to which the tongue is attached. The **appendicular skeleton** includes the upper extremities: shoulder girdles, arms, wrists, hands; and the lower extremities: hip girdle, legs, ankles and feet, Figure 6-3.

AXIAL SKELETON

Skull

The skull is composed of the cranium and facial bones. The cranium houses and protects the delicate brain, while the facial bones guard and support the eyes, ears, nose, and mouth. Some of the facial bones, such as the nasal bones, are made of bone and cartilage. For

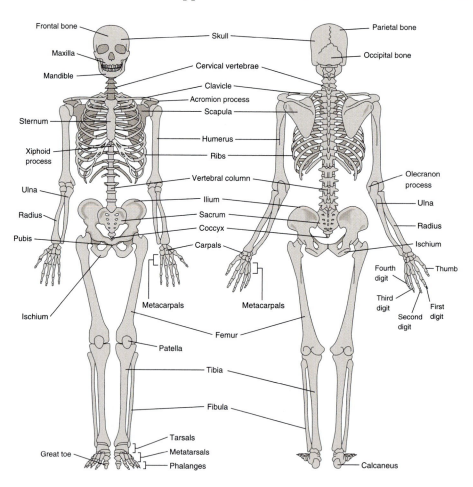

Labels (front view, top to bottom): Frontal bone, Maxilla, Mandible, Sternum, Xiphoid process, Ulna, Radius, Pubis, Ischium

Center labels: Skull, Cervical vertebrae, Clavicle, Acromion process, Scapula, Humerus, Ribs, Vertebral column, Ilium, Sacrum, Coccyx, Carpals, Metacarpals, Metacarpals, Femur, Patella, Tibia, Fibula, Great toe, Tarsals, Metatarsals, Phalanges

Labels (back view): Parietal bone, Occipital bone, Olecranon process, Ulna, Radius, Ischium, Fourth digit, Third digit, Second digit, Thumb, First digit, Calcaneus

FIGURE 6-3 *Bones of the skeleton*

example, the upper part of the nose (bridge) is bone, while the lower part is cartilage.

Cranial bones are thin and slightly curved. During infancy, these bones are held snugly together by an irregular band of connective tissue called a suture. As the child grows, this connective tissue ossifies and turns into hard bone. Thus the cranium becomes a highly efficient, dome-shaped shield for the brain. The dome shape affords better protection than a flat surface, deflecting blows directed toward the head. However, it is not invulnerable and a particularly hard blow may fracture it. This can lead to a concussion: if the bone is depressed, serious injury to brain tissue may result. A depressed fracture may require surgery to relieve the pressure from the brain.

Collectively, there are twenty-two bones in the skull, Figure 6-4. There are eight bones in the cranium:

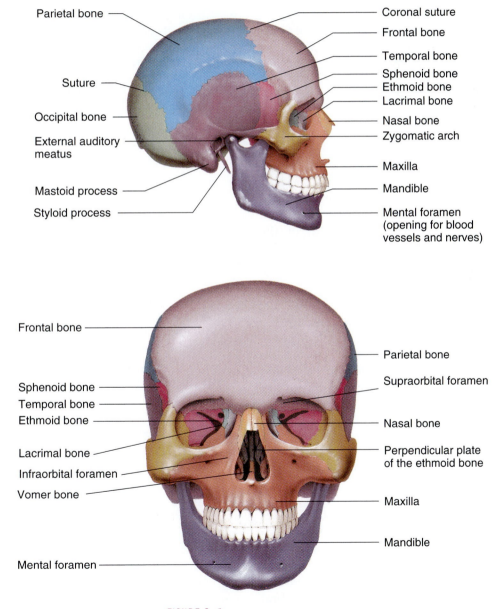

FIGURE 6-4 *Bones of the skull*

1 **frontal** forms the forehead,

2 **parietal** form the roof and sides of the skull,

2 **temporal** house the ears,

1 **occipital** forms the base of the skull and contains the foramen magnum

1 **ethmoid** (located between the eyes) forms part of the nasal septum,

1 **sphenoid** (which resembles a bat) is considered the key bone of the skull; all other bones connect to it.

There are fourteen facial bones:

5 nasal (2 are **nasal** bones which form the bridge of the nose [your glasses sit on this bone]; 1 is the **vomer** bone which forms the lower part, or midline, of the nasal septum; and 2 are **inferior concha** bones which make up the side walls of the nasal cavity),

2 **maxilla** make up the upper jaw,

2 **lacrimal** (in the inner aspect of the eyes) contain the tear ducts,

2 **zygomatic** form the prominence of the cheek,

2 **palatine** form the hard palate of the mouth,

1 **mandible** which is the lower jaw and the only movable bone in the face.

The skull contains large spaces within the facial bones, referred to as paranasal sinuses. These sinuses are lined with mucous membranes. When a person suffers from a cold, flu or hayfever, the membranes become inflamed and swollen, producing a copious amount of mucus. This may lead to sinus pain and a "stuffy" nasal sensation.

Spinal Column/Vertebra

The spine, or vertebral column, is strong and flexible. It supports the head and provides for the attachment of the ribs. The spine also encloses the spinal cord of the nervous system.

The spine consists of small bones called vertebrae which are separated from each other by pads of cartilage tissue called intervertebral disks, Figure 6-5. These disks serve as cushions between the vertebrae and act as shock absorbers. During our lifetime these disks become thinner, which accounts for a loss of height as we age.

The vertebral column is divided into five sections named according to the area of the body where they are located, see Figure 6-5(a).

1. **Cervical vertebrae** (7) are located in the neck area. The **atlas**, Figure 6-5(b), is the first cervical vertebra which articulates, or is jointed, with the occipital bone of the skull. This permits us to nod our heads. On the **axis**, Figure 6-5(c), the second cervical vertebra is the odontoid process which forms a pivot on which the atlas rotates; this permits us to turn our heads.

2. **Thoracic vertebrae** (12) are located in the chest area. They articulate with the ribs.

3. **Lumbar vertebrae** (5) are located in the back. They have large bodies which bear most of the body's weight.

4. **Sacrum** is a wedge-shaped bone formed by five fused bones. It forms the posterior pelvic girdle and serves as an articulation point for the hips.

5. **Coccyx** is also known as the tailbone. It is formed by four fused bones.

The spinal nerves enter and leave the spinal cord through the openings (foramen) between the vertebrae.

When you study a model of the human skeleton, you will notice that the spine is curved instead of straight. A curved spine has more strength than a straight one would have. Before birth, the thoracic and sacral regions are convex curves. As the infant learns to hold up its head, the cervical region becomes concave. When the child learns to stand, the lumbar region also becomes concave. This completes the four curves of a normal, adult human spine.

A typical vertebra, as seen in Figure 6-6, contains three basic parts: body, foramen, and (several) processes. The large, solid part of the vertebra is known as the body; the central opening for the spinal cord is called the foramen. Above the foramen protrude two wing-like bony structures called transverse processes.

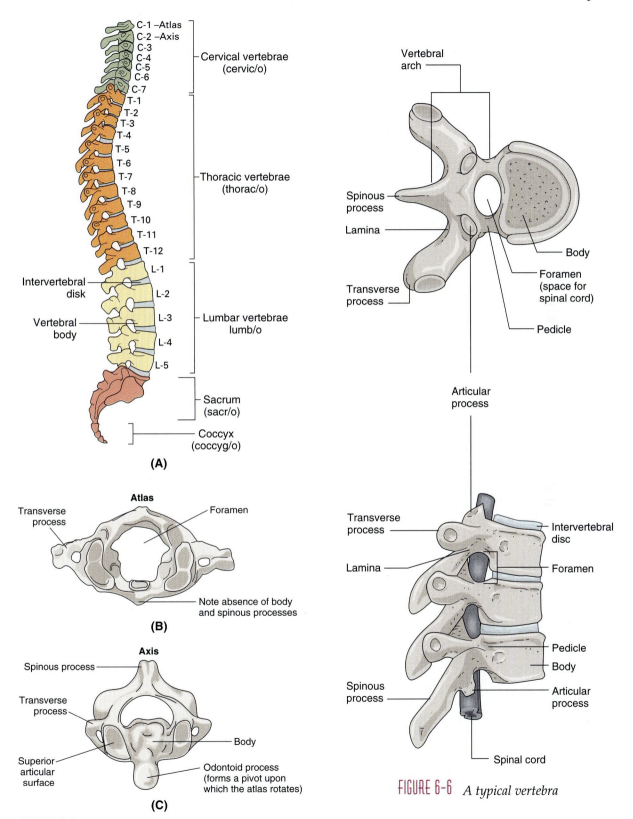

C-1 –Atlas
C-2 –Axis
C-3
C-4
C-5
C-6
C-7

Cervical vertebrae
(cervic/o)

T-1
T-2
T-3
T-4
T-5
T-6
T-7
T-8
T-9
T-10
T-11
T-12

Thoracic vertebrae
(thorac/o)

Intervertebral disk

Vertebral body

L-1
L-2
L-3
L-4
L-5

Lumbar vertebrae
lumb/o

Sacrum
(sacr/o)

Coccyx
(coccyg/o)

(A)

Atlas

Transverse process

Foramen

Note absence of body and spinous processes

(B)

Axis

Spinous process

Transverse process

Superior articular surface

Body

Odontoid process (forms a pivot upon which the atlas rotates)

(C)

FIGURE 6-5 *(A) Lateral view of the spine; (B) View of the atlas; (C) View of the axis*

Vertebral arch

Spinous process

Lamina

Transverse process

Body

Foramen (space for spinal cord)

Pedicle

Articular process

Transverse process

Lamina

Spinous process

Intervertebral disc

Foramen

Pedicle

Body

Articular process

Spinal cord

FIGURE 6-6 *A typical vertebra*

The roof of the foramen contains the spinous process (spine) and the articular processes.

Ribs and Sternum

The thoracic area of the body is protected and supported by the thoracic vertebrae, ribs, and sternum.

The sternum (breastbone) is divided into three parts: the upper region (manubrium), the body, and a lower cartilaginous part called the xiphoid process. Attached to each side of the upper region of the sternum, by means of ligaments, are the two clavicles (collar bones).

Seven pairs of costal cartilages join seven pairs of ribs directly to the sternum. These are known as **true ribs**, Figure 6-7. The human body contains twelve pairs of ribs. The first seven pairs are true ribs. The next three pairs are "false ribs" because their costal cartilages are attached to the seventh rib instead of directly to the sternum. Finally, the last two pairs of ribs, connected neither to the costal cartilages nor the sternum, are floating ribs.

THE APPENDICULAR SKELETON

The appendicular skeleton includes the bones in the upper and lower extremities. There are 126 bones in the appendicular skeleton.

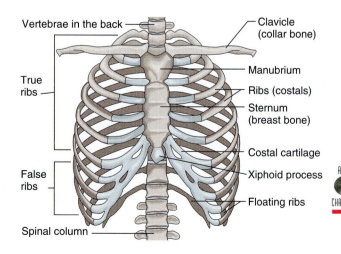

Vertebrae in the back
Clavicle (collar bone)
True ribs
Manubrium
Ribs (costals)
Sternum (breast bone)
Costal cartilage
Xiphoid process
False ribs
Floating ribs
Spinal column

FIGURE 6-7 *Ribs and sternum*

Shoulder Girdle

The shoulder girdle (also called pectoral girdle) consists of four bones: two curved **clavicles** (collar bones) and two triangular **scapulae** (shoulder bones). Using a model of the human skeleton, we observe two broad, flat triangular surfaces (scapulae) on the upper posterior surface. They permit the attachment of muscles which assist in arm movement, while also serving as a place of attachment for the arms. The two clavicles, attached at one end to the scapulae and at the other to the sternum, help to brace the shoulders and prevent excessive forward motion.

Arm

The bone structure of the arm consists of the humerus, the radius, and the ulna. The humerus is located in the upper arm and the radius and ulna in the forearm.

The **humerus**, the only bone in the upper arm, is the second largest bone in the body. The upper end of the humerus has a smooth, round surface called the head, which articulates with the scapula. The upper humerus is attached to the scapula socket (glenoid fossa) by muscles and ligaments. These muscles are the biceps and triceps brachii.

The forearm is composed of two bones: the radius and the ulna. The **radius** is the bone running up the thumb side of the forearm. Its name derives from the fact that it can rotate around the ulna. This is an important characteristic, permitting the hand to rotate freely and with great flexibility. The ulna, by contrast, is far more limited. It is the largest bone in the forearm: at its upper end, it produces a projection called the olecranon process, forming the elbow, Figure 6-8. When you bang your elbow (the olecranon process) it is usually referred to as "hitting your funny bone." The olecranon process articulates with the humerus.

Hand

The human hand is a remarkable piece of skeletal engineering and dexterity. It contains more bones for its size than any other part of the body. Collectively, the hand has twenty-seven bones, Figure 6-9.

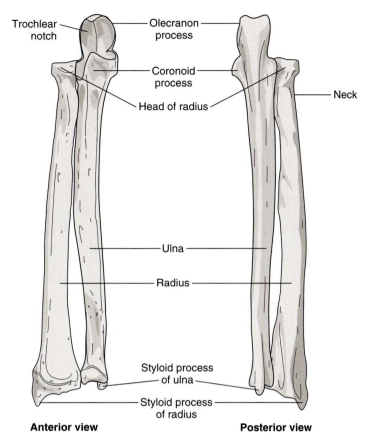

FIGURE 6-8 *Radius and ulna*

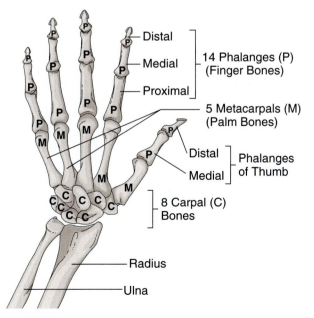

FIGURE 6-9 *The twenty-seven bones of the left hand*

The wrist bone, or **carpals**, is comprised of eight small bones arranged in two rows. They are held together by ligaments which permit sufficient movement to allow the wrist a great deal of mobility and flexion. However, there is very little lateral (side) movement of these carpal bones. On the palm side of the hand are attached a number of short muscles which supply mobility to the little finger and thumb.

The hand is composed of two parts: the palmer surface with five **metacarpal** bones, and five fingers comprised of fourteen **phalanges** (singular, phalanx). Each finger, except for the thumb, has three phalanges, whereas the thumb has two. There are hinge joints between each phalanx, allowing the fingers to be bent easily. The thumb is the most flexible finger because the end of the metacarpal bone is more rounded, and there are muscles attached to it from the hand itself. Thus the thumb can be extended across the palm of the hand. Only man and other primates possess such a digit known as an opposable thumb.

Pelvic Girdle

In youth, the pelvic girdle (innominate bones) consists of three bones. Found on either side of the midline of the body, the innominate bones include the ilium, the ischium and the pubis. However, these bones eventually fuse with the sacrum to form a bowl-shaped structure called the pelvic girdle, Figure 6-10. Eventually these two sets of innominate bones form a joint with the bones in front, called the symphysis pubis and with the sacrum in back, as the sacroiliac joint.

The pelvic girdle serves as an area of attachment for the bones and muscles of the leg. It also provides support for the viscera (soft organs) of the lower abdominal region.

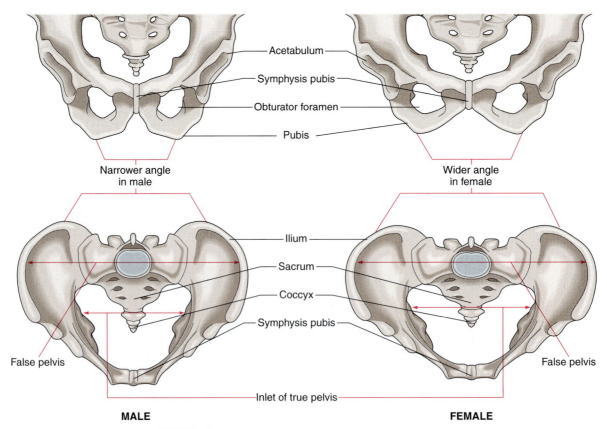

- Acetabulum
- Symphysis pubis
- Obturator foramen
- Pubis

Narrower angle in male

Wider angle in female

- Ilium
- Sacrum
- Coccyx
- Symphysis pubis

False pelvis

False pelvis

Inlet of true pelvis

MALE

FEMALE

FIGURE 6-10 *Comparison of the male and female pelvises*

There is an obvious anatomical difference between the male and female pelvis. The female pelvis is much wider than that of the male. This is necessary for childbearing (pregnancy) and childbirth. In addition, the *pelvic inlet* is wider in the female, and the pelvic bones are lighter and smoother than those of the male.

Upper Leg

The upper leg contains the longest and strongest bone in the body, the thigh bone or **femur**. The upper part of the femur has a smooth rounded head, Figure 6-11. It fits neatly into a cavity of the ilium known as the acetabulum, forming a ball-and-socket joint. The femur is an amazingly strong bone. A direct compressible force applied to the *top* of the femur of from 15,000-19,000 pounds per square inch is required to break it.

Lower Leg

The lower leg consists of two bones: the **tibia** and the **fibula**. The tibia is the largest of the two lower leg bones. The **patella** (kneecap) is found in front of the knee joint. It is a flat, tri-

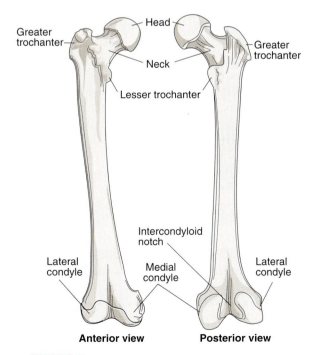

FIGURE 6-11   *Anterior/posterior view of the femur*

angular, sesamoid bone, Figure 6-3. The patella is formed in the tendons of the large muscle in front of the femur (quadriceps femoris). In females, it appears at around two or three years of age; in males, at about six. The patella, attached to the tibia by a ligament, ossifies as early as puberty. Surrounding the patella are four bursae, which serve to cushion the knee joint.

Ankle

The ankle (tarsus) contains seven **tarsal** bones. These bones provide a connection between the foot and leg bones. The largest ankle bone is the heel bone or **calcaneus**. The tibia and fibula articulate with a broad tarsal bone called the talus. Ankle movement is a sliding motion, allowing the foot to extend and flex when walking.

Foot

The foot has five **metatarsal** bones which are somewhat comparable to the metacarpals of the hand. But, there is an important difference between the metatarsals and the metacarpals within the palm of the hand. The metatarsal and tarsal bones are arranged to form two distinct arches, which of course are not found in the palm of the hand. One arch runs longitudinally from the calcaneus to the heads of the metatarsals: it is called the longitudinal arch. The other, which lies perpendicular to the longitudinal arch in the metatarsal region, is known as the transverse arch. Strong ligaments and leg muscle tendons help to hold the foot bones in place to form those two arches. In turn, arches strengthen the foot and provide flexibility and springiness to the stride. In certain cases, these arches may "fall" due to weak foot ligaments and tendons. Then downward pressure by weight of the body slowly flattens them, causing "fallen arches" or "flatfeet." Flatfeet cause a good deal of stress and strain on the foot muscles, leading to pain and fatigue. Factors which may lead to flatfeet include improper prenatal nutrition, dietary or hormonal imbalances, fatigue, overweight, poor posture, and shoes which do not fit properly.

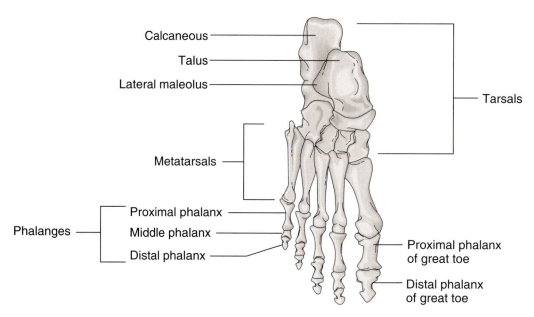

Calcaneous

Talus

Lateral maleolus

Tarsals

Metatarsals

Phalanges

Proximal phalanx

Middle phalanx

Distal phalanx

Proximal phalanx of great toe

Distal phalanx of great toe

FIGURE 6-12   *The foot—dorsal view.*

The toes are similar in composition to the fingers. There are three phalanges in each, with the exception of the big toe which has only two. Since the big toe is not opposable like the thumb, it cannot be brought across the sole. There are a total of fourteen phalanges in each foot, Figure 6-12.

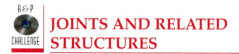

JOINTS AND RELATED STRUCTURES

Joints, or articulations, are points of contact between two bones. They are classified into three main types according to their degree of movement: diarthroses (movable) joints, amphiarthroses (partially movable) joints, and synarthroses (immovable) joints, Figure 6-13.

Most of the joints in our body are **diarthroses.** They tend to have the same structure. These movable joints consist of three main parts: articular cartilage, a bursa (joint capsule), and a synovial (joint) cavity.

When two movable bones meet at a joint, their surfaces do not touch one another. The two articular (joint) surfaces are covered with a smooth, slippery cap of cartilage known as **articular cartilage**. This articular cartilage

helps to absorb shocks and prevent friction between parts.

Enclosing two articular surfaces of the bone is a tough, fibrous connective tissue capsule called an articular capsule. Lining the articular capsule is a **synovial membrane** which secretes **synovial fluid** (a lubricating substance) into the **synovial cavity** (an area between the two articular cartilages). The synovial fluid reduces the friction of joint movement.

The clefts in connective tissue between muscles, tendons, ligaments, and bones contain **bursa sacs**. An inflammation of this area is called **bursitis**. The synovial fluid secreted serves as a lubricant to prevent friction between a tendon and a bone. If this sac becomes irritated or injured, a condition known as bursitis develops. The synovial fluid can be aspirated (withdrawn) from the bursa sacs to examine for diagnostic purposes.

As we advance in age, the joints undergo degenerative changes. The synovial fluid is not secreted as quickly, and the articular cartilaginous surfaces of the two bone ends become ossified. This results in excess bone outgrowths along the joint edges, which tend to stiffen joints, causing inflammation, pain and a decrease in mobility.

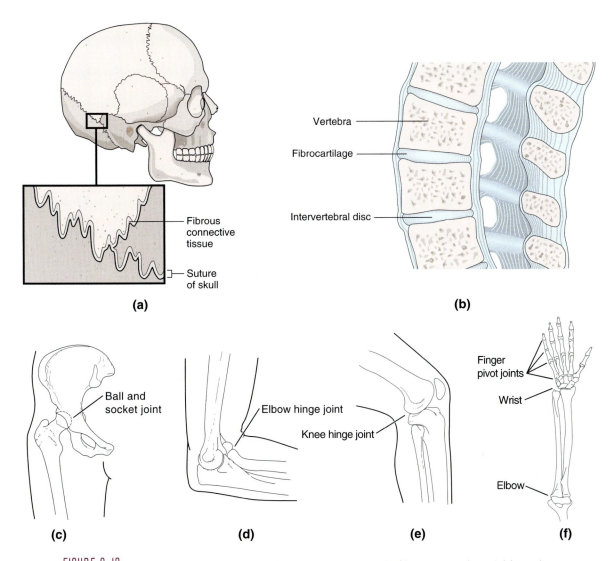

FIGURE 6-13 *Types of joints: (a) a synarthrosis, an immovable fibrous joint (cranial bones); (b) an amphiarthrosis, a slightly movable cartilaginous joint (ribs or vertebra); (c-f) diarthroses, freely movable hinge or ball-and-socket joints*

Diarthroses Joints

There are four types of diarthroses joints:

1. **Ball-and-socket joints** allow the greatest freedom of movement. Here, one bone has a ball-shaped head which nestles into a concave socket of the second bone. Our shoulders and hips have ball-and-socket joints.

2. **Hinge joints** move in one direction or plane, as in the knees, elbows and outer joints of the fingers.

3. **Pivot joints** are those with an extension rotating in a second, arch-shaped bone. The radius and ulna (long bones of the forearm) are pivot joints. Another example is the joint between the **atlas** (first cervical vertebra in the neck) which supports the head, and the **axis** (second cervical vertebra) which allows the head to rotate.

4. **Gliding joints** are those in which nearly flat surfaces glide across each other, as in the vertebrae of the spine. These joints

enable the torso to bend forward, backward and sideways, as well as rotate.

Between each body of the vertebrae are found fibrous disks. At the center of each fibrous disk is a pulpy, elastic material which loses its resiliency with increased usage and/or age. Disks can be compressed by sudden and forceful jolts to the spine. This may cause a disk to protrude from the vertebrae and impinge upon the spinal nerves resulting in extreme pain. Such a condition is known as a *herniated* or *slipped disk*.

Amphiarthroses Joints

Amphiarthroses are partially movable joints. These joints have cartilage between their articular surfaces. Two examples are : (1) the attachment of the ribs to the spine and (2) symphysis pubis, the joint between the two pubic bones.

Synarthroses Joints

Synarthroses are immovable joints connected by tough, fibrous connective tissue. These joints are found in the adult cranium. The bones are fused together in a joint which forms a heavy protective cover for the brain. Such cranial joints are commonly called **sutures**.

Ligaments are fibrous bands which connect bones and cartilages and serve as support for muscles. Joints are also bound together by ligaments. Tendons are fibrous cords which connect muscles to bones.

CAREER PROFILES

PHYSICAL THERAPIST (PT)

The physical therapist improves mobility, relieves pain, and prevents or limits permanent disability of patients suffering from injuries or disease. Therapists evaluate history, test and measure patient's strength and range of motion, and develop a treatment plan. Treatment often includes exercises to increase flexibility and range of motion. Physical therapists need to have moderate strength, since the job can be physically demanding. Job prospects are excellent. Education required is preparation in a Bachelor's or Master's program in Physical Therapy. Entry is highly competitive; some schools require volunteer activity in therapy departments in a hospital or a clinic prior to admission. All states require the physical therapist to pass the licensure examination.

PHYSICAL THERAPY ASSISTANTS

The physical therapy assistant works under the supervision of a physical therapist. They instruct patients in a wide variety of treatment plans to prevent permanent disability and help the patient resume the activities of daily living. The PT assistant needs to have a moderate degree of strength because of the physical demands of the job. Education requirement for the PT assistant is an Associate degree from an accredited program for Physical Therapy Assistants. Education requires a clinical component. At the present time, forty-one states require licensure of certification. Job prospects are excellent because of the aging population.

TYPES OF MOTION

Joints can move in many directions, Figure 6-14. **Flexion** is the act of bringing two bones closer together which decrease the angle between two bones.

Extension is the act of increasing the angle between two bones which results in a straightening motion. **Abduction** is the movement of an extremity away from the midline (an imaginary line which divides the body from head to toe). **Adduction** is movement toward the midline. **Circumduction** includes flexion, extension, abduction and adduction.

A **rotation** movement allows a bone to move around one central axis. This type of pivot motion occurs when you turn your head from side to side (just say "no"). In **pronation**,

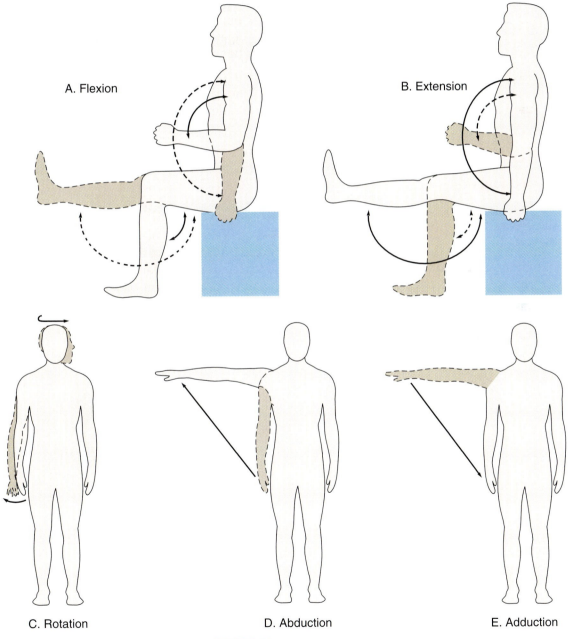

A. Flexion

B. Extension

C. Rotation

D. Abduction

E. Adduction

FIGURE 6-14 *Joint movements*

the forearm turns the hand so the palm is downward or backward. In **supination**, the palm is forward or upward.

DISORDERS OF THE BONES AND JOINTS

The most common injury to a bone is a **fracture**, or break. When this occurs, there is swelling due to injury and bleeding tissues. The process of restoring bone is done through three main methods:

1. *Closed Reduction*—the bony fragments are brought into alignment by manipulation, and a cast or splint is applied.

2. *Open Reduction*—through surgical intervention, devices such as wires, metal plates or screws are used to hold the bone in alignment and a cast or splint may be applied.

3. *Traction*—a pulling force is used to hold the bones in place (used for fractures of the long bone).

The following outline identifies the common types of fractures, Figure 6-15.

- *Closed/Simple*—The bone is broken, but the broken ends do not pierce through the skin forming an external wound.

- *Open/Compound*—This is the most serious type of fracture, where the broken bone ends pierce and protrude through the skin. This can cause infection of the bone and of the neighboring tissues.

- *Greenstick*—Here we have the simplest type of fracture. The bone is partly bent, but it never completely separates. The break is similar to that of a young, sap-filled wood-stick where the fibers separate lengthwise when bent. Such fractures are common among children because their bones contain flexible cartilage.

- *Comminuted*—The bone is splintered or broken into many pieces that can become embedded in the surrounding tissue.

Bone and Joint Injuries

A **dislocation** occurs when a bone is displaced from its proper position in a joint. This may result in the tearing and stretching of the ligaments. Reduction or return of the bone to

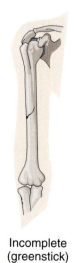 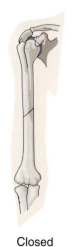 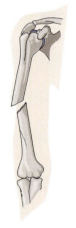 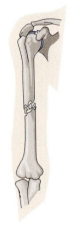

| Incomplete (greenstick) | Closed or simple | Open or compound | Comminuted |

FIGURE 6-15 *Types of fractures*

its proper position is necessary, along with rest to allow the ligaments to heal.

A **sprain** is an injury to a joint caused by any sudden or unusual motion, such as "turning the ankle." The ligaments are either torn from their attachments to the bones or torn across, but the joint is not dislocated. A sprain is accompanied by rapid swelling and acute pain in the area and is treated with non steroid anti-inflammatory drugs.

DISEASES OF THE BONES

Arthritis is an inflammatory condition of one or more joints, accompanied by pain and often by changes in bone position. There are at least twenty different types, the most common being rheumatoid arthritis and osteoarthritis:

- **Rheumatoid arthritis** is a chronic, autoimmune (when the body's immune system attacks the tissue) disease which affects the connective tissue and joints. There is acute inflammation of the connective tissue, thickening of the synovial membrane, and ankylosis (joints become fused) of joints. The joints are badly swollen and painful. The pain, in turn, causes muscle spasms which may lead to deformities in the joints. In addition, the cartilage that separates the joints will degenerate, and hard calcium fills the spaces. When the joints become stiff and immobile, muscles attached to these joints slowly atrophy (shrink in size). This disease affects approximately three times more women than men. Its cause is unknown, although everything from emotional factors to endocrine and metabolic disorders has been cited.

- **Osteoarthritis** is known as degenerative joint disease. It occurs with aging; about 80% of all Americans are affected. In this disease the articular cartilage degenerates and a bony spur formation occurs at the joint. The joints may enlarge; there is pain and swelling, especially after activity.

Treatment for arthritis includes many folk remedies such as wearing a copper bracelet, using special tonic mixtures, and eating vitamins and certain foods. At the present time, arthritis has no known cure. Treatment with non-steroid anti-inflammatory drugs may alleviate pain and swelling. Hip and knee replacement (arthroplasty) may be done for the affected joints. Researchers are working on a new class of arthritic drugs since they now have a better understanding of how the body produces inflammation.

Gout is an increase of uric acid in the bloodstream. Uric acid crystals are deposited in joint cavities and kidneys; the site most commonly affected is the great toe. There is severe pain. More males are affected than females.

Rickets is usually found in children and caused by a lack of vitamin D. Bones become soft, due to lack of calcification, causing such deformities as bowlegs and pigeon breast. The disease may be prevented with sufficient quantities of calcium, vitamin D, and exposure to sunshine.

Slipped (herniated) disc is a condition where a cartilage disc (one of which is between each vertebra and acts as a shock absorber for the spine) ruptures or protrudes out of place and places pressure on the spinal nerve. This usually occurs in the lower back (lumbarsacral) area. It may be treated by a chiropractor or with bed rest, traction, or surgery.

Whiplash injury is trauma to the cervical vertebra, usually the result of an automobile accident. The force generated by the car's speed whips the head backward, putting tremendous strain on the cervical spine and neck muscles. Treatment depends on the extent of the injury.

Abnormal Curvatures of the Spine

Kyphosis ("hunchback") is a humped curvature in the thoracic area of the spine, Figure 6-16.

Lordosis ("swayback") is an exaggerated inward curvature in the lumbar region of the spine just above the sacrum.

Scoliosis is a side-to-side or lateral curvature of the spine.

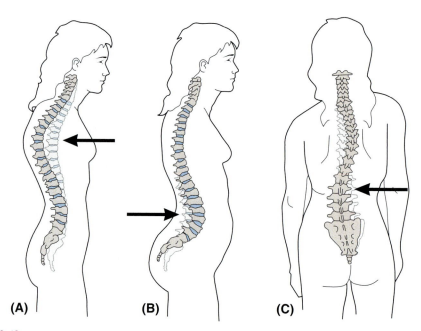

FIGURE 6-16 *Abnormal curvatures of the spine: (A) Kyphosis, (B) Lordosis, (C) Scoliosis*

OTHER MEDICALLY RELATED DISORDERS

Osteoporosis is a disease which affects twenty-five million Americans—according to the National Osteoporosis Foundation, 80% are women. In osteoporosis, the mineral density of the bone is reduced from 65% to 35%. By age fifty-five, the average woman has lost about 30% of her bone mass. This loss of bone mass leaves the bone thinner, porous, and susceptible to fracture, Figure 6-17. An x-ray of the bone is said to resemble swiss cheese. Treatment is aimed at preventing or slowing down osteoporosis. Average intake of calcium in the diet and regular exercise helps to build bone mass and prevent osteoporosis. Post-menopausal women may take estrogen to help maintain bone mass. Diets which are too high in sodium and potassium contribute to the loss

MEDICAL HIGHLIGHT: TECHNOLOGY

Arthroscopy and Microdiskectomy

Arthroscopy is the examination into a joint using an arthroscope. The arthroscope is a small fiber optic viewing instrument made up of a tiny lens, light source, and video camera. Through an incision about 1/4" long, a physician may examine, diagnose, and treat injuries of joint areas. Most knee injuries are treated through arthroscopic technique.

Microdiskectomy is an operation to remove a prolapsed or damaged intervertebral disc through a tiny incision. The surgeon uses a bone plug to replace the damaged disc, which can either be a graft from the patient's hip bone or from a bone bank. Another option is to fill the space with coralline, which is obtained from sea coral. The patient may be out of bed the next day.

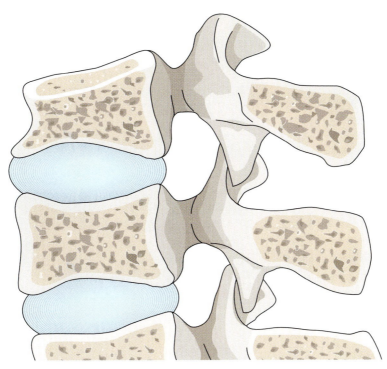

FIGURE 6-17 *Artist's conception of progressive osteoporotic bone loss and compression fractures (Courtesy of Ayerst Laboratories, New York, New York)*

of calcium from the body. Women are encouraged to have bone density studies done to detect early onset of osteoporosis.

Osteomyelitis is an infection which may involve all parts of the bone. It may result from injury or systemic infection and most commonly occurs in children between the ages of five and fourteen years.

Osteosarcoma, or bone cancer, may occur in younger people. The most common site of affliction is just above the knee.

● REVIEW QUESTIONS

Select the letter of the choice that best completes the statement.

1. Supination is one type of:
    a. extension
    b. abduction
    c. adduction
    d. rotation

2. The bones found in the skull are:
    a. irregular bones
    b. flat bones
    c. short bones
    d. long bones

3. The cranium protects the:
   a. lungs
   b. brain
   c. heart
   d. stomach

4. Pivot joints may be found in the:
   a. vertebral column
   b. skull
   c. wrist
   d. shoulder

5. Bones are a storage place for minerals such as:
   a. calcium and sodium
   b. calcium and potassium
   c. sodium and potassium
   d. calcium and phosphorous

6. The site of blood cell formation is:
   a. yellow marrow
   b. periosteum
   c. articular cartilage
   d. red marrow

7. Immovable joints are found in the:
   a. infant's skull
   b. adult cranium
   c. adult spinal column
   d. child's spinal column

8. Flexion means:
   a. bending
   b. rotating
   c. extending
   d. abduction

9. The degree of motion at a joint is determined by:
   a. the amount of synovial fluid
   b. the number of bursa
   c. the unusual amount of exercise
   d. bone shape and joint structure

10. The bone that forms the base of the skull is the:
    a. parietal
    b. temporal
    c. occipital
    d. frontal

11. The key bone of the skull is the:
    a. ethmoid
    b. frontal
    c. parietal
    d. sphenoid

12. The only moveable bone of the face is the:
    a. lacrimatic
    b. mandible
    c. maxilla
    d. palatine

13. The central opening on the vertebrae for passage of the spinal cord is the:
    a. transverse process
    b. intervertebral disc
    c. foramen
    d. spinous process

14. The shoulder girdle is composed of two bones:
    a. radius and ulna
    b. clavicle and scapula
    c. tibia and fibula
    d. metatarsal and tarsal

15. The ribs which are attached directly to the sternum are called:
    a. floating
    b. true
    c. false
    d. humerus

16. The bone of the arm located on the thumb side is called:
    a. ulna
    b. radius
    c. humerus
    d. carpal

17. The bones of the wrist are called:
    a. tarsal
    b. metatarsals
    c. carpals
    d. metacarpals

18. The longest, strongest bone in the body is the:
    a. humerus
    b. tibia
    c. femur
    d. fibula

19. The heel bone is known as the:
    a. calcaneus
    b. patella
    c. fibula
    d. talus

20. An inflammation of the bone is known as:
    a. arthritis
    b. bursitis
    c. osteomyelitis
    d. osteoarthritis

● MATCHING

Match each term in Column I with its correct description in Column II.

Column I	Column II
_____ 1. osteoarthritis	a. first cervical vertebra
_____ 2. closed fracture	b. shock absorbers
_____ 3. fontanel	c. moveable joint
_____ 4. endosteum	d. degeneration of articular cartilage
_____ 5. bursa	e. bone broken, skin intact
_____ 6. epiphysis	f. joint capsule
_____ 7. periosteum	g. area in infant skull where bone is not yet formed
_____ 8. atlas	h. lining of the marrow cavity
_____ 9. intervertebral disc	i. calcium and phosphorous
_____ 10. diarthrosis joint	j. end structure of long bone
	k. bone cells or osteocytes
	l. bone covering which contains blood vessels

● APPLYING THEORY TO PRACTICE

1. What type of joint movement is used:
   - to shut off a light?
   - to comb your hair?

2. If someone you know has broken the long bone of his leg skiing, what type of treatment will be used?

3. You are running and you have "turned your ankle." Name the bones involved. What is the best way to treat a sprain?

4. Your grandmother tells you her bones are stiff. Explain what causes this condition.

5. More Americans are living longer, which means more people will be susceptible to a condition called osteoporosis. Define this condition and its treatment. How will this condition affect Medicare costs?

● LABELING

1. Label the parts of the skeleton.

2. Label the parts of the long bone.

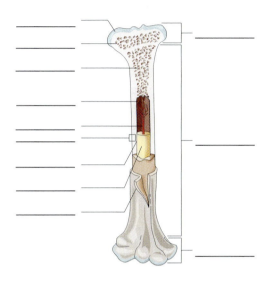

CHAPTER

7

Muscular System

KEY WORDS

abdominal hernia
acetylcholine
action potential
antagonist
atrophy
belly
biceps
cardiac muscle
contractibility
deltoid
diaphragm
dilator muscle
elasticity
ergonomics
excitability
extensibility
fibromyalgia
flatfeet (talipes)
flexor
gastrocnemius

hernia
hiatal hernia
hypertrophy
inguinal hernia
insertion
intramuscular
irritability
isometric
isotonic
motor unit
muscle dystrophy
muscle fatigue
muscle spasm
muscle tone
muscular dystrophy
myalgia
myasthenia gravis
neuromuscular
    junction
neurotransmitter

origin
pectoralis major
prime mover
physiotherapy
rehabilitation
rotator cuff disease
sarcolemma
sarcoplasm
shin splints
skeletal muscle
smooth muscle
sphincter muscle
sternocleidomastoid
strain
strength
synergists
tennis elbow
tetanus
torticollis
triceps

The ability to move is an essential activity of the living human body which is made possible by the unique function of contractility in muscles. Muscles comprise a large part of the human body: nearly half our body weight comes from muscle tissue. If you weigh 140 pounds, about 60 pounds of it comes from the muscles attached to your bones. Collectively, there are over 650 different muscles in the human body. Muscles are responsible for all body movement. They allow us to move from place to place, as well as perform involuntary functions such as the heart beating and breathing. Muscles give our bodies form and shape; just think what you would look like if all your muscles "collapsed." Muscles are responsible for producing most of our body heat.

There are three main functions of the muscle system:

1. responsible for all body movement.

2. responsible for body form and shape (helps us maintain our posture).

3. responsible for body heat which maintains our body temperature.

TYPES OF MUSCLES

All body movements are determined by three principle types of muscles. They are skeletal, smooth, and cardiac muscle. These muscles are also described as striated, spindle-shaped, and nonstriated because of the way their cells look under the ordinary compound light microscope.

Skeletal muscles are attached to the bone of the skeleton. They are called striped or striated because they have cross bandings (striations) of alternating light and dark bands running perpendicular to the length of the muscle, Figure 7-1. Skeletal muscle is also called voluntary muscle, because it contains nerves under voluntary control. Skeletal muscle is composed of bundles of muscle cells. Each cell is multinucleate (containing many nuclei). Each muscle cell is known as a muscle fiber. The cell membrane is **sarcolemma** and the cytoplasm is **sarcoplasm** (refer to page 97 for further explanation of sarcolemma).

The fleshy body parts are made of skeletal muscles. They provide movement to the limbs, but contract quickly, fatigue easily and lack the ability to remain contracted for prolonged periods. Blinking the eye, talking, breathing, dancing, eating, and writing are all produced by the motion of these muscles. This chapter focuses on skeletal muscle.

Smooth (visceral) **muscle** cells are small and spindle-shaped. There is only one nucleus, located at the center of the cell. They are called smooth muscles because they are unmarked by

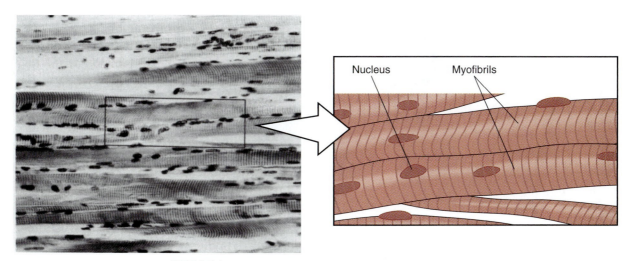

FIGURE 7-1 *Voluntary or striated (skeletal) muscle cells*
(photograph courtesy of Armed Forces Institute of Pathology, negative 72-13786)

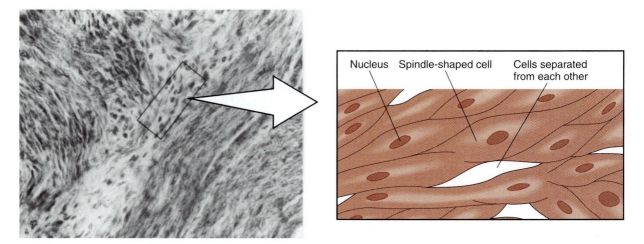

FIGURE 7-2 *Involuntary or smooth muscle cells*
(photograph courtesy of Armed Forces Institute of Pathology, negative 71-9163)

any distinctive striations. Unattached to bones, they act slowly, do not tire easily, and can remain contracted for a long time, Figure 7-2.

Smooth muscles are not under conscious control; for this reason they are also called involuntary muscles. Their actions are controlled by the autonomic (automatic) nervous system. Smooth muscles are found in the walls of the internal organs, including the stomach, intestines, uterus, and blood vessels. They help push food along the length of the alimentary canal, contract the uterus during labor and childbirth, and control the diameter of the blood vessels as the blood circulates throughout the body.

Cardiac muscle is found only in the heart. Cardiac muscle cells are striated and branched, and they are involuntary, Figure 7-3. Cardiac cells are joined in a continuous network without a sheath separation. The membranes of

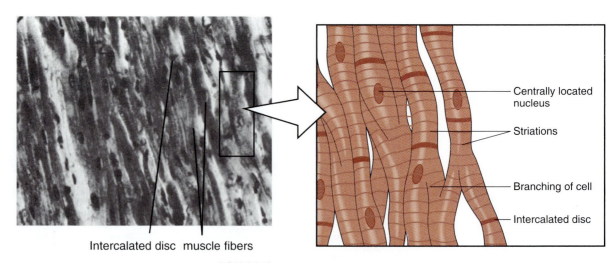

FIGURE 7-3 *Cardiac muscle cells*
(photograph reprinted, by permission, from Joan G. Creager, Human Anatomy and Physiology, 97)

adjacent cells are fused at places called intercalated disks. A communication system at the fused area will not permit independent cell contraction. When one cell receives a signal to contract, all neighboring cells are stimulated and they contract together to produce the heart beat. Healthy cardiac muscle contracts rapidly and is very strong. When the heart beats normally, it holds a rhythm of about seventy-two beats per minute. However, the activity of various nerves leading to the heart can increase or decrease its rate. Cardiac muscle requires a continuous supply of oxygen to function. Should its oxygen supply be cut off for as little as thirty seconds, the cardiac muscle would die.

Sphincter, or dilator, muscles are special circular muscles in the openings between the esophagus and stomach, and the stomach and small intestine. They are also found in the walls of the anus, the urethra, and mouth. They open and close to control the passage of substances.

Table 7-1 summarizes the characteristics of the three major muscle types.

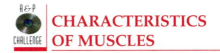

CHARACTERISTICS OF MUSCLES

All muscles, whether they are skeletal, smooth or cardiac, have four characteristics in common. One is contractibility, a quality possessed by no other body tissue. When a muscle shortens or contracts, it reduces the distance between the parts of its contents, or the space it surrounds. The contraction of skeletal muscles which connect a pair of bones brings the attachment points closer together. This causes the bone to move. When cardiac muscles contract, they reduce the area in the heart chambers, pumping blood from the heart into the blood vessels. Likewise, smooth muscles surround blood vessels and the intestines, causing the diameter of these tubes to decrease upon contraction.

Excitability (irritability), another characteristic of both muscle and nervous cells (neurons), is the ability to respond to certain stimuli by producing electric signals called action potentials (impulses).

Another property of muscles is extensibility (the ability to be stretched). When we bend our forearm, the muscles on the back of it are

TABLE 7-1 • *Names, Formulas, Locations or Uses of Some Common Acids*

MUSCLE TYPE	LOCATION	STRUCTURE	FUNCTION
Skeletal muscle (striated voluntary)	Attached to the skelton and also located in the wall of the pharynx and esophagus.	A skeletal muscle fiber is long, cylindrical, multinucleated, and contains alternating light and dark striations. Nuclei located at edge of fiber.	Contractions occur voluntarily and may be rapid and forceful. Contractions stabilize the joints.
Smooth muscle (nonstriated, involuntary)	Located in the walls of tubular structures and hollow organs, such as in the digestive tract, urinary bladder, and blood vessels.	A smooth muscle fiber is long and spindle-shaped with no striations.	Contractions occur involuntarily and are rhythmic and slow.
Cardiac (heart) muscle	Located in the heart.	Short, branching fibers with a centrally located nucleus; striations not distinct.	Contractions occur involuntarily and are rhythmic and automatic.

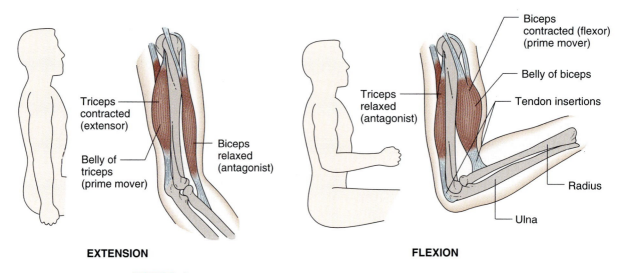

EXTENSION

FLEXION

FIGURE 7-4 *Coordination of prime mover and antagonistic muscles*

extended or stretched. Finally, muscles exhibit **elasticity** (ability of a muscle to return to its original length when relaxing). Collectively, these four properties of muscles—contractibility, excitability, extensibility, and elasticity—produce a veritable mechanical device capable of complex, intricate movements.

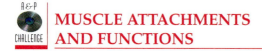

MUSCLE ATTACHMENTS AND FUNCTIONS

There are over 600 different muscles in the body. For any of these muscles to produce movement in any part of the body, it must be able to exert its force upon a movable object. Muscles must be attached to bones for leverage in order to have something to pull against. Muscles only pull, never push.

Muscles are attached to the bones of the skeleton by nonelastic cords called tendons. Bones are connected by joints. Skeletal muscles are attached in such a way as to bridge these joints. When a skeletal muscle contracts, the bone to which it is attached will move.

Muscles are attached at both ends to bones, cartilage, ligaments, tendons, skin, and sometimes to each other. The **origin** is the part of a skeletal muscle that is attached to a fixed struc-

ture or bone; it moves least during muscle contraction. The **insertion** is the other end, attached to a movable part; it is the part that moves most during a muscle contraction. The **belly** is the central body of the muscle, Figure 7-4.

The muscles of the body are arranged in pairs. One produces movement in a single direction called the **prime mover**, the other does so in the opposite direction called the **antagonist**. This arrangement of muscles with opposite actions is known as an antagonist pair.

By example, upper arm muscles are arranged in antagonist pairs, Figure 7-4. The muscle located on the front part of the upper arm is the **biceps**. One end of the biceps is attached to the scapula and humerus (its origin). When the biceps contracts, these two bones remain stationary. The opposite end of the biceps is attached to the radius of the lower arm (its insertion); this bone moves upon contraction of the biceps.

The muscle on the back of the upper arm is the **triceps**. Try this simple demonstration: Bend your elbow. With your other hand, feel the contraction of the belly of the biceps. At the same time, stretch your fingers out (around the arm) to touch your triceps; it will be in a relaxed state. Now extend your forearm; feel the simultaneous contraction of the triceps and relaxation of the biceps. Now bend the forearm halfway and contract the biceps and triceps. They cannot move, since both sets of muscles are contracting at the same time. In some muscle activity, the role of prime mover and antagonist may be reversed. When you flex your arm, the biceps brachii is the prime mover and triceps is the antagonist. When you extend your arm, the triceps is the prime mover and the biceps is the antagonist.

There is also another group of muscles called the synergists, which help steady a movement or stabilize joint activity.

SOURCES OF ENERGY AND HEAT

When muscles do their work, they not only move the body but also produce the heat which our bodies need. To get warm on a cold day, you jump up and down. Human beings must maintain their body temperatures within a narrow range (98.6°F to 99.8°F). For muscles to contract and do their work they need energy. The major source of this energy is adenosine triphosphate (ATP), a compound found in the muscle cell. To make ATP, the cell requires oxygen, glucose, and other material which is brought to the cell by the circulating blood. Extra glucose can be stored in the cell in the form of glycogen. When a muscle is stimulated the ATP is released, producing the heat our bodies need and the energy the muscle needs to contract. During this process, lactic acid, which is a by-product of cell metabolism, builds up.

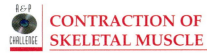

CONTRACTION OF SKELETAL MUSCLE

Movement of muscles occurs as a result of two major events: myoneural stimulation and contraction of muscle proteins. Skeletal muscles must be stimulated by nerve impulses to contract. A motor neuron (nerve cell) stimulates all of the skeletal muscles within a motor unit. A motor unit is a motor neuron plus all the muscle fibers it stimulates. The junction between the motor neuron's fiber (axon) which transmits the impulse, and the muscle cell's sarcolemma (muscle cell membrane) is the neuromuscular junction. The gap between the axon and the muscle cell is known as the synaptic cleft.

When the nerve impulses reach the end of the axon, the chemical neurotransmitter acetylcholine is released. Acetylcholine diffuses across the synaptic cleft and attaches to receptors on the sarcolemma. The sarcolemma then becomes temporarily permeable to sodium ions (Na+) which go rushing into the muscle cell. This gives the muscle cell excessive positive ions which upset and change the electrical condition of the sarcolemma. This electrical upset causes an action potential (an electric current).

Skeletal muscle contraction begins with the action potential which travels along the muscle fiber length. The basic source of energy is from glucose and the energy derived is stored in the form of ATP and phosphocreatinine. The latter serves as a trigger mechanism by allowing energy transfer to the protein molecules, actin and myosin, within the muscle fibers. Once begun, the action potential travels over the entire surface of the sarcolemma conducting the electric impulse from one end of the cell to the other. This results in the contraction of the muscle cell. The movement of electrical current along the sarcolemma causes calcium ions (Ca++) to be released from storage areas inside the muscle cell. When calcium ions attach to the action myofilaments (contractile elements of skeletal muscle) the sliding of the myofilaments is triggered and the whole cell shortens. The sliding of the myofilaments is energized by ATP.

The events that return the cell to a resting phase include the diffusion of potassium and sodium ions cell back to their initial positions outside the cell. When the action potential ends, calcium ions are reabsorbed into their storage areas and the muscle cell relaxes and returns to its original length. The amazing part is that this entire activity takes place in just a few thousandths of a second.

While the action potential is occurring, acetylcholine (which began the process) is broken down by enzymes on the sarcolemma. For this reason, a single nerve impulse produces

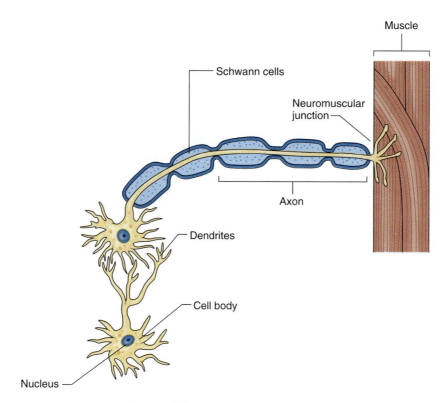

Muscle

Schwann cells

Neuromuscular
junction

Axon

Dendrites

Cell body

Nucleus

FIGURE 7-5 *A neuron stimulating muscle*

only one contraction at a time. The muscle cell relaxes until it is stimulated by the next release of acetylcholine, Figure 7-5.

MUSCLE FATIGUE

Muscle fatigue is caused by an accumulation of lactic acid in the muscles. During periods of vigorous exercise, the blood is unable to transport enough oxygen for the complete oxidation of glucose in the muscles. This causes the muscles to contract anaerobically (without oxygen).

The lactic acid normally leaves the muscle, passing into the bloodstream. But if vigorous exercise continues, the lactic acid level in the blood rises sharply. In such cases, lactic acid accumulates within the muscle. This impedes muscular contraction, causing muscle fatigue and cramps. After exercise, a person must stop, rest, and take in enough oxygen to change the

lactic acid back to glucose and other substances to be used by the muscle cells. The amount of oxygen needed is called the oxygen debt. When the debt is paid back, respirations resume a normal rate.

MUSCLE TONE

In order to function muscles should always be slightly contracted and ready to pull. This is **muscle tone**. Muscle tone can be achieved through proper nutrition and regular exercise. Muscle contractions may be **isotonic** or **isometric**. When muscles contract and shorten, it is called an isotonic contraction. This occurs when we walk, talk, and so on. When the tension in a muscle increases but the muscle does not shorten, it is called an isometric contraction. This occurs with exercises such as tensing the abdominal muscles. If we fail to exercise, our muscles become weak and flaccid. Muscles may also shrink from disuse. This is called atrophy. If we overexercise, muscles will become enlarged. This is known as hypertrophy. In hypertrophy, the size of the muscle fiber (cell) enlarges.

PRINCIPLE SKELETAL MUSCLES

The skeletal or voluntary muscles are made up of all the muscles that are attached to and help to move the skeleton. These muscles line the walls of the oral, abdominal, and pelvic cavities. Skeletal muscles also control the movement of the following structures—the eyeballs, the eyelids, the lips, the tongue, and the skin.

Naming of Skeletal Muscles

Muscles are named by location, size, direction, number of origins, location of origin and insertion, and action; however, not *all* muscles are named in this manner.

- location   frontalis—forehead

- size   gluteus maximus—largest muscle in buttock

- direction of fibers   external abdominal oblique—edge of the lower rib cage

- number of origins   biceps—two-headed muscle in humerus

- location of origin and insertion   sternocleidomastoid—origin in sternum

- action
  flexor   flexor carpi ulnaris—flexes the wrist
  extensor   extensor carpi ulnaris—extends the wrist
  levator and depressor   raises or lowers body parts; depressor anguli oris—depresses the corner of the mouth

Look at Figures 7-6 and 7-7 and find other muscles named by location, size, direction, number of origins, and action.

There are 656 muscles in the human body. This breaks down to 327 antagonistic muscle pairs and two unpaired muscles. These two unpaired muscles are the orbicularis oris and the diaphragm. The 656 muscles can be divided and subdivided into the following muscle regions.

A. *Head muscles*
   1. Muscles of expression
   2. Muscles of mastication (chewing)
   3. Muscles of the tongue
   4. Muscles of the pharynx
   5. Muscles of the soft palate

B. *Neck muscles*
   1. Muscles moving the head
   2. Muscles moving the hyoid bone and the larynx
   3. Muscles moving the upper ribs

C. *Trunk and extremity muscles*
   1. Muscles that move the vertebral column
   2. Muscles that move the scapula
   3. Muscles of breathing
   4. Muscles that move the humerus
   5. Muscles that move the forearm
   6. Muscles that move the wrist, hand, and finger digits
   7. Muscles that act on the pelvis
   8. Muscles that move the femur
   9. Muscles the move the leg
   10. Muscles that move the ankles, the foot, and the toe digits

Tables 7-2 through 7-7 on the following pages give a listing of some representative skeletal muscles that are involved in various types of bodily movements.

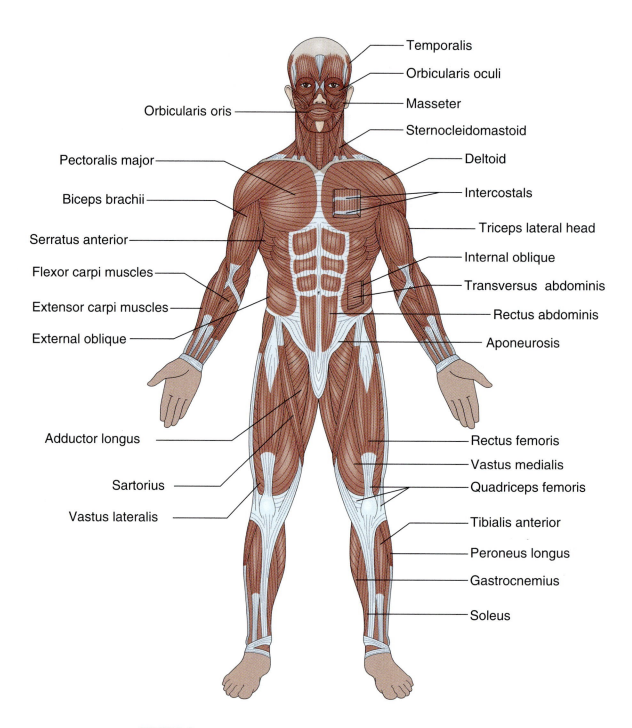

Temporalis

Orbicularis oculi

Masseter

Sternocleidomastoid

Deltoid

Intercostals

Triceps lateral head

Internal oblique

Transversus abdominis

Rectus abdominis

Aponeurosis

Rectus femoris

Vastus medialis

Quadriceps femoris

Tibialis anterior

Peroneus longus

Gastrocnemius

Soleus

Orbicularis oris

Pectoralis major

Biceps brachii

Serratus anterior

Flexor carpi muscles

Extensor carpi muscles

External oblique

Adductor longus

Sartorius

Vastus lateralis

FIGURE 7-6 *Principal skeletal muscles of the body—anterior view*

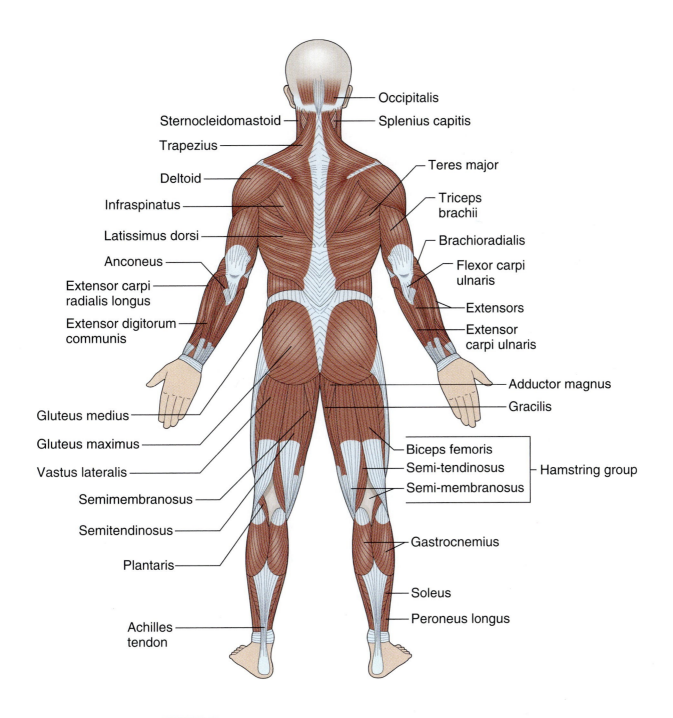

Occipitalis

Sternocleidomastoid

Splenius capitis

Trapezius

Deltoid

Teres major

Infraspinatus

Triceps brachii

Latissimus dorsi

Brachioradialis

Anconeus

Flexor carpi ulnaris

Extensor carpi radialis longus

Extensors

Extensor digitorum communis

Extensor carpi ulnaris

Adductor magnus

Gracilis

Gluteus medius

Gluteus maximus

Biceps femoris

Vastus lateralis

Semi-tendinosus

Hamstring group

Semimembranosus

Semi-membranosus

Semitendinosus

Gastrocnemius

Plantaris

Soleus

Peroneus longus

Achilles tendon

FIGURE 7-7 *Principal skeletal muscles of the body—posterior view*

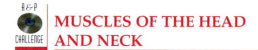

MUSCLES OF THE HEAD AND NECK

Muscles controlling facial expression, Figure 7-8. These control human facial expressions such as anger, fear, grief, joy, pleasure, and pain. Refer to Table 7-2.

Muscles of mastication, Figure 7-8. These muscles control the mandible (lower jaw), raising it to close the jaw and lowering it to open the jaw. Refer to Table 7-3.

Muscles that move the head, Figure 7-8. Extension, flexion, and rotation are the major movements of the head. Refer to Table 7-4.

TABLE 7-2 • *Representative Muscles of Facial Expression*

MUSCLE	EXPRESSION	LOCATION	FUNCTION
Frontalis	Surprise	On either side of the forehead	Raises eyebrow and wrinkles forehead
Depressor anguli oris	Doubt, disdain, contempt	Found along the side of the chin	Depresses corner of mouth
Orbicularis oris	Doubt, disdain, contempt	Ring-shaped muscle found around the mouth	Compresses and closes the lips
Platysma (broad sheet muscle)	Horror	Broad, thin muscular sheet covering the side of the neck and lower jaw	Draws corners of mouth downward and backward
Zygomaticus major	Laughing or smiling	Extends diagonally upward from corner of mouth	Raises corner of mouth
Nasalis	Muscles of the nose	Found over the nasal bones	Closes and opens the nasal openings
Orbicularis oculi	Sadness	Surrounds the eye orbit underlying the eyebrows	Closes the eyelid and tightens the skin on the forehead

TABLE 7-3 • *Representative Muscles of Mastication*

MUSCLE	LOCATION	FUNCTION
Masseter	Covers the lateral surface of the ramus (angle) of the mandible	Closes the jaw
Temporalis	Located on the temporal fossa of the skull	Raises the jaw and closes the mouth and draws the jaw backward

TABLE 7-4 • *Representative Muscles of the Neck*

MUSCLE	LOCATION	FUNCTION
Sternocleidomastoid (two heads)	Large muscles extending diagonally down sides of neck	Flexes head; rotates the head toward opposite side from muscle

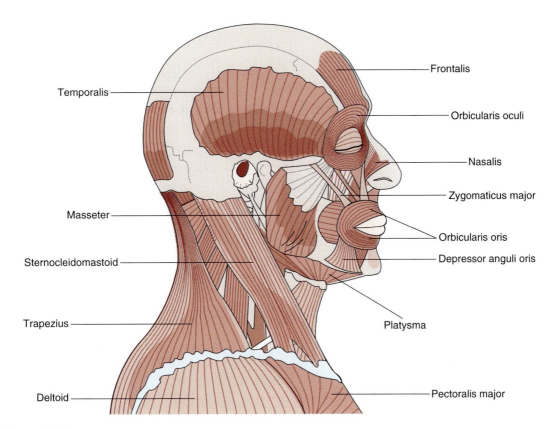

FIGURE 7-8 *Head and neck muscle arrangement: muscles controlling facial expression, mastication, and movement of the head*

MUSCLES OF THE UPPER EXTREMITIES

These muscles help to move the shoulder (scapula) and arm (humerus) and the forearm, wrist, hand, and fingers. Refer to Table 7-5 and Figure 7-9.

MUSCLES OF THE TRUNK

The trunk muscles control breathing and the movements of the abdomen and the pelvis. Refer to Table 7-6 and Figure 7-10, page 105.

MUSCLES OF THE LOWER EXTREMITIES

The muscles of the lower extremities, Figure 7-11, page 106, assist in the movement of the thigh (femur), the leg, the ankle, the foot, and the toes. Refer to Table 7-7, page 106. Athletes often pull what are known as the "hamstrings." The group of muscles which make up the "hamstrings" are the semitendinosus, biceps femoris, and semimembranosus. The tendons of these muscles attach posteriorly to the tibia and fibula. They can be felt behind the knee. The "hamstring" muscle group is responsible for flexing the knee.

Exercise and training will alter the size, structure, and strength of a muscle.

HOW EXERCISE AND TRAINING CHANGE MUSCLES

Exercise and training will alter the size, structure, and strength of a muscle.

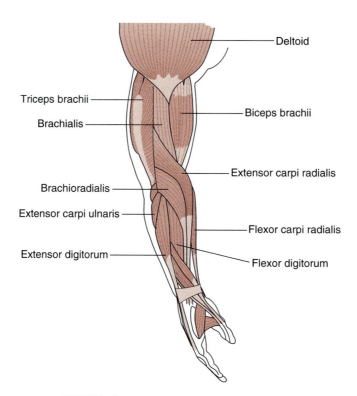

Deltoid

Triceps brachii

Brachialis

Biceps brachii

Extensor carpi radialis

Brachioradialis

Extensor carpi ulnaris

Flexor carpi radialis

Extensor digitorum

Flexor digitorum

FIGURE 7-9 *Muscles of the upper extremity*

TABLE 7-5 ● *Representative Muscles of the Upper Extremities*

MUSCLE	LOCATION	FUNCTION
*Trapezius	A large triangular muscle located on upper surface of back	Moves the shoulder; extends the head
*Deltoid	A thick triangular muscle that covers the shoulder joint	Abducts the upper arm
*Pectoralis major	Anterior part of the chest	Flexes the upper arm and helps to abduct the upper arm
Serratus	Anterior chest	Moves scapula forward and helps to raise the arm
*Biceps brachii	Upper arm to radius	Flexes the lower arm
*Triceps brachii	Posterior arm to ulna	Extends the lower arm
Extensor and flexor carpi muscle groups	Extends from the anterior and posterior forearm to the hand	Moves the hand
Extensor and flexor digitorum muscle groups	Extends from the anterior and posterior forearm to the fingers	Moves the fingers
*Major Prime Movers		

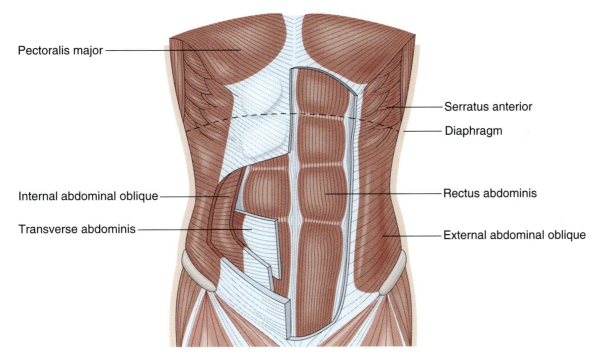

FIGURE 7-10 *Muscles of the trunk*

TABLE 7-6 ● *Representative Muscles of the Trunk*

MUSCLE	LOCATION	FUNCTION
External intercostals	Found between the ribs	Raises the ribs to help in breathing
Diaphragm	A dome-shaped muscle separating the thoracic and abdominal cavities	Helps to control breathing
Rectus abdominis	Extends from the ribs to the pelvis	Compresses the abdomen
External oblique	Anterior inferior edge of the last eight ribs	Depresses ribs, flexes the spinal column, and compresses the abdominal cavity
Internal oblique	Found directly beneath the external oblique, its fibers running in the opposite direction	Same as above

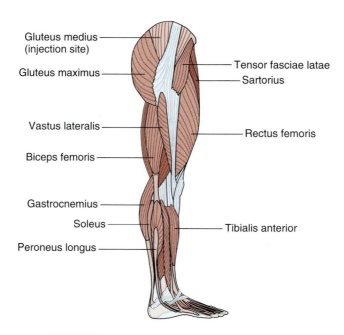

Gluteus medius
(injection site)

Gluteus maximus

Tensor fasciae latae

Sartorius

Vastus lateralis

Rectus femoris

Biceps femoris

Gastrocnemius

Soleus

Peroneus longus

Tibialis anterior

FIGURE 7-11 *Muscles of the lower extremity*

TABLE 7-7 ● *Representative Muscles of the Lower Extremities*

MUSCLE	LOCATION	FUNCTION
*Gluteus maximus	Buttocks	Extends femur and rotates it outward
Gluteus medius	Extends from the deep femur to the buttocks; injection site	Abducts and rotates the thigh
Tensor faciae latae	A flat muscle found along the upper lateral surface of the thigh	Flexes, abducts, and medially rotates the thigh
*Rectus femoris	Anterior thigh	Flexes thigh and extends the lower leg
*Sartorius (Tailor's muscle)	A long, straplike muscle that runs diagonally across the anterior and medial surface of the thigh	Flexes and rotates the thigh and leg
*Tibialis anterior	In front of the libia bone	Dorsiflexes the foot; permits walking on the heels
*Gastrocnemius	Calf muscle	Points toes and flexes the lower leg
*Soleus	A broad flat muscle found beneath the gastrocnemius	Extends foot
Peroneus logus	A superficial muscle found on the lateral side of the leg	Extends and everts the foot and supports arches
*Major Prime Movers		

Size and Muscle Structure

Skeletal muscles that are not used will atrophy and those that are used excessively will hypertrophy. The hypertrophy is caused by change in the sarcoplasm (cytoplasm found in the individual skeletal muscle fibers) and *not* to an increase in the number of muscle fibers (cells). Muscles that have been injured can regenerate only to a limited degree. If the muscle damage is extensive, then the muscle tissue is replaced by connective (scar) tissue. Muscles that are overexercised or worked will have a tremendous increase of connective tissue between the muscle fibers. This causes the skeletal muscle to become tougher.

Effect of Training on Muscle Efficiency

The following will occur:

- Improved coordination of all muscles involved in a particular activity

- Improvement of the respiratory and circulatory system to supply the needs of an active muscular system

- Elimination or reduction of excess fat

- Improved joint movement involved with that particular muscle activity.

MEDICAL HIGHLIGHT

Massage Therapy

Massage: Does it have therapeutic value or does it just make you feel good? Tiffany Field, a psychologist at the University of Miami's School of Medicine's Touch Institute has been documenting with her colleagues that massage's feel-good effects can translate into striking improvements in medical conditions ranging from asthma to rheumatoid arthritis to burns.

The researchers are also shedding light on what massage can do for healthy people who want to ward off colds and viruses, cope more effectively with stress and pain, and sleep more soundly. Stress causes a flight or fight response from the body. Massage intervenes by convincing the body that the emergency is over. "Massage mechanically forces muscle tension to decrease," says Robert Sapolsky, a Stanford University neurobiologist. As the pressure of the therapist's hands loosens tight muscles, the body produces few of the stress hormones, such as cortisol and norepinephrine. Once the muscles start to relax, tension seems to ease.

Massage therapists believe that a regular laying-on of hands can tune up the immune system, making people less susceptible to colds and viruses. The theory is that deep massage strokes push lymph fluid more quickly through the network of vessels that deliver it throughout the body. Since lymph fluid carries immune cells, massage is thought to give those cells more opportunities to seek out and neutralize disease invaders.

Massage can help produce sound sleep by turning off the sympathetic nervous system, which makes us alert and vigilant, and switching on the parasympathetic, which calms things down. Massage seems to help relieve serious back pain as well as pain associated with rheumatoid arthritis, fibromyalgia, and burns. The theory seems to be that massage may raise the levels of enkephalins, one of the body's natural painkillers. As more research is done, massage may be an alternative way to treat some common diseases.

Effect of Training on Muscle Strength

Strength (capacity to do work) is increased by proper training. Training can have the following effects on skeletal muscles:

● Increase in muscle size

● Improved antagonistic muscle coordination, where antagonistic muscles are relaxed at the right moment and do not interfere with the functioning of the working muscle.

● Improved functioning in the cortical brain region, where the nerve impulses that start muscular contraction

MASSAGE MUSCLES

Occasionally a health care professional must give either a total body massage or a massage to a specific body area to a patient. The correct type of massage is essential in either providing the proper **physiotherapy** or a general sense of comfort and well-being to a patient.

The health care professional must be aware of the specific skeletal muscles involved in therapeutic massage. The importance of these skeletal muscles comes from their proximity to the body's surface and their relatively large size. Table 7-8 gives the names of these superficial skeletal muscles and their general locations. It is essential for the health care professional to be able to locate these skeletal muscles not only on the muscle diagrams but also on the living bodies of patients with different physiques: scrawny, muscular, thin, fat, male, and female.

A&P CHALLENGE INTRAMUSCULAR INJECTIONS

A health care professional occasionally has to administer an **intramuscular** (into the muscle) injection into the patient. Therefore, a working knowledge of the major skeletal muscles and the underlying anatomy of the area to be injected is needed. The most common sites for an intramuscular injection are the **deltoid** muscle of the upper arm, vastus lateralis (anterior thigh), or gluteus medius (buttocks.)

TABLE 7-8 ● *Skeletal Muscles Involved in Massage*

NAME OF SKELETAL MUSCLE	LOCATION
Sternocleidomastoid	Side of neck
Trapezius	Back of the neck and upper back
Latissimus dorsi	Lower back
Pectoralis major	Chest
Serratus anterior	Lateral ribs
External oblique	Anterior and lateral abdomen
Deltoid	Shoulder
Biceps brachii	Anterior aspect of arm
Triceps brachii	Posterior aspect of arm
Brachioradialis	Anterior and proximal forearm
Gluteus maximus	Buttock
Tensor fascia latae	Lateral and Proximal Thigh
Sartorius	Anterior thigh
Quadriceps femoris group (rectus femoris, vastus lateralis, vastus medialis, vastus intermedius)	Anterior thigh
Hamstring group (biceps, femoris, semitendinosus, semimembranosus)	Posterior thigh
Gracilis	Medial thigh
Tibialis anterior	Anterior leg
Gastrocnemius	Posterior leg
Soleus	Posterior (Deep) leg
Peroneus longus	Lateral leg

CAREER PROFILES

CHIROPRACTORS

Chiropractors, also known as chiropractic doctors, diagnose and treat patients whose health problems are associated with the body's muscular, nervous, or skeletal systems. The chiropractic approach to health care is holistic, stressing the patient's overall well-being. Chiropractors use natural, non-surgical health treatments such as water, heat, light, and massage. With difficulties involving the muscular system, the chiropractor manually manipulates or adjusts the spinal column.

Education required is a bachelor's degree or at least two years of college in addition to completion of a four year course of study at a chiropractic college. All states require licensure. To qualify, a candidate must meet educational requirements and pass the state boards. Job prospects are excellent and employment is expected to grow faster than the average for all other occupations until the year 2005.

MUSCULO-SKELETAL DISORDERS

Muscle and skeletal systems work as a team to move the body. Muscular coordination is very important if a person is to perform his/her daily functions efficiently. Injuries and diseases, which may affect the musculo-skeletal system, sometimes interfere with these functions. The retraining of injured or unused muscles is a type of rehabilitation called therapeutic exercise.

Muscle atrophy can occur to muscles which are infrequently used; they shrink in size and lose muscle strength, an example is in a stroke (cerebro-vascular accident). The muscles are understimulated, and gradually waste away. Muscle atrophy due to nerve paralysis may reduce a muscle up to 25% of its normal size. Muscle atrophy can also be caused by prolonged bedrest or the immobilization of a limb in a cast. Muscle atrophy can be minimized by massage or special exercise.

A muscle strain is a tear in the muscle resulting from excessive use. Limited bleeding inside the muscle can result in pain and swelling. Ice packs will help to stop bleeding and reduce swelling.

Muscle spasm, or cramp, is a sustained contraction of the muscle. These contractions may occur because of overuse of the muscle.

Myalgia is a term used to describe muscle pain. Fibromyalgia disease is a collection of symptoms (syndrome). In fibromyalgia, the most definite symptom is chronic muscle pain lasting three or more months in specific muscle points. Other symptoms may include fatigue, headache, feelings of numbness and tingling, and feelings of joint pain. Treatment is directed at pain relief and counseling.

Hernia occurs when an organ protrudes through a weak muscle. Abdominal hernia occurs when organs protrude through the abdominal wall. Inguinal hernia occurs in the inguinal area (see Figure 1-4, Chapter 1) and hiatal hernia occurs when the stomach pushes through the diaphragm.

Flatfeet (talipes) result from a weakening of the leg muscles that support the arch. The downward pressure on the foot eventually flattens out the arches. The condition can be helped by exercise, massage, and corrective shoes.

Tetanus (lockjaw) is an infectious disease characterized by continuous spasms of the voluntary muscles. It is caused by a toxin from the bacillus, *clostridium tetani*, a bacterium that can enter the body through a puncture wound. This disease can be prevented by a tetanus anti-toxoid vaccine.

Torticollis, or wry neck, may be due to an inflammation of the trapezius and/or sternocleidomastoid muscle.

Muscular dystrophy is a group of diseases in which the muscle cells deteriorate. The most common type is Duchenne Muscular Dystrophy caused by a genetic defect. At birth, the child appears normal; as growth occurs and muscle cells die, the child becomes weak. The child loses the ability to walk between the ages of nine and eleven. There is progressive deterioration of muscle and death will occur in the late teens or early twenties unless mechanical breathing is instituted.

Myasthenia gravis leads to progressive muscular weakness and paralysis, sometimes even death. The cause is still unknown, but many researchers believe it may be due to a defect in the immune system, affecting myoneural function. In extreme cases, it can be fatal due to the paralysis of the respiratory muscles.

Recreation Injuries

The need to exercise can sometimes lead to excessive stress on the tendons. The tendons are cords of connective tissue that attach the muscles to bone. They are not able to contract and return to their original place; therefore, they are more susceptible to straining and tearing. For example, a sudden severe muscle contraction needed for playing tennis can cause the tendons to tear.

Tennis elbow, or lateral epicondylitis, occurs at the bony prominence (lateral epicondyle) on the sides of the elbow. The tendon that connects the arm muscle to elbow becomes inflamed because the repetitive use of the arm and under conditioning, Figure 7-12. This can occur from carrying luggage, playing tennis, swinging a golf club, or pounding a hammer. Treatment consists of relief of pain and ice packs to reduce the inflammation. Sleeping on the affected arm should be avoided. Surgery is used as a last resort.

Shin splints occur when there is injury to the muscle tendon in the front of the shin. This occurs when jogging. To prevent shin splints, choose the correct running shoe—one that is comfortable and has proper arch support.

Rotator cuff disease is an inflammation of a group of tendons that fuse together and surround the shoulder joint. This injury can occur because of repetitive overhead swinging, such as swinging a tennis racquet or pitching a ball. The most common complaint is aching in the top and front of the shoulder. Pain increases when the arm is lifted overhead. Treatment includes rest and physical therapy.

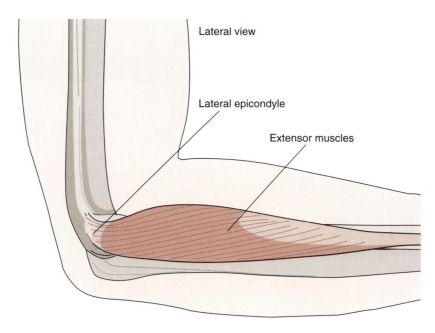

Lateral view

Lateral epicondyle

Extensor muscles

FIGURE 7-12 *Tennis elbow*

MEDICAL HIGHLIGHT: TECHNOLOGY
Cumulative Trauma Disorders

Computerization of the workplace has created not only a new way of life for many workers, but it has also contributed to one of the fastest growing occupational disorders. *Cumulative trauma disorders* (CTD) or *repetitive motion disorder* results from the repeated type of muscle use required for an activity such as using a computer keyboard.

A United States Bureau of Labor statistics report shows that CTD accounted for more than half of all occupational illnesses in the United States. This tissue inflammation and pain occurs in workers who spend many hours of the day making the same motion over and over. This disorder has given rise to a new area of expertise called **ergonomics**, which is the study of the application of biology and engineering to the relationship between workers and their environment.

Workers must be educated in the causes and symptoms of CTD. Additionally, workers must be educated in the proper use of tools and lifting techniques to prevent this disorder. For example, wrist disorders may be prevented by making changes in the computer work station such as adjusting the height of the keyboard and screens, and making sure that chairs are well suited to both the job and the individual worker.

● REVIEW QUESTIONS

Select the letter of the choice that best completes the statement.

1. The muscle system is responsible for:
   a. producing red blood cells
   b. providing a framework
   c. moving the body
   d. conducting impulses

2. Skeletal muscle is also known as:
   a. involuntary
   b. voluntary
   c. cardiac
   d. smooth

3. The muscle responsible for action in a single direction is called:
   a. prime mover
   b. antagonist
   c. synergistic
   d. adduction

4. Muscles are always in a state of partial contraction called:
   a. muscle atrophy
   b. muscle tone
   c. tetanus
   d. muscle hypertrophy

5. The muscle you use to turn your head is the:
   a. trapezius
   b. sternocleidomastoid
   c. orbicularis
   d. temporalis

6. The muscle in the upper arm which is used as an injection site is the:
   a. triceps
   b. biceps
   c. trapezius
   d. deltoid

7. The muscle used in breathing is the:
   a. oblique
   b. diaphragm
   c. rectus abdominus
   d. serratus

8. A muscle located on the chest wall is the:
   a. trapezius
   b. frontalis
   c. pectoralis major
   d. rectus abdominus

9. Muscle fatigue is caused by a buildup of:
   a. glycogen
   b. oxygen
   c. lactic acid
   d. ATP

10. The muscle on the calf portion of the leg is the:
    a. gastrocnemius
    b. sartorius
    c. rectus femoris
    d. tibialis anterior

●APPLYING THEORY TO PRACTICE

1. Your body feels very warm after exercising. What has happened?

2. After running up a hill, you are out of breath and have a cramp in your leg. What caused the cramp? How can you relieve it? When will your breathing get back to normal?

3. While looking at yourself in the mirror, look surprised. Name and locate the muscle you used. Place your fingers on the muscle and feel it contract. Do the same exercise making a frown and a smile.

4. Name the leg muscles that you would use to kick a soccer ball.

5. A friend has had an accident and has a leg cast on. Describe the condition which will occur without exercise. How can you prevent this condition?

6. A patient comes to the office and explains that she is on the school "all star" tennis team; but her right shoulder and arm is hurting all over. The doctor states that her condition is known as rotator cuff disease. Explain recreation injuries to the patient and rotator cuff disease.

CHAPTER

8

Central Nervous System

OBJECTIVES

- Describe the functions of the central nervous system
- List the main divisions of the central nervous system
- Identify the parts of the brain
- Describe the structure of the brain and spinal cord
- Describe the functions of the parts of the brain
- Describe the functions of the spinal cord
- Describe disorders of the brain and spinal cord
- Define the key words that relate to this chapter

KEY WORDS

Alzheimer's disease
anticonvulsant
arachnoid (mater)
associative neuron
autonomic nervous
    system
axons
blood-brain barrier
brain stem
central nervous
    system
cerebellum
cerebral aqueduct
cerebral cortex
cerebral palsy
cerebral ventricles
cerebrospinal fluid
cerebrum
chorea
choroid plexus
corpus callosum
dementia
dendrites
diencephalon
dura mater

encephalitis
epilepsy
exudate fissures
fibers
fourth ventricle
frontal lobe
glioma
gyri (convolutions)
hematoma
hydrocephalus
hypothalamus
interventricular
    foramen
interneuron
lateral ventricle
lumbar puncture
medulla oblongata
membrane
    excitability
memory
meninges
meningitis
motor neuron
    (efferent)
multiple sclerosis

myelin sheath
    (neurilemma)
neuroglia
neuron
nystagmus
occipital lobe
paraplegia
parietal lobe
Parkinson's disease
peripheral nervous
    system
pia mater
poliomyelitis
pons
sensory neuron
    (afferent)
spastic quadriplegia
spinal cord
sulci
synapse
synaptic cleft
temporal lobe
thalamus
third ventricle

INTRODUCTION TO THE CENTRAL NERVOUS SYSTEM

The study of body functions reveals that the body is made up of millions of small structures that perform a multitude of different activities; these are coordinated and integrated into one harmonious whole. The two main communications systems are the endocrine system and the nervous system. They send chemical messengers and nerve impulses to all of the structures. The endocrine system and hormonal regulation are discussed in other chapters. Hormonal regulations are slow, while neural regulation is comparatively rapid.

Functions of the central nervous system:

1. It is the communication and coordination system in the body.

    - it receives messages from stimuli all over the body
    - the brain interprets the message
    - the brain responds to the message and carries out an activity

2. The brain is also the seat of intellect and reasoning.

The central nervous system is the most highly organized system of the body, consisting of the brain, spinal cord, and nerves. The nerve cell, or **neuron**, is specially constructed to carry out its function, that being transmitting a message from one cell to the next. In addition to the nucleus, cytoplasm, and cell membrane, the neuron has extensions of cytoplasm from the cell body. These extensions, or *processes*, are called **dendrites** and **axons**. There may be several dendrites, but only one axon. These processes, or **fibers**, as they are often called, are paths along which nerve impulses travel, Figure 8-1. The axon has a specialized covering called **neurilemma** or **myelin sheath**, Figure 8-1. This covering speeds up the nerve impulse as it travels along the axon. The myelin sheath produces a fatty substance called myelin which protects the axon; this substance is also called "white matter." The Nodes of Ranvier is the area which has no myelin present. This is important in the conduction of a nerve impulse. Axons carry messages away from the cell body. Dendrites carry messages to the cell body.

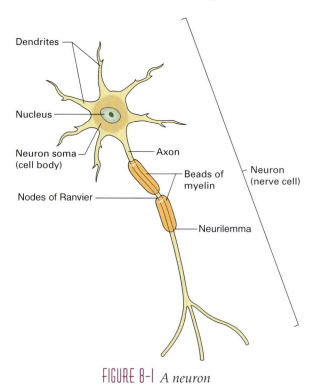

Dendrites

Nucleus

Neuron soma (cell body)

Nodes of Ranvier

Axon

Beads of myelin

Neurilemma

Neuron (nerve cell)

FIGURE 8-1 *A neuron*

Nervous Tissue

Nerve tissue is made up of two major types of nerve cells: **neuroglia** and neurons. Neuroglia is the type of cells that insulate, support, and protect the neurons. They are sometimes referred to as "nerve glue."

All neurons possess the characteristics of being able to react when stimulated and of being able to pass the nerve impulse generated on to other neurons. These characteristics are irritability (the ability to react when stimulated) and conductivity (the ability to transmit a disturbance to distant points). The dendrites receive the impulse and transmit it to the cell body, and then to the axon where it is passed on to another neuron or to a muscle or gland. There are three types of neurons:

1. **Sensory neurons** or **afferent** neurons which emerge from the skin or sense organs and carry messages, or impulses, toward the spinal cord and brain.

2. **Motor neurons** or **efferent** neurons which carry messages from the brain and spinal cord to the muscles and glands.

3. **Associative neurons** or **interneurons**, which carry impulses from the sensory neuron to the motor neuron.

Function of the Nerve Cell/ Membrane Excitability

Nerves carry impulses by creating electric charges in a process known as **membrane excitability**. Neurons have a membrane that separates the cytoplasm inside from the extracellular fluids outside the cell, thereby creating two chemically different areas. Each area has differing amounts of potassium and sodium ions and some other charged substances, with the inside being the more negatively charged. When a neuron is stimulated, ions move across the membrane creating a current, which if large enough, will briefly change the inside of the neuron to be more positive than the outside area. This state is known as action potential. Neurons and other cells that produce action potentials are said to have membrane excitability.

To understand how impulses are carried along nerves or throughout a muscle when it contracts, we need to learn a little more about membrane excitability. Ions cross a membrane through channels, some of which are open and allow ions to "leak" (diffuse) continuously. Other channels are called "gated" and open only during action potential. Another membrane opening is called a sodium-potassium pump which, by active transport, maintains the flow of ions from higher to lower concentrations levels across the membrane and restores the cytoplasm and extracellular fluid to their original value, after an action potential occurs. This action is in response to the fact there is an imbalance between the cytoplasm and the extracellular fluid. When diffusion takes place, particles move from an area of greater concentration to an area of lesser concentration.

The following simplified description explains how this whole process works.

1. A neuron membrane is "at rest." There are large amounts of potassium (K+) ions inside the cells but not very many sodium (NA+) ions. The reverse is true outside the cell in the extracellular fluid. Most of the open channels are for potassium to pass through, so it leaks out of the cell.

2. As the K+ ions leave, the inside becomes relatively more negative until some K+ ions are attracted back in and the electrical force balances the diffusion force and movement stops. The inside is still more negative and the amount of energy between the two differently charged areas is ready to work (carry an impulse). This state is called *resting membrane potential*, Figure 8-2(a). The membrane is now polarized. The sodium ions are not able to move "in" since their channels are closed during the resting state; however, if a few leak in, the membrane pump sends an equal number out.

3. Now suppose a sensory neuron receptor is stimulated by something, a sound for instance. This will cause a change in the

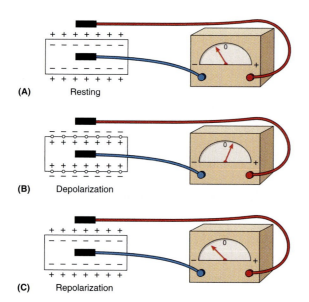

(A) Resting

(B) Depolarization

(C) Repolarization

FIGURE 8-2 *Sequence of events in membrane potential and relative positive and negative states: (a) Normal resting potential (negative inside/positive outside); (b) Depolarization (positive inside/negative outside); (c) Repolarization (negative inside/positive outside)*

membrane potential. The stimulus energy is converted to an electrical signal and if it is strong enough, it will depolarize a portion of the membrane and allow the gated sodium ion channels to open initiating an action potential, Figure 8-2(b).

4. The sodium ions move through the gated channels into the cytoplasm and the inside becomes more positive until the membrane potential is reversed and the gates close to sodium ions.

5. Next the potassium gates open and large amounts of potassium leave the cytoplasm resulting in the repolarization of the membrane, Figure 8-2(c). After repolarization, the sodium-potassium pump restores the initial concentrations of sodium and potassium ions inside and outside the neuron.

This whole process occurs in a few milliseconds. When this action occurs in one part of the cell membrane, it spreads to adjacent membrane regions, continuing away from the original site of stimulation, sending "messages" over the nerve. This cycle is completed millions of times a minute throughout the body, day after day, year after year.

Synapse

A **synapse** is where the messages go from one cell to the next cell. The nerve cell has both an axon and a dendrite. Messages go from the axon of one cell to the dendrite of another; they never actually touch. The space between them is known as the **synaptic cleft**. The conduction is accomplished through neurotransmitters at the end of each axon, which are special chemicals, namely epinephrine, norepinephrine, and acetylcholine.

An impulse travels along the axon to the end where the neurotransmitter is released. This helps the impulse to "jump" the space between and the impulse is sent to the dendrite of the next nerve cell. The neurotransmitter between muscle cells and the nervous system is acetylcholine.

DIVISIONS OF THE NERVOUS SYSTEM

The nervous system can be divided into three divisions: the central, peripheral, and the autonomic nervous system.

1. The **central nervous system** consists of the brain and spinal cord

2. The **peripheral nervous system** is made up of the nerves of the body consisting of twelve pairs of cranial nerves extending out from the brain and thirty-one pairs of spinal nerves extending out from the spinal cord

3. The **autonomic nervous system** includes peripheral nerves and ganglia (a group of cell bodies outside the central nervous system that carry impulses to involuntary muscles and glands)

Where decision is called for and action must be considered, the central and peripheral nervous systems are involved. They carry information to the brain where it is interpreted, organized, and stored. An appropriate command is sent to

MEDICAL HIGHLIGHT: DISCOVERY

Connection Between Nerves and Muscles

Scientists have unraveled the secret of how a nerve communicates with a muscle. Dr. George Yancopoulos and another team working independently have produced the most detailed picture of this incredibly complex system. Their reports were published in the journal *CELL*.

Nerve cells communicate with each other as well as give orders to muscles by sending messages across gaps called *synapses*. Nerves and muscles create chemically intricate synapses in just the right places. The secret is two proteins: one is called agrin and another is known as muscle-specific receptor kinase, or MuSK. In working with mice, the researchers found that both proteins were necessary during embryonic development to make working connections between nerves and muscles. If either protein was missing, the mice were unable to breathe and died soon after birth.

During development it appears that nerve cells grow toward muscles and release agrin. On the muscle side of the gap, the agrin is received by MuSK which works in combination with another protein called muscle-associated-specificity component. This connection starts a complicated chain reaction that eventually results in changes in both the nerve and the muscle, which add up to a working synapse. The nerve cells talk to the muscle cells by releasing the neurotransmitter acetylcholine. Agrin is the first step; it signals the muscle to pull together the chemicals it needs to construct acetylcholine receptors so that it can receive these messages.

This discovery may offer insight into how cell-to-cell communication goes on inside the brain and it could also lead to new treatments for nerve injuries and a variety of diseases.

---

organs or muscles. The autonomic nervous system supplies heart muscle, smooth muscle, and secretory glands with nervous impulses as needed. It is usually involuntary in action.

THE BRAIN

A&P CHALLENGE

The adult human brain is a highly developed, complex, and intricate mass of soft nervous tissue. It weighs about 1400 grams (3 lbs) and is composed of 100 billion neurons. The brain is protected by the bony cranial cavity; further protection is afforded by three membranous coverings called **meninges**, and the cerebrospinal fluid. The brain is composed of white and gray matter. The outer cortex, known as the **cerebral cortex**, is gray. This is

the highest center of reasoning and intellect. You may have heard people say when trying to resolve a problem, "I need to use my gray matter." The deeper part of the cerebral cortex is composed of myelinated nerve tracts and it is called the white matter. An adequate blood supply to the brain is critical. Without oxygen, brain damage will occur within four to eight minutes. The brain is divided into four major parts: the cerebrum, diencephalon, cerebellum, and brain stem, see Figure 8-3.

Memory

The brain is our warehouse which stores information we have learned and packages and stores new information. We call this process **memory**. In order to create a memory,

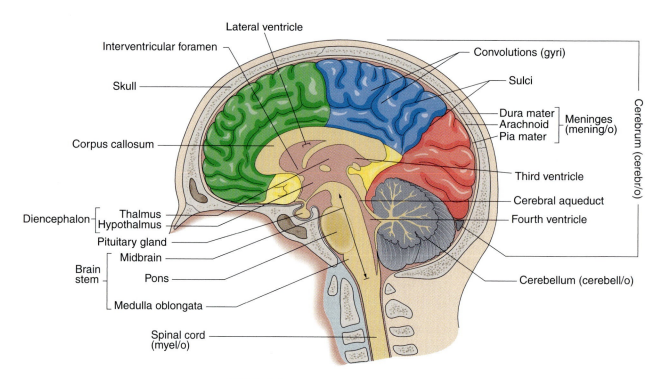

FIGURE 8-3 *Cross-section of the brain*

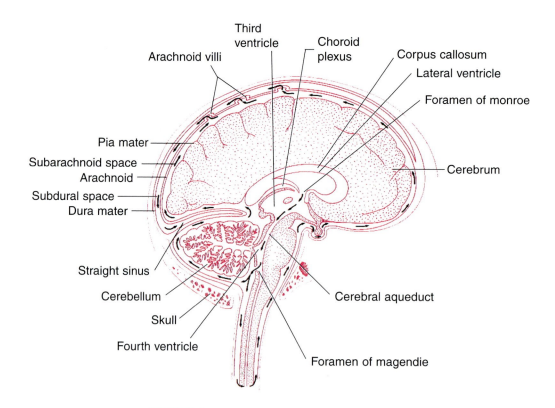

FIGURE 8-4 *Circulation of the cerebrospinal fluid*

nerve cells are thought to form new interconnections. No one area of the brain stores all memories because the storage site depends on the type of memory. For example, how to swim would be held in the motor area of the brain, while visual memories would be stored in the visual area of the brain. Scientists believe that the hippocampus of the limbic system acts like a receptionist, deciding the significance of the event and determining which part of the brain the information should be stored in.

Memory may be short term or long term. It depends on how much attention we paid to an event, how many times we repeated an activity, and what the memory is associated with. People frequently recall what took place during a traumatic event, such as their first day at school. Compare that with how many times you see a commercial before you can remember it.

Coverings of the Brain

The three meninges are the dura mater, arachnoid, and the pia mater, see Figure 8-3. The **dura mater** is the outer brain covering, which lines the skull on the inside. This is a tough dense membrane of fibrous connective tissue containing an abundance of blood vessels. The **arachnoid** (**mater**) is the middle layer. It resembles a fine cobweb with fluid-filled spaces. Covering the brain surface itself is the **pia mater**, comprised of blood vessels held together by fine areolar connective tissue. The space between the arachnoid and pia mater is filled with cerebrospinal fluid, produced within the ventricles of the brain. This fluid acts both as a shock absorber and a source of nutrients for the brain.

VENTRICLES OF THE BRAIN

The brain contains four lined cavities filled with cerebrospinal fluid. These cavities are called **cerebral ventricles**, Figure 8-4. The ventricles lie deep within the brain. The two largest, located within the cerebral hemispheres, are known as the right and left **lateral ventricles**.

The **third ventricle** is placed behind and below the lateral ventricles. It is connected to the two lateral ventricles via the **interventricular foramen**. The **fourth ventricle** is situated below the third, in front of the cerebellum, and behind the pons and the medulla oblongata. The third and fourth ventricles are interconnected via a narrow canal called the **cerebral aqueduct**.

Each of the four ventricles contains a rich network of blood vessels of the pia mater referred to as the **choroid plexus**. The choroid plexus is in contact with the cells lining the ventricles, which helps in the formation of cerebrospinal fluid.

Cerebrospinal Fluid and its Circulation

Cerebrospinal fluid is a substance that forms inside the four brain ventricles from the blood vessels of the choroid plexuses. This fluid serves as a liquid shock absorber protecting the delicate brain and spinal cord. It is formed by filtration from the intricate capillary network of the choroid plexuses. The fluid transports nutrients to, and removes metabolic waste products from, the brain cells.

Choroid plexus capillaries differ significantly in their selective permeability from capillaries in other areas of the body. As a result drugs carried in the bloodstream may not effectively penetrate brain tissue, rendering infections (such as meningitis) difficult to cure. This phenomenon is commonly referred to as the **blood-brain barrier**.

After filling the two lateral ventricles of the cerebral hemispheres, the cerebrospinal fluid seeps into the third ventricular through the foramen (opening). From here it flows through the cerebral aqueduct into the fourth ventricle. The fluid then passes through the foramen of the 4th ventricle and the two lateral foramina of the 4th ventricle into the small, tubelike central canal of the cord and into the subarachnoid spaces. The subarachnoid spaces are thus filled with cerebrospinal fluid which bathes the brain and the spinal cord. Ultimately the cerebrospinal fluid returns to the bloodstream via the venous structures in the brain, called arachnoid villi.

The formation and circulation of cerebrospinal fluid is used by members of the health team to detect some defects or disease of the brain. For example, inflammation of the cranial meninges quickly spreads to the meninges of the spinal cord. This leads to an increased secretion of cerebrospinal fluid which collects in the confined bony cavity of the brain and spinal column. The accumulation of excess fluid causes headaches, reduced pulse rate, slow breathing, and partial or total unconsciousness.

Removal of cerebrospinal fluid for diagnostic purposes is accomplished with a **lumbar puncture**. The needle used to withdraw the cerebrospinal fluid is inserted between the third and fourth lumbar vertebrae. The fluid, or exudate withdrawn contains by-products of the inflammation and organisms causing it. Therefore, a lumbar puncture is helpful in diagnosing such diseases as cerebral hemorrhage, increased pressure, intracranial tumors, meningitis, and syphilis. It also serves to alleviate the pressure caused by meningitis, and especially hydrocephalus.

A & P
CHALLENGE

CEREBRUM

The **cerebrum** is the largest and highest part of the brain. It occupies the whole upper part of the skull and weighs about two pounds. Covering the upper and lower surfaces of the cerebrum is a layer of gray matter called the **cerebral cortex**.

The cerebrum is divided into two hemispheres right and left, by a very deep groove known as the longitudinal fissure. The cerebral surface is completely covered with furrows and ridges. The deeper furrows, or grooves are referred to as **fissures**, and the shallower ones, **sulci**.

The elevated ridges between the sulci are the **gyri**, also known as **convolutions**, Figure 8-5. These convolutions serve to increase the surface area of the brain, resulting in a proportionately larger amount of gray matter. The arrangement of the gyri and sulci on the brain's surface varies from one brain to another. Certain fissures,

however, are constant and represent important demarcations. They help to localize specific functional areas of the cerebrum, and to divide each hemisphere into, four lobes.

Each cerebral hemisphere is divided into a frontal, parietal, occipital, and temporal lobe. These lobes correspond to the cranial bones by which they are overlaid, see Figure 8-5.

The five major fissures dividing the cerebral hemispheres include:

1. *Longitudinal fissure*—a deep groove divides the cerebrum into two hemispheres. The middle region of the two hemispheres is held together by a wide band of axonal fibers called the **corpus callosum**.

2. *Transverse fissure*—divides the cerebrum from the cerebellum.

3. *Central fissure*, or *fissure of Rolando*—located beneath the coronal suture of the skull, dividing the frontal from the parietal lobes.

4. *Lateral fissure* or *fissure of Sylvius*—situated on the side of the cerebral hemispheres, dividing the frontal and temporal lobes.

5. *Parieto-occipital fissure*—the least obvious of all the fissures, serves to separate the occipital lobe from the parietal and temporal lobes. There is, however, no definite demarcation between these two lobes.

Cerebral Functions

Each lobe of the cerebral hemispheres controls different types of functions, Figure 8-6.

1. *Frontal lobe*—The cerebral cortex of the frontal lobe controls the motor functions of humans. The motor area occupies a long band of cortex, just in front of the central fissure in the posterior part of the frontal lobe. This motor area controls the voluntary muscles. Cells in the right hemisphere activate voluntary movements which occur in the left side of the body; the left hemisphere controls voluntary movements of the right side. The frontal lobe also includes two areas

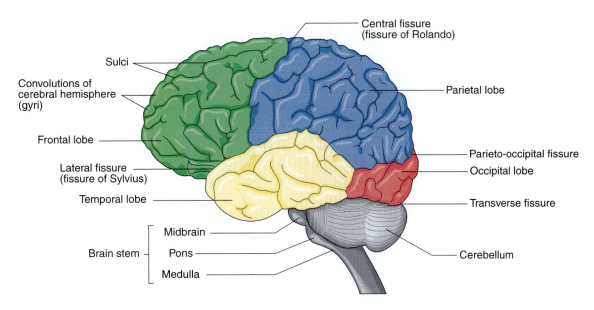

FIGURE 8-5 *Lateral view of the brain*

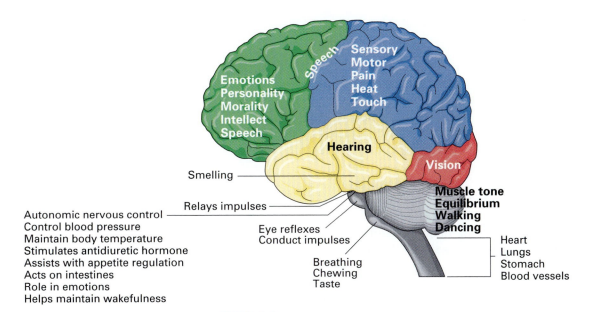

FIGURE 8-6 *Cerebral functions*

which control speech. The *speech area*, located anterior to the central fissure usually in the left hemisphere, is also called *Broca's area*. This area is associated with our ability to speak. Damage to this area means that you may know what to say, but you cannot vocalize the words.

The speech area which allows us to recognize words and to interpret the meaning, spoken or read, is located at the junction of the temporal, parietal, and occipital lobes.

2. *Parietal lobe*—the parietal lobe comprises the sensory (somesthetic) area. It is found

behind the fissure of Rolando, in front of the parietal lobe. This area receives and interprets nerve impulses from the sensory receptors for pain, touch, heat, and cold. It further helps in the determination of distances, sizes, and shapes.

3. *Occipital lobe*—The occipial lobe, located over the cerebellum, houses the visual area, controlling eyesight.

4. *Temporal lobe*—The upper part of the temporal lobe contains the auditory area (including specific tones) the anterior part of the lobe is occupied by the olfactory (smell) area.

The cerebral cortex also controls conscious thought, judgment, memory, reasoning, and will power. This high degree of development makes the human the most intelligent of all animals.

DIENCEPHALON

The **diencephalon** is located between the cerebrum and the midbrain. It is composed of two major structures, the **thalamus** and the hypothalamus. The thalamus is a spherical mass of gray matter. It is found deep inside each of the cerebral hemispheres, lateral to the third ventricle. The thalamus acts as a relay station for incoming and outgoing nerve impulses. It receives direct or indirect nerve impulses from the various sense organs of the body (with the exception of olfactory sensations). These nerve impulses are then relayed to the cerebral cortex. The thalamus also receives nerve impulses from the cerebral cortex, cerebellum, and other areas of the brain. Damage to the thalamus may result in increased sensibility to pain, or total loss of consciousness.

The **hypothalamus** lies below the thalamus. It forms part of the lateral walls and floor of the third ventricle. A bundle of nerve fibers connects the hypothalamus to the posterior pituitary gland, the thalamus, and the midbrain. The *limbic system* is that part of the brain which is associated with emotional control. The hippocampal gyri of the limbic system

helps to store and retain short term memory. The hypothalamus is part of the limbic system and is considered to be the "brain" of the brain. Through the use of feedback, the hypothalamus stimulates the pituitary to release its hormones. Nine vital functions are performed by the hypothalamus:

1. *Autonomic nervous control*—Regulates the parasympathetic and sympathetic systems of the autonomic nervous system.

2. *Cardiovascular control*—controls blood pressure regulating the constriction and dilation of blood vessels and the beating of the heart.

3. *Temperature control*—Helps in the maintenance of normal body temperature (37°C or 98.6°F).

4. *Appetite control*—Assists in regulating the amount of food we ingest. The "feeding center," found in the lateral hypothalamus is stimulated by hunger "pangs," which prompt us to eat. In turn, the "satiety center" in the medial hypothalamus becomes stimulated when we have eaten enough.

5. *Water balance*—Within the hypothalamus, certain cells respond to the osmotic pressure of the blood. When osmotic pressure is high, due to water deficiency, the antidiuretic hormone (ADH) is secreted. A "thirst area" is found near the satiety area, becoming stimulated when the blood's osmolality is high. This causes us to consume more liquids.

6. *Manufacture of oxytocin*—Contracts the uterus during labor.

7. *Gastrointestinal control*—Increases intestinal peristalsis and secretion from the intestinal glands.

8. *Emotional state*—Plays a role in the display of emotions such as fear and pleasure.

9. *Sleep control*—Helps keep us awake when necessary.

MEDICAL HIGHLIGHT: TECHNOLOGY

Limbic System

The limbic system relates to the primitive behavior of mankind. It influences unconscious, instinctive behaviors that relate to survival. This behavior is modified by the action of the cerebral cortex. Our primitive brain says, "I want it now"; our higher functioning brain says, "You can't have it now. You have to wait until later."

The limbic system encircles the top of the brain stem almost like a covering (the word limbic means "border"), linking the cerebral cortex and the midbrain areas with the lower centers that control the automatic functions of the body.

The limbic system plays a role in the expression of instincts, drives, and emotions, mediates the effects of the moods on external behavior, and influences internal changes in bodily functions. The association of feelings with sensations such as sight and smell and the formation of memories are influenced by the limbic system.

Parts of the limbic system include:

- *Septum pellucidum*—connects the fornix to the corpus callosum.

- *Mammillary body*—this nucleus transmits messages between the fornix and thalamus.

- *Olfactory bulbs*—this connection may explain why the sense of smell evokes forgotten memories (think of good smells from your childhood).

- *Amygdala*—this structure influences behavior appropriate to meet the body's needs, which include feeding, sexual interest, and emotional reactions such as anger.

- *Parahippocampal gyrus*—helps to modify strong emotions such as rage and fright.

- *Hippocampus*—involved with learning and memory, recognizes new information and recalls spatial relationships.

- *Fornix*—pathway of nerve fibers transmits information from the hippocampus to the mammillary body.

- *Cingulate gyrus*—this area, with others, comprises the limbic cortex which modifies behavior and emotion.

CEREBELLUM

A&P CHALLENGE

The **cerebellum** is located behind the pons and below the cerebrum (see Figure 8-5). It is composed of two hemispheres or wings: the right cerebellar hemisphere and the left cerebellar hemisphere. These two hemispheres are connected to a central portion called the vermis. The cerebellum consists of gray matter on the outside the white matter on the inside. The white matter on the inside of the cerebellum is marked with a tree-like pattern. This pattern is called *arbor vitae* (tree of life).

The cerebellum communicates with the rest of the central nervous system by three pairs of tracts called peduncles. These three peduncles are composed of "incoming" axons that carry nerve messages into the cerebellum and "outgoing" axons that transmit messages out of the cerebellum. The incoming axons carry messages to the cerebellum regarding movement within joints, muscle tone, position of the body, and the tightness of ligaments and tendons. Any and all information relating to skeletal muscle activity is carried to the cerebellum. This information reaches the cerebellum directly from sensory receptors including the inner ear, the eye, and the proprioceptors of the skeletal muscle. The "outgoing" axons carry nerve messages to the different parts of the brain that control skeletal muscles.

Cerebellar Function

The cerebellum controls all body functions that have to do with skeletal muscles.

● *Maintenance of balance.* If the body is imbalanced, sensory receptors in the inner ear send nerve messages to the cerebellum. There the cerebellum carries impulses to the motor controlling areas of the brain. These brain areas, in turn, stimulate muscle contraction that restores balance.

● *Maintenance of muscle tone.* The cerebellum transmits nerve impulses to the red nucleus that, in turn, relays them to the spinal cord and then to the skeletal muscles.

● *Coordination of muscle movements.* Any voluntary movement is initiated in the cerebral cortex. However, once the movement is started, its smooth execution is the role of the cerebellum. The cerebellum allows each muscle to contract at the right time, with the right strength, and for the right amount of time so that the overall movement is smooth and flowing. This is important when doing complex or skilled movements such as speaking, walking, writing; even simple movements need the coordinating abilities of the cerebellum. A simple action such as raising the hand to the face to avoid a blow requires the synchronized action of 50 or more muscles. These muscles then act on 30 separate bones of the arm and hand.

The removal of or injury to the cerebellum results in motor impairment.

BRAIN STEM

The **brain stem** is made up of three parts: the midbrain, pons, and the medulla. The brain stem provides a pathway for the ascending and descending tracts (messages going to the cerebrum and messages coming back from the cerebrum). Extending the length of the brain stem is the gray matter of the reticular formation system. These are the neurons that are involved in the sleep-wake cycle. If there is damage to this area, coma results. The **pons** is located in front of the cerebellum, between the midbrain and the medulla oblongata. It contains interlaced transverse and longitudinal myelinated, white nerve fibers mixed with gray matter. The pons serves as a two-way conductive pathway for nerve impulses between the cerebrum, cerebellum, and other areas of the nervous system. The pons is also the site for the emergence of four pairs of cranial nerves, and it contains a center that controls respiration.

The midbrain extends from mammillary bodies to the pons. The cerebral aqueduct travels through the midbrain. It contains the nuclei for reflex centers involved with vision and hearing.

The **medulla oblongata** is a bulb-shaped structure found between the pons and the spinal cord. It lies inside the cranium and above the foramen magnum of the occipital bone. The medulla is white on the outside, just like the pons, because of the myelinated nerve fibers which serve as a passageway for nerve impulses between the brain and spinal cord. It contains the nuclei for vital functions such as the heart rate, the rate and the depth of respiration, the vasoconstrictor center which affects blood pressure, and the center for swallowing and vomiting.

SPINAL CORD

The **spinal cord** continues down from the brain. The spinal cord begins at the foramen magnum of the occipital bone and continues to the second lumbar vertebrae. It is white and soft and lies within the vertebrae of the spinal column. Like the brain, the spinal cord is submerged in cerebrospinal fluid and is surrounded by the three meninges. The gray matter in the spinal cord is located in the internal section; the white matter composes the outer part, Figure 8-7. In the gray matter of the cord, connections can be made between incoming and outgoing nerve fibers which provide the basis for reflex action. The spinal cord functions as a reflex center and as a conduction pathway to and from the brain.

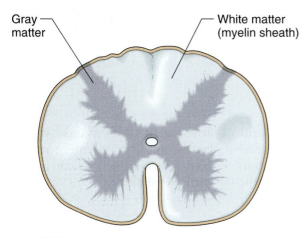

Gray matter

White matter (myelin sheath)

FIGURE 8-7 *Cross-section of the spinal cord*

DISORDERS OF THE CENTRAL NERVOUS SYSTEM

Meningitis is the inflammation of the linings of brain and spinal cord. The cause may be bacterial or viral. The disease does have outbreaks at times, appearing in high school or college age students. Symptoms include headache, fever, and stiff neck. In severe form, it may lead to paralysis, coma, and death. If the cause is bacterial, it may be treated with antibiotics.

Encephalitis is an inflammation of the brain. The disease may be caused by a virus; in certain conditions, the cause may be chemical. The symptoms of this disorder usually are fever, lethargy, extreme weakness, and visual disturbances.

Epilepsy is a seizure disorder of the brain, characterized by a recurring and excessive discharge from neurons. Approximately one person out of 200 in the United States suffers from some form of epilepsy. Epileptic seizures are believed to be a result of spontaneous, uncontrolled, cycles of electrical activity in the neurons of the brain. The cause is uncertain. One portion of the brain stimulates another, setting off a cycle of activity that accelerates and runs its course until the neurons become fatigued. The subject may suffer hallucinations and a seizure (convulsion) and a loss of consciousness. Grand mal, or severe seizure, is less frequent than the petit mal (milder seizure). In petit mal, some victims seem to be staring or daydreaming. Medications used to control seizures are referred to as **anticonvulsants**. Examples are phenobarbital, dilantin, and tegretol.

Cerebral palsy is a disturbance in voluntary muscular action due to brain damage. Definite causes are unknown; it may be due to birth injury or abnormal brain development. The most pronounced characteristic is **spastic quadriplegia**, which involves spastic paralysis of all four limbs. The person with cerebral palsy frequently exhibits head rolling, grimacing, and difficulty in speech and swallowing. In cerebral palsy, there is usually no impairment of the intellect; the person frequently has normal or above normal intelligence.

Poliomyelitis is a disease of the nerve pathways of the spinal cord which causes paralysis. Since the Sabin and Salk vaccines are now used, this disease has been almost eliminated in the United States. However, the disease still occurs in other countries.

Hydrocephalus is a condition in which there is an increased volume of cerebrospinal fluid within the ventricles of the brain. The usual cause is a blockage somewhere in the third or fourth ventricles. There is an enlargement of the head and this condition is usually noted at birth. A bypass or shunt operation is performed which diverts the cerebrospinal fluid around the blocked area. This operation prevents a buildup of pressure on brain tissue.

Parkinson's disease is a characterized by tremors, a shuffling gait, pill-rolling (movement of the thumb and index finger) and muscular rigidity. The patient with Parkinson's has difficulty initiating movement. The cause may be a decrease of the neurotransmitter dopamine. Persons with Parkinson's disease are treated with the drug L-dopa and other drugs which help to control the symptoms of the disease.

Multiple sclerosis (MS) is a chronic inflammatory disease of the central nervous system in which immune cells attack the myelin sheath of nerve cell axons. The myelin sheaths are destroyed, leaving scar tissue on the nerve cells.

This destruction delays or completely blocks the transmission of nerve impulses in the affected areas. The cause is unknown. There is no definitive test for MS. The diagnosis for multiple sclerosis is symptoms and signs of impairment to more than one area of the central nervous system, occurring at more than one time.

Symptoms include weakness of extremities, numbness, double vision, **nystagmus** (tremorous movement of the eye), speech problems, loss of coordination, and possible paralysis. It typically strikes young adults between the ages of twenty and forty; about two-thirds are women. With MS there are outbreaks of the symptoms and then the disease may go into remission for a long period of time. This disease is classified in the autoimmune category and the drug *interferon* has been used. In May of 1996, the Food and Drug Administration approved the use of a drug called Avonex, which tests have shown can slow progression of multiple sclerosis and decrease the number of flare-ups. Adequate rest, exercise, and minimal stress may also lessen the effects of multiple sclerosis.

Dementia is a general term that includes specific disorders such as Alzheimer's disease, vascular dementia and others. Dementia is defined as a loss in at least two areas of complex behavior, such as language, memory, visual, and spatial abilities. or judgment that significantly interferes with a person's daily life. *Note:* Everyone has areas that they are weak in and people are frequently forgetful. This does not necessarily mean that the person is experiencing dementia.

Alzheimer's disease is a progressive disease in which the initial symptom is usually a problem with remembering recently learned information. With Alzheimer's disease, the nerve endings in the cortex of the brain degenerate and block the signals that pass between nerve cells. These areas of degeneration have a unique appearance which are called plaques. The nerve cells undergo further change and abnormal fibers build up, creating neurofibrillary tangles, like a group of telephone lines getting tangled.

The cause of Alzheimer's is unknown. The cells that produce the neurotransmitter acetylcholine are sometimes destroyed in this disease. The cause of the disease may be virus related, environmental factors may play a role, or it may be associated with a gene defect on chromosome 21 which is also involved with Down's syndrome.

Alzheimer's disease usually has three stages. The first may last from two to four years and involves confusion, short-term memory loss, anxiety, and poor judgment. In the second stage, which may last from two to ten years, there is an increase in memory loss, difficulty in recognizing people, motor problems, logic problems, and loss of social skills. The third stage includes the inability to recognize oneself, weight loss, seizures, mood swings, and aphasia (loss of speech). This stage may last from one to three years.

Factors that may help prevent Alzheimer's disease are continued education, cardiovascular exercise, estrogen replacement therapy, antioxidants such as Vitamins C, E, and betacarotene, and the use of anti-inflammatory agents.

Brain tumors may develop in any area of the brain. the symptoms depend on which area of the brain is involved. Early detection, surgery, and chemotherapy may cure some cases of brain tumors.

Hematoma is a localized mass of blood collection and may occur in the spaces between the meninges. The cause may be a blow to the head; the person may have a sub-dural hematoma (located between the dura mater and arachnoid layer).

MEDICAL HIGHLIGHT: TECHNOLOGY
Low Back Pain

Richard Deyo of the University of Washington is a physician who heads a team of researchers studying back pain and its treatment. Deyo says that back pain "is a lot like the common cold, a condition that we're all going to get, and most of the time don't even need to see the doctor for it."

The exact cause of low back pain remains a mystery. Since the 1950s, the assumption was that low back pain was caused by a slipped disc. When the cushions between discs bulge, they press on a spinal nerve, causing back pain. New studies show that when people with no back pain are examined with magnetic resonance imaging scans, about one-third of younger adults and virtually all older ones have some bulging discs. A back full of completely "normal" discs is the exception, not the rule. Other possible explanations for lower-back pain—also still speculative—are muscle spasms or the result of the spinal nerve roots being compressed by arthritic spurs or bony overgrowth.

More studies have now documented that most cases of acute lower back pain will get better all by themselves, usually in a couple of weeks.

In 1995, a United States Public Health Service panel of experts issued a clinical guideline advising doctors not to prescribe more than four days of bed rest for people with acute lower back pain. Studies show that staying in bed more than a few days actually slows recovery because it reduces muscle tone and cardiovascular fitness. More severe problems with back pain involve pain going down the leg (sciatica), numbness and weakness in the leg or groin, or intense pain for more than two weeks. If a person has any of these symptoms, they must see a doctor.

The only treatment established to relieve symptoms temporarily is spinal manipulation, which is performed by osteopaths, physicians, physical therapists, and chiropractors. Before seeking manipulative treatments, see your regular doctor first to rule to any serious disease.

● REVIEW QUESTIONS

Select the letter of the choice that best completes the statement.

1. Each nerve cell has only one:
   a. axon
   b. neurilemma
   c. dendrite
   d. myelin

2. The fatty substance which helps to protect the axon is called:
   a. neurotransmitter
   b. myelin
   c. dendrite
   d. Nodes of Ranvier

3. The junction between the axon of one cell and the dendrite of another is called:
   a. neurilemma
   b. myelin
   c. synaptic cleft
   d. Nodes of Ranvier

4. The neurons which carry messages to the brain are called:
   a. motor
   b. associate
   c. connective
   d. sensory

5. The nervous system which is composed of twelve pairs of cranial nerves and thirty-one pairs of spinal nerves is called:
   a. central
   b. peripheral
   c. sympathetic
   d. parasympathetic

6. The outermost covering of the meninges is:
   a. arachnoid
   b. arachnoid villa
   c. dura mater
   d. pia mater

7. The lumbar puncture must be done below the:
   a. first lumbar vertebrae
   b. second lumbar vertebrae
   c. third lumbar vertebrae
   d. sacrum

8. The front, parietal, temporal, and occipital lobes make up:
   a. the cerebrum
   b. the cerebellum
   c. the midbrain
   d. brain stem

9. The part of the brain associated with muscle movement is:
   a. midbrain
   b. thalamus
   c. cerebrum
   d. medulla

10. The thalamus and hypothalamus are parts of the:
    a. cerebrum
    b. cerebellum
    c. diencephalon
    d. brain stem

● MATCHING

Match each term in Column I with its correct description in Column II.

Column I	Column II
_____ 1. frontal lobe—cerebrum	a. auditory
_____ 2. occiptal lobe—cerebrum	b. receptor for pain, touch, and so on
_____ 3. hypothalamus	c. reflex center
_____ 4. temporal lobe	d. speech area
_____ 5. parietal lobe	e. maintain balance
_____ 6. cerebellum	f. eyesight
_____ 7. thalamus	g. respiratory center
_____ 8. spinal cord	h. appetite control
_____ 9. medulla	i. site for four pairs of cranial nerves
_____ 10. pons	j. relay station for nerve impulses

● APPLYING THEORY TO PRACTICE

1. The central nervous system serves as the communication center of our bodies. Explain how your hand touches something cold and you know it; refer to a sensory neuron and the correct lobe of the cerebrum.

2. A blow to the head can cause a loss of consciousness. What centers in the brain are associated with alertness?

3. You frequently hear the expression "I have early Alzheimer's"; explain what this means. Do you think this illness will have an impact on the cost of health care? Explain your answer.

CHAPTER

9

The Peripheral and Autonomic Nervous System

OBJECTIVES

- Describe a mixed nerve
- Describe the functions of the cranial and spinal nerves
- Relate the functions of the sympathetic and parasympathetic nervous system
- Explain the simple reflex arc pattern
- Describe common disorders of the peripheral nervous system
- Define the key words that relate to this chapter

KEY WORDS

analgesic
Bell's palsy
carpal tunnel
  syndrome
cranial nerves
electromyograph
  (EMG)
effector
femoral nerve
mixed nerve
motor (efferent)
  nerve

neuralgia
neuritis
parasympathetic
  system
paresthesia
phrenic nerve
plexus
pruritus
radial nerve
receptor
reflex
reflex arc

sciatic nerve
sciatica
sensory (afferent)
  nerve
shingles (herpes
  zoster)
spinal nerves
stimulus
sympathetic system
trigeminal neuralgia
visceral organs

PERIPHERAL NERVOUS SYSTEM

The peripheral nervous system includes all the nerves of the body and ganglia (groups of cell bodies), see Figure 9-1. It connects the central nervous system to the various body structures. The autonomic nervous system is a specialized part of the peripheral system; it controls the involuntary, or automatic, activities of the vital internal organs.

Functions of the peripheral nervous system:

1. To control the automatic or involuntary activities of the body.

2. Act as the reflex center of the body.

NERVES

A nerve is composed of bundles of nerve fibers enclosed by connective tissue. If the nerve is composed of fibers that carry impulses from the sense organs to the brain or spinal cord it is called a **sensory**, or **afferent**, nerve; if it is composed of fibers carrying impulses from the brain or spinal cord to muscles or glands, it is known as a **motor**, or **efferent**, nerve; and if it contains both sensory and motor fibers, it is referred to as a **mixed nerve**.

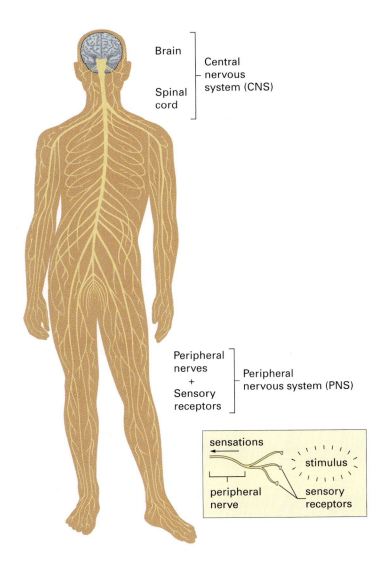

Brain

Spinal cord

Central nervous system (CNS)

Peripheral nerves + Sensory receptors

Peripheral nervous system (PNS)

sensations

stimulus

peripheral nerve

sensory receptors

FIGURE 9-1 *Peripheral nervous system. This connects the central nervous system to the structures of the body.*

CRANIAL AND SPINAL NERVES

Cranial and spinal nerves are part of the peripheral nervous system.

The cranial nerves are twelve pairs which begin in areas of the brain. The cranial nerves are designated by number and name; the name may give a clue to its function, Table 9-1. For example, the olfactory nerve, cranial nerve I, is responsible for the sense of smell. The optic nerve, cranial nerve II, is responsible for vision. The functions of the cranial nerves are concerned mainly with the activities of the head and neck, with the exception of the vagus nerve. The vagus nerve, cranial nerve X, is responsible for activities involving the throat as well as regulating the heart rate; it also affects the smooth muscle of the digestive tract. Most of the cranial nerves are mixed nerves: they carry both sensory and motor fibers. But the olfactory, optic, and vestibulococchlear carry only the sensory fibers. They only pick up the stimuli.

The spinal nerves originate at the spinal cord and go through openings in the vertebrae. There are thirty-one pairs of spinal nerves. All spinal nerves are mixed nerves. The spinal nerves are named in relation to their location on the spinal cord. Since spinal nerves carry messages to and from the spinal cord, when there is a spinal cord injury there is no sensation as well as no movement. The spinal nerves carry messages to and from the spinal cord and brain and to all parts of the body. Each of these spinal nerves divides and branches. They go either directly to a particular body segment or they form a network with adjacent spinal nerves and veins called a plexus, Figure 9-2 and Table 9-2.

AUTONOMIC NERVOUS SYSTEM

The autonomic nervous system includes nerves, ganglia, and plexuses which carry impulses to all smooth muscle, secretory glands, and heart muscle, Figure 9-3, page 134. It regulates the activities of the visceral organs (heart and blood vessels, respiratory organs, alimentary canal, kidneys and urinary bladder, and reproductive organs). The activities of these organs are usually automatic and not subject to conscious control

The autonomic system is comprised of two divisions: the sympathetic and the parasympathetic. These two divisions may be antagonistic in their action. The sympathetic system may

TABLE 9-1 • *Cranial Nerves*

NUMBER	NAME	FUNCTION
I	Olfactory	Smell
II	Optic	Vision, eyesight
III	Oculomotor	Movement of eye muscle
IV	Trochlear	Movement of eye muscle
V	Trigeminal	Face and teeth muscles, chewing
VI	Abducens	Movement of eye muscle
VII	Facial	Facial expressions, taste
VIII	Vestibulocochlear	Hearing and balance
IX	Glossopharyngeal	Movement of throat muscle, taste
X	Vagus	Movement of throat, affects heart, digestive system
XI	Accessory	Movement of neck muscles
XII	Hypoglossal	Movement of tongue muscles

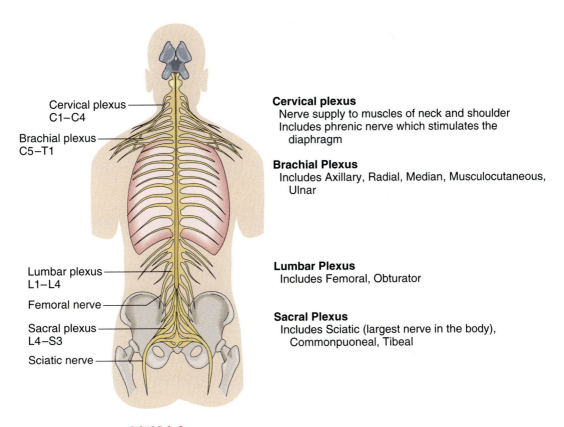

Cervical plexus
C1–C4

Brachial plexus
C5–T1

Lumbar plexus
L1–L4

Femoral nerve

Sacral plexus
L4–S3

Sciatic nerve

Cervical plexus
Nerve supply to muscles of neck and shoulder
Includes phrenic nerve which stimulates the
   diaphragm

Brachial Plexus
Includes Axillary, Radial, Median, Musculocutaneous,
   Ulnar

Lumbar Plexus
Includes Femoral, Obturator

Sacral Plexus
Includes Sciatic (largest nerve in the body),
   Commonpuoneal, Tibeal

FIGURE 9-2 *Spinal nerve plexus and important nerves*

TABLE 9-2 • *Spinal Nerve Plexus*

NAME	LOCATION	FUNCTION
Cervical plexus	C1-C4	Supplies motor movement to muscles of neck and shoulders and receives messages from these areas. **Phrenic nerve** is part of this group and stimulates the diaphragm.
Brachial plexus	C5-C8, T1	Supplies motor movement to shoulder, wrist, and hand and receives messages from these areas. **Radial nerve** is part of this group and stimulates the wrist and hand.
Lumbar plexus	T12, L1-L4	Supplies motor movement to buttocks, anterior leg, and thighs and receives messages from these areas. **Femoral nerve** is part of this group and stimulates the hip and leg.
Sacral plexus	L4-L5, S1-S2	Supplies motor movement to posterior of leg and thighs and receives messages from these areas. **Sciatic nerve** is the largest nerve in the body and is part of this group. It passes through the gluteus maximums and down the back of the thigh and leg. It extends the hip and flexes the knee. (You must avoid this nerve when you are giving an IM injection.)

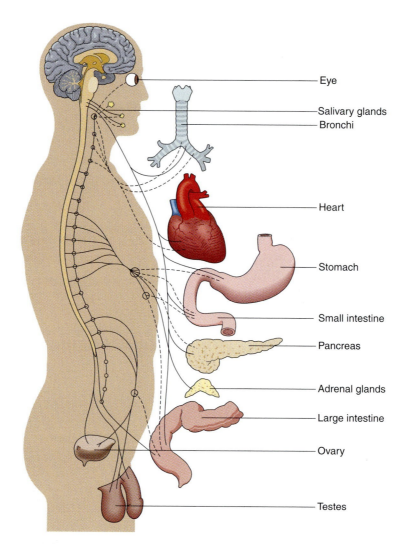

FIGURE 9-3 *Autonomic nervous system and target organs*

accelerate the heartbeat in response to fear, whereas the parasympathetic slows it down. Normally the two divisions are in balance; the activity of one or the other becomes dominant as dictated by the needs of the organism.

The **sympathetic system** consists primarily of two cords, beginning at the base of the brain and proceeding down both sides of the spinal column. These are made up of nerve fibers and ganglia of nerve cell bodies. The cord between the ganglia is a cable of nerve fibers, closely associated with the spinal cord. Sympathetic nerves extend to all the vital internal organs, including the liver and pancreas, heart, stomach, intestines, blood vessels, the iris of the eye,

sweat glands, and the bladder. The sympathetic nervous system is often referred to as the "fight or flight system." When the body perceives it is in danger or under stress it prepares to run away or stand and fight. The sympathetic nervous system sends the message to the adrenal medulla which secretes its hormones to prepare our body for this action. Think about how you feel when you are facing a major test, or think about the patient waiting in the doctor's office for test results. You can feel your heart beating faster and your mouth going dry—all results of the automatic response to danger. When the danger passes, the parasympathetic nervous system will help restore the balance to the body system. If our system gets too much of the "stress hormones," health problems may result. Learning to live with stress is the key to a healthier person.

The parasympathetic system is composed of two important active nerves: the vagus and the pelvic nerves. The vagus nerve, which extends from the medulla and proceeds down the neck, sends branches to the chest and neck. The pelvic nerve, emerging from the spinal cord around the hip region sends branches to the organs in the lower part of the body.

Both the sympathetic and parasympathetic are strongly influenced by emotion. During periods of fear, anger, or stress, the sympathetic division acts to prepare the body for action. The effects of the parasympathetic are generally to counteract the effects of the sympathetic. For example, the sympathetic nervous system increases the rate of heart muscle contraction, and the parasympathetic decreases the rate. The two systems operate as a pair, striking a nearly perfect balance when the body is functioning properly.

The Reflex Act

The simplest type of nervous response is the **reflex** act, which is unconscious and involuntary. The blinking of the eye when a particle of dust touches it, the removing of the finger from a hot object, the secretion of saliva at the sight or smell of food, the movements of the heart, stomach, and intestines, are all examples of reflex actions.

Every reflex act is preceded by a stimulus. Any change in the environment is called a **stimulus**. Examples of stimuli are sound waves, light waves, heat energy, and odors. Special structures called **receptors** pick up these stimuli. For example, the retina of the eye is the receptor for light; special cells in the inner ear are receptors for sound waves; and special structures in the skin are the receptors for heat and cold.

A simple reflex is one in which there is only a sensory nerve and a motor nerve involved. The classic example is the "knee-jerk" reflex. The knee is tapped and the leg extends, Figure 9-4. This test is used by physicians to test both the muscle and nervous system.

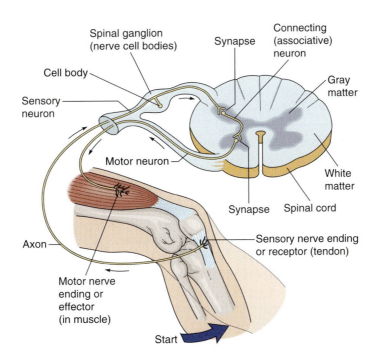

FIGURE 9-4 *In this example, tapping the knee (patellar tendon) results in extension of the leg, producing the knee jerk reflex.*

Reaction to a stimulus is called the response. The response may be in the form of movement; in which case, the muscles are the **effectors**, or responding organs. If the response is in the form of a secretion, the glands are the effectors. Reflex actions, also known as autonomic reflexes, involving the skeletal muscles are controlled by the spinal cord. They also may be called somatic reflexes.

DISORDERS OF THE PERIPHERAL NERVOUS SYSTEM

Neuritis is an inflammation of a nerve or a nerve trunk. The symptoms may be severe pain, hypersensitivity, loss of sensation, muscular atrophy, weakness, and **paresthesia** (tingling, burning, and crawling of the skin). The causes of neuritis may be infectious, chemical, or occur because of other conditions such as chronic alcoholism. In the alcoholic patient, neuritis usually occurs because of a lack of Vitamin B or improper diet.

In the treatment of neuritis it is necessary to determine the cause to eliminate the symptoms. The pain of neuritis may be relieved with **analgesics** (painkillers).

Sciatica is a form of neuritis which affects the sciatic nerve. The cause may be a rupture of a lumbar disc or arthritic changes. The most common symptom is pain which radiates through the buttock and behind the knee down to the foot. The person may have difficulty walking. Treatment includes traction, physiotherapy, exercises, and possible surgery to alleviate the symptoms.

Neuralgia is a sudden severe, sharp, stabbing pain along the pathway of a nerve. The pain is often brief; it may be a symptom of a disease. The various forms of neuralgia are named according to the nerve they affect.

Trigeminal neuralgia is a condition which involves the fifth cranial nerve (trigeminal). The cause is unknown and the onset is very rapid. The pain is severe. The spasm of pain can be brought on by so slight a stimulus as a breeze, or a piece of food in the mouth, or even

a change in temperature. The term "tic douloureux" is sometimes applied to this condition, since the pain only lasts two to five seconds. The treatment may be analgesics or partial removal of the fifth cranial nerve.

Bell's palsy is a condition which involves the seventh cranial nerve (facial). The patient seems to have had a stroke on one side of the face. Bell's palsy only affects one side of the face. They eye does not close properly, the mouth droops, and there is numbness on the effected side. The cause is unknown. The treatment consists of massage and heat application. The patient must do exercises such as whistling to prevent atrophy of the cheek muscles. The symptoms usually disappear within a few weeks, with no residual effects.

Shingles or **herpes zoster** is an acute viral nerve infection. It is characterized by a unilateral (one-sided) inflammation of a cutaneous nerve. The intercostal nerves are the ones most commonly affected. The course of nerve inflammation can spread to any nerve. Symptoms include extremely painful vesicular eruptions of the skin and mucous membrane along the route of the inflamed nerve. Shingles is frequently seen in the elderly or the debilitated. The causative organism herpes zoster is the same virus that causes chickenpox in children. Treatment consists of analgesics for the pain and medications which relieve the **pruritus** (itching).

Carpal tunnel syndrome is a condition which affects the median nerve and the flexor tendons that attach to the bones of the wrist (carpal). The syndrome develops because of repetitive movement of the wrist, in which the hands are held in an unusual position. Swelling (edema) develops around the carpal tunnel. This is where the median nerve passes through. The edema causes pressure on the nerve, which results in pain, muscle weakness, and tingling sensations of the hand. The diagnostic test for carpal tunnel syndrome is an **electromyograph** (EMG). An EMG is a record of muscle electric activity. Treatment consists of immobilizing the wrist joint. If this treatment is not effective, surgery may be done.

● REVIEW QUESTIONS

Select the letter of choice that best completes the statement.

1. A nerve which contains fibers that both send and receive messages is called:
   a. sensory nerve
   b. afferent nerve
   c. efferent nerve
   d. mixed nerve

2. The cranial nerve which is responsible for chewing is:
   a. trochlear
   b. facial
   c. glossopharyngeal
   d. trigeminal

3. The cranial nerves responsible for eye muscle movement are the oculomotor, trochlear, and:
   a. abducens
   b. vestibulocochlear
   c. accessory
   d. hypoglossal

4. A network of spinal nerves is called:
   a. mixed
   b. efferent
   c. plexus
   d. afferent

5. The autonomic nervous system is also called:
   a. voluntary
   b. involuntary
   c. neuralgic
   d. carpal

6. The autonomic nervous system is part of the:
   a. central nervous system
   b. peripheral nervous system
   c. sympathetic nervous system
   d. parasympathetic nervous system

7. The sympathetic nervous system which acts in the same manner as adrenalin, does the following:
   a. increases the heart rate and dilates the pupils
   b. increases the heart rate and constricts the pupils
   c. slows the heart rate and dilates the pupils
   d. slows the heart rate and constricts the pupils

8. The nerve which activates the diaphragm is called:
   a. sciatic
   b. phrenic
   c. radial
   d. femoral

9. The simplest type of nervous system response is called:
    a. stimulus
    b. effector action
    c. reflex
    d. affector action

10. The acute viral infection which usually affects the intercostal nerves is called:
    a. Bell's palsy
    b. neuralgia
    c. sciatica
    d. shingles

● COMPLETION

Complete the following statements.

1. A nerve is composed of small blood vessels and of bundles of fibers called _____.

2. A nerve composed of fibers carrying impulses from sense organs to the brain or spinal cord is called a _____ or _____ nerve.

3. A nerve composed of fibers which carry impulses from the brain or spinal cord to muscles or glands is called a _____ or _____ nerve.

4. A mixed nerve contains both _____ and _____ fibers.

5. The autonomic nervous system is a specialized part of the peripheral system and controls _____.

6. The autonomic nervous system has two parts which counterbalance each other; these are the _____ and _____ systems.

● LABELING

Identify the structures on the following figure. Enter your answers in the spaces provided.

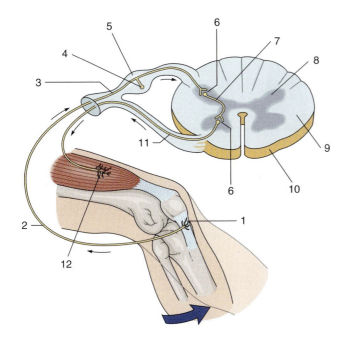

1. _____
2. _____
3. _____
4. _____
5. _____
6. _____
7. _____
8. _____
9. _____
10. _____
11. _____
12. _____

● APPLYING THEORY TO PRACTICE

1. You are passing by a pizzeria and smell the pizza cooking. Describe what happens to your salivary glands. What else do you notice you are feeling? Relate these reactions to your peripheral nervous system.

2. The knee jerk is the most common reflex we know about in health care. You are born with certain reflexes and you learn some reflexes. Name at least five reflexes that you are born with and five reflexes you have learned.

3. A doctor has a patient who is experiencing facial and cheek pain, sometimes called trigeminal neuralgia. Describe this condition and the appropriate treatment.

4. After a lengthy car ride, your elderly uncle gets out of the car and complains, "I can hardly walk. It must be sciatica." Explain what this means.

5. Carpal tunnel syndrome is affecting many middle-aged Americans. What are the types of jobs which increase the risk of this disease, and what are some of the treatments?

CHAPTER

10

Special Senses

KEY WORDS

amblyopia
anterior chamber
anvil (incus)
aqueous humor
astigmatism
cataracts
choroid coat
ciliary body
cochlea
cochlear duct
cones
conjunctivitis
cornea
detached retina
deviated nasal
  septum
diplopia
eustachian tube
extrinsic muscle
fovea centralis
glaucoma

hammer (malleus)
hyperopia (far
  sightedness)
intrinsic muscle
iris
lacrimal gland
lens
macular degenera-
  tion nasal polyp
Meniere's disease
miotic
myringotomy
myopia (near
  sightedness)
optic disc (blind
  spot)
organ of Corti
otitis media
otosclerosis
pinna
posterior chamber

presbyopia
presbycusis
pupil
retina
rhinitis
rods
sclera
semicircular canals
stapes mobilization
stirrup (stapes)
strabismus ("cross
  eyes")
sty
suspensory
  ligament
tonometer
tinnitus
tympanic
  membrane
vertigo
vitreous humor

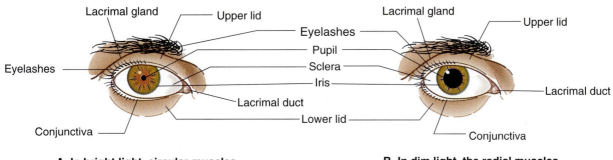

A. In bright light, circular muscles contract and constrict the pupil.

B. In dim light, the radial muscles contract and dilate the pupil.

FIGURE 10-1 *External view of the eye*

The special senses are those organs and receptors that are associated with touch (sensory receptors), vision, hearing, smell, and taste. Functions of the special senses:

> To receive stimuli from the sensory receptors, the eye, the ear, the nose, and the tongue and to transmit these impulses to the brain for interpretation.

SENSORY RECEPTORS

Sensory receptors are special structures which are stimulated by changes in the environment. Sensory receptors (touch, pain , temperature, and pressure) are found all over the body, located either in the skin or connective tissues. Special sensory receptors include the taste buds of the tongue, special cells in the nose, the retina of the eye, and the special cells in the inner ear which make up the organ of Corti. When a sense organ is stimulated, the impulse travels along nerve pathways to the brain, where it is registered in a certain area. Sensation actually takes place in the brain, but it is mentally referred back to the sense organ. This is called projection of the sensation.

THE EYE

The human eye is a tender sphere about 1″ in diameter (about 2.5 cm). It is protected by the orbital socket of the skull. The eyeball is moved by muscles. The eye is protected by the bone surrounding it and by the eyebrows, eyelids, and eyelashes, Figure 10-1. The eyes are continuously bathed in fluid by tears secreted by lacrimal glands, which are located above the lateral area of each eye. The tears flow across the eye into the lacrimal duct. The lacrimal duct is located in the corner of the eye and empties into the nasal cavity, causing an increase in fluids. This explains why, when we cry, we may also need to blow our noses. Lacrimal secretions have some antibiotic properties: tears cleanse and moisten the eyes on a continuous basis.

Along the border of each eyelid are glands that secrete an oily substance which lubricates the eye. An infection of this gland is called a **sty**.

The conjunctiva is the thin membrane that lines the eyelids and covers part of the eye. The conjunctiva secretes mucous which helps to lubricate the eye.

The location of the eyes in front of the head allows for superimposition of images from each eye. This enables us to see stereoscopically in three dimensions (length, width, and depth). The eye's optical system for detecting light is similar to that of a camera.

The wall of the eye is made up of three concentric layers, or coats, each with its specific function. These three layers are the sclera, the choroid, and the retina, Figure 10-2.

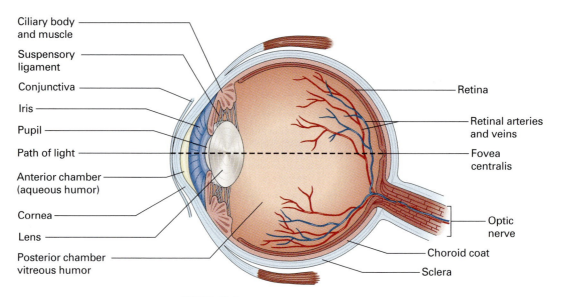

Ciliary body and muscle

Suspensory ligament

Conjunctiva

Iris

Pupil

Path of light

Anterior chamber (aqueous humor)

Cornea

Lens

Posterior chamber vitreous humor

Retina

Retinal arteries and veins

Fovea centralis

Optic nerve

Choroid coat

Sclera

FIGURE 10-2 *Internal view of the eye*

Sclera

The outer layer is called the sclera, or white of the eye. It is a tough, unyielding fibrous capsule which maintains the shape of the eye and protects the delicate structures within. Muscles responsible for moving the eye within the orbital socket are attached to the outside of the sclera. These muscles are referred to as the extrinsic muscles, Figure 10-3. They include the superior, inferior, lateral, medial rectus, and the superior and inferior oblique. See Table 10-1 for a listing of the extrinsic eye muscles and their functions.

Cornea

In the very front center of the sclerotic coat lies a circular clear area called the cornea. The cornea is sometimes referred to as the "window" of the eye. It is transparent to permit

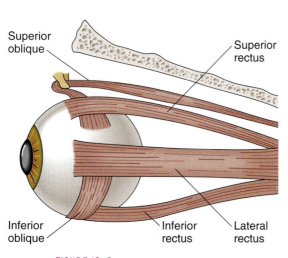

Superior oblique

Superior rectus

Inferior oblique

Inferior rectus

Lateral rectus

FIGURE 10-3 *Extrinsic eye muscles*

TABLE 10-1 • *Extrinsic and Intrinsic Eye Muscles*

EYE MUSCLE	FUNCTION
A. Extrinsic	
1. Superior rectus	Rolls eyeball upward
2. Inferior rectus	Rolls eyeball downward
3. Lateral rectus	Rolls eyeball laterally
4. Medial rectus	Rolls eyeball medially
5. Superior oblique	Rolls eyeball on its axis, moves cornea downward and laterally
6. Inferior oblique	Rolls eyeball on its axis, moves cornea upward and laterally
B. Intrinsic	
1. Sphincter pupillae	Constricts pupil
2. Dilator pupillae	Dilates pupil

light rays to pass through it. This transparency is due to the lack of blood vessels. Thus corneal cells are fed by the movement of lymph through interstitial, or lymph spaces. The cornea is composed of five layers of flat cells arranged much like sheets of plate glass. Possessing pain and touch receptors, it is sensitive to any foreign particles that come in contact with its surface. An injury to the cornea causes scarring and impaired vision.

Choroid Coat and the Iris

The middle layer of the eye is the **choroid coat**. It contains blood vessels to nourish the eye, and a non-reflective pigment rendering it dark and opaque. The pigment provides the choroid coat with a deep, red-purple color; this darkens the eye chamber, preventing light reflection within the eye. In front, the choroid coat has a circular opening called the **pupil**. A colored, muscular layer surrounds the pupil; this is the **iris**, or colored part of the eye. The iris may be blue, green, gray, brown, or black.

Eye color is related to the number and size of melanin pigment cells in the iris. If there is little melanin present, the eye is blue, because light is scattered to a greater extent. With increasing quantities of melanin, eye color ranges from green to black. The total absence of melanin results in a pink eye color, characteristic of albinism. Such irises are pink because the blood inside the choroid blood vessels shows through the iris.

Within the iris are two sets of antagonistic, smooth muscles, the sphincter and the dilator pupillae. These **intrinsic muscles** help the iris to control amounts of light entering the pupil. When the eye is focused on a close object or stimulated by bright light, the sphincter pupillae muscle contracts, rendering the pupil smaller. Conversely, when the eye is focused on a distant object or stimulated by dim light, the dilator pupillae muscle contracts. This causes the pupil to grow larger, permitting as much light as possible to enter the eye. In this way the eye may be compared to a camera; the iris corresponds to the diaphragm.

MEDICAL HIGHLIGHT: TECHNOLOGY AND SENSES

Eyestrain and Computers

There is no scientific evidence that computers cause damage to the eyes. Computer eyestrain, however, can result from too much light coming from behind the computer causing a glare on the monitor or a strong light source behind the user. These problems can be resolved by repositioning the monitor, using a glare screen, or wearing dark clothing to reduce glare caused by reflection. If the computer is by a window, the use of shades may be helpful.

Another cause of eyestrain is dry eyes, which comes form staring at the computer and forgetting to blink. Symptoms of dry eyes include redness, burning, itching, gritty watery eyes, and eye fatigue. In this case, the computer monitor should be positioned just below eye level so that the eyes are not open too widely, which increases evaporation of tears from the eyes and causes computer users to raise their brows unnaturally, leading to fatigue and headaches. If you wear glasses, use those which allow for near, intermediate (computer use) and far vision. Give your eyes a break; look away from the computer monitor periodically.

Lens and Related Structures

The **lens** is a crystalline structure located behind the iris and pupil. It is composed of concentric layers of fibers and crystal-clear proteins in solution. It is an elastic, disc-shaped structure with anterior and posterior convex surfaces, thus forming a biconvex lens. However, the posterior surface is more curved than that of the anterior. The curvature of each surface alters with age. During infancy, the lens is spherical; in adulthood, medium convexed; and almost flattened in old age. The capsule surrounding the lens also loses it elasticity over a period of time. The lens is held in place behind the pupil by **suspensory ligaments** from the **ciliary body** of the choroid body.

The lens is situated between the **anterior** and **posterior chambers**. The anterior chamber is filled with a watery fluid referred to as the **aqueous humor**, and it is constantly replenished by blood vessels behind the iris, Figure 10-4. **Vitreous humor**, a transparent jellylike substance, fills the posterior chamber. Both of these substances help to maintain the eyeball's spherical shape, refracting (bending) light rays as they pass through the eye.

Retina

The **retina** of the eye is the innermost, or third coat of the eye. It is located between the posterior chamber and the choroid coat. The retina does not extend around the front portion of the eye. It is upon this light-sensitive layer that light rays from an object form an image. After the image is focused on the retina, it travels via the optic nerve to the visual part of the cerebral cortex (occipital lobe). If light rays do not focus correctly on the retina, the condition may be corrected with properly fitted contact lenses, or eyeglasses, which bend the light rays as required.

The retina contains pigment and specialized cells known as **rods** and **cones**, Figure 10-5, which are sensitive to light. The rod cells are sensitive to dim light and the cones are sensitive to bright light. The cones are also responsible for color vision. There are three varieties of cone cells. Each type is sensitive to a special color. The part of the retina where the nerve fibers enter the optic nerve to go to the brain does not have these specialized cells.

The Optic Disc and the Fovea. Viewing the retina through an ophthalmoscope, one can observe a yellow disc known as the macula lutea. Within this disc is the **fovea centralis**, which contains the cones for color vision, see

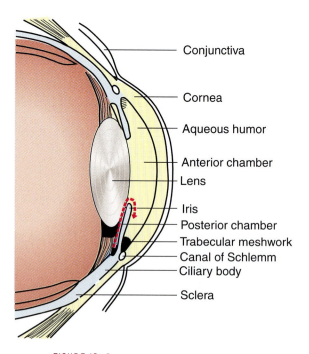

Conjunctiva

Cornea

Aqueous humor

Anterior chamber

Lens

Iris

Posterior chamber

Trabecular meshwork

Canal of Schlemm

Ciliary body

Sclera

FIGURE 10-4 *Flow of the aqueous humor*

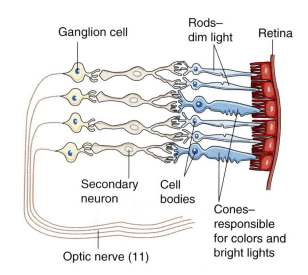

Ganglion cell

Rods– dim light

Retina

Secondary neuron

Cell bodies

Cones– responsible for colors and bright lights

Optic nerve (11)

FIGURE 10-5 *Diagram of visual neurons showing rods and cones*

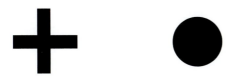

1. Close your left eye and focus your right eye on the <u>cross</u>.
2. Move the page slowly away from your eye and then slowly toward your eye.
3. At a distance of about 6–8 inches the black <u>circle</u> "disappears."

FIGURE 10-6 *Testing for the blind spot*

Figure 10-2. The area around the fovea centralis is the extrafoveal or peripheral region. This is where the rods for dim and peripheral vision can be found.

Slightly to the side of the fovea lies a pale disc called the **optic disc** or **blind spot**. Nerve fibers from the retina gather here to form the nerve. The optic disc contains no rods or cones; therefore, it is devoid of visual reception.

See Figure 10-6 to help you locate your blind spot.

PATHWAY OF VISION

Images in the light $\longrightarrow$ *pupil* $\longrightarrow$ *cornea* $\longrightarrow$ *lens* $\longrightarrow$ where the light rays are bent or refracted $\longrightarrow$ *retina* $\longrightarrow$ rods and cones (nerve cells) pick up the stimulus $\longrightarrow$ *optic nerve* $\longrightarrow$ *optic chiasma* (where the two optic nerves cross) $\longrightarrow$ *optic tracts* $\longrightarrow$ *occipital lobe* of the brain for interpretation, Figure 10-7.

EYE DISORDERS

Conjunctivitis is an inflammation of the conjunctival membranes in front of the eye. Redness, pain, swelling, and discharge of mucous occur. Conjunctivitis, or "pink eye," usually begins in one eye and spreads rapidly to the other by a wash cloth or hands. Since it is highly contagious, other family members should not share the same washcloths or towels with the infected person. Good handwashing is important to prevent the spread to others. Treatment includes eye washes or eye irrigations which will cleanse the conjunctiva and relieve the inflammation and pain. Bacterial conjunctivitis responds to antibiotic and sulfa drug therapy.

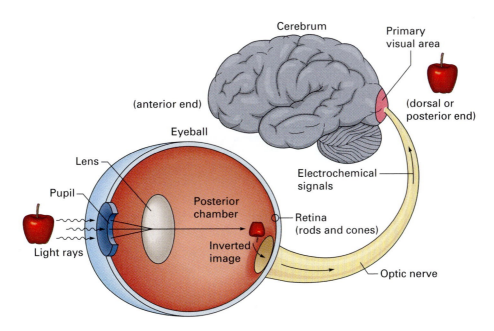

FIGURE 10-7 *Pathway of vision*

Glaucoma is a condition of excessive intraocular pressure resulting in the destruction of retina and atrophy of the optic nerve. The condition results from overproduction of aqueous humor, or the obstruction of its outflow through the canal of Schlemm for absorption into the venous circulation. Symptoms are gradual. They include mild aching, a loss of peripheral vision, and a halo around the light.

Glaucoma may occur with aging and has no initial symptoms. It is important for people to be tested for glaucoma annually after age forty. Intraocular eye pressure is measured by a **tonometer**. A puff of air is directed onto the eye or a pressure-sensitive tip is placed gently near the eye to measure the intraocular pressure. The diagnosis is confirmed by viewing through an ophthalmoscope characteristic changes in the optic disk.

Treatment involves **miotic** drugs which constrict the pupil and thus increase the outflow of aqueous humor, or drugs which reduce the amount of aqueous fluid produced by the eye. Today, laser surgery or incisional surgery helps to increase the flow of aqueous humor. All treatments are focused on lowering the intraocular pressure.

Cataracts is a condition where the lens of the eye gradually becomes cloudy. This frequently occurs in people over seventy years of age. The condition causes a painless, gradual blurring and loss of vision. The pupil turns from black to milky white. People with cataracts may complain of seeing halos around lights or being blinded at night by oncoming headlights.

Cataracts are treated by the surgical removal of the lens and postoperative substitution of contact lenses or eyeglasses. There may also be an intraocular lens implanted directly behind the cornea.

Macular degeneration is another eye disorder that occurs as a person ages. In the central part of the retina is the macula which is responsible for sharp central vision. Symptoms include a dimming or distortion of vision that is most obvious when reading. In one form of the disease straight lines look wavy and blind spots may develop in the visual field. There are two types of macular degeneration: dry and wet. In the dry type, the main defect is a gradual thinning of the retina. This is slowly progressive and there is no known treatment. Central vision will be greatly reduced but usually there is not total blindness.

In the wet type, leakage develops under the retina causing blister formation which may involve blood vessels. Laster treatment may be used with this type of macular degeneration. The good news about macular degeneration is that the majority of people who develop it will be able to maintain their independence of movement with low-vision aids.

Detached retina is another problem which may occur with aging. It may also occur as the result of an accident at a younger age. The vit-

MEDICAL HIGHLIGHT: TECHNOLOGY

Lasers

Laser, short for **l**ight **a**mplification by **s**timulated **e**mission of **r**adiations, is based on the principle that certain atoms, molecules, or ions can be excited by absorption of thermal, electrical, or light energy. After such energy absorptions, the atoms, molecules, or ions give off a beam of synchronized light waves. The laser beam is a narrow, intense and monochromatic (single color) light beam that can be used for a variety of purposes. For example, it can stop bleeding, make incisions, or remove tissue.

reous fluid contracts as it ages and pulls on the retina, causing a tear. Symptoms include loss of peripheral vision and then loss of central vision. Early detection is important since it can be repaired with laser or a freezing technique. *NOTE:* It is important to have annual eye examinations. Early detection of eye problems can save your vision.

Sty (hordeolum) is a tiny abscess at the base of an eyelash. The eye is red, painful, and swollen. It is due to the inflammation of one of the tiny sebaceous glands of the eyelid. Treatment consists of warm, wet compresses to relieve pain and promote drainage.

Eye Injuries

In most cases of simple eye irritation the natural flow of tears will help to cleanse the eye. In cases where pieces of glass or other fragments get into the eye, do not attempt to remove the object. Patch both eyes and get medical treatment.

Corneal abrasions and scarring may occur as a result of an accident or irritation. The cornea is avascular; that is, there are no blood vessels present. Therefore, corneal transplants can be done readily without fears of tissue rejection.

Eye irritations can be caused by chemicals or fragments that get into the eye. Rinse eyes with water for at least fifteen minutes and seek medical treatment.

Night blindness is a condition that makes it difficult to see at night. The rod cells in the retina are affected in this condition.

Color blindness is the inability to distinguish colors. There are three specific types of cone cells in the retina related to the primary colors: blue, red, and green. The cone cells are affected in color blindness. Color blindness is a genetic disorder carried by the female and transmitted only to the male children.

Vision Defects

Presbyopia is a condition in which the lenses lose their elasticity resulting in a

decrease in ability to focus on close objects. It usually occurs after age forty. There is difficulty in focusing with this condition.

Hyperopia (hypermetropia far sightedness) is a condition in which the focal point is beyond the retina because the eyeball is shorter than normal, Figure 10-8. Objects must be moved further away from the eye to be seen clearly. Convex lenses help correct this situation.

Myopia (near sightedness) is a condition in which the focal point is in front of the retina, because the eyeball is elongated, see Figure 10-8. Objects must be brought very close to the eye to be seen clearly. Concave lenses help correct this condition.

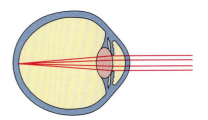

Normal eye
Light rays focus on the retina

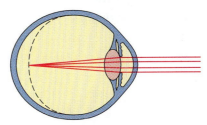

Myopia (nearsightedness)
Light rays focus in front of the retina

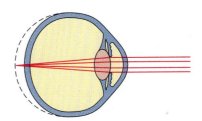

Hyperopia (farsightedness)
Light rays focus beyond the retina

FIGURE 10-8 *Vision defects*

Amblyopia is a reduction, or dimness, of vision.

Astigmatism is a condition in which there is an irregular curvature of the cornea or lens, which causes blurred vision and possible eyestrain. A special prescription eyeglass helps this condition.

Diplopia is blurred vision.

Strabismus (**"cross-eyes"**) is a condition in which the muscles of the eyeball do not coordinate their action. This condition is usually seen early in children and can be corrected by eye exercises or surgery.

THE EAR

The ear is a special sense organ which is especially adapted to pick up sound waves and send these impulses to the auditory center of the brain. The auditory center is located in the temporal area just above the ears. The receptor for hearing is the delicate **organ of Corti**, which is located within the cochlea of the inner ear.

The ear is also involved with equilibrium. The receptors in the inner ear send a message to the cerebellum in the brain about the position of our heads to help us maintain our bal-

ance. Other receptors include propioceptors in our eyes and receptors located around our joints. The information picked up by these receptors is processed by the cerebellum and cerebral cortex to enable the body to cope with changes in our equilibrium. For example, if you become drowsy and feel yourself sliding off a chair, your body will become alert and make you sit up straight again.

The ear has three parts: the outer or external ear, the middle ear, and the inner ear, see Figure 10-9.

The Outer Ear

The **pinna**, or outer ear, collects sound waves and directs them into the auditory canal. The auditory canal is lined with sebaceous glands also called ceruminous which secrete a waxlike or oily substance called cerumen. This substance protects the ear. The auditory canal leads to the eardrum or **tympanic membrane**, which separates the outer and middle ear.

The Middle Ear

The middle ear is really the cavity in the temporal bone. It connects with the pharynx by

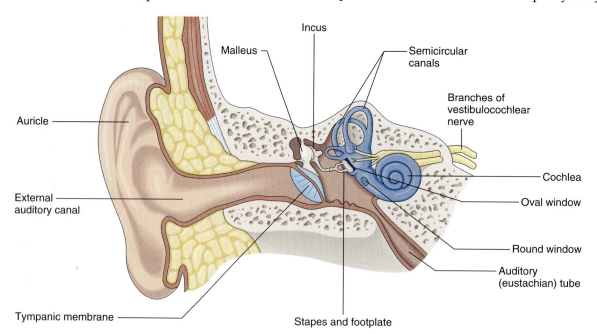

FIGURE 10-9 *The ear and its structures*

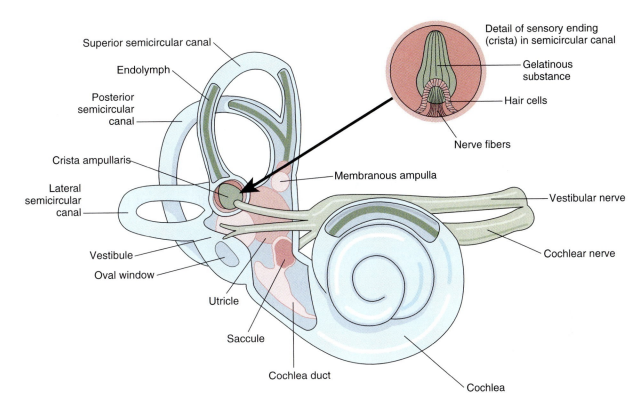

Superior semicircular canal

Endolymph

Posterior semicircular canal

Crista ampullaris

Lateral semicircular canal

Vestibule

Oval window

Utricle

Saccule

Cochlea duct

Detail of sensory ending (crista) in semicircular canal

Gelatinous substance

Hair cells

Nerve fibers

Membranous ampulla

Vestibular nerve

Cochlear nerve

Cochlea

FIGURE 10-10 *Enlargement of the inner ear showing the three semicircular canals*

means of a tube called the **eustachian tube**. This tubes serves to equalize the air pressure in the middle ear with that of the outside atmosphere. A chain of three tiny bones is found in the middle ear: the **hammer** (**malleus**), the **anvil** (**incus**), and the **stirrup** (**stapes**); they transmit sound waves from the ear drum to the inner ear.

The Inner Ear

The inner ear consists of several membrane-lined channels which lie deep within the temporal bone. The special organ of hearing is a spiral-shaped passage known as the **cochlea**, which contains a membranous tube called the **cochlear duct**. The duct is filled with fluid that vibrates when the sound waves from the stirrup bone strike against it. Located in the cochlear duct are delicate cells which make up the organ of Corti. These *hairlike* cells pick up the vibrations caused by sound waves against the fluid, then they transmit them through the auditory nerve to the hearing center of the brain.

Three **semicircular canals** also lie within the inner ear, Figure 10-10. They contain a liquid, and delicate hairlike cells which bend when the liquid is set in motion by head and body movements. These impulses are sent to the cerebellum, helping to maintain body balance, or equilibrium. They have nothing to do with the sense of hearing.

PATHWAY OF HEARING

Sound waves ⟶ *Pinna*, or outer ear ⟶ *auditory canal* ⟶ *tympanic membrane* ⟶ *ear ossicles* (hammer, anvil and stirrup) ⟶ stimulate the receptors in the *cochlea* ⟶ *cochlear nerve* (part of the vestibulocochlear nerve) ⟶ *temporal lobe* of the brain for interpretation, Figure 10-11.

When the same sound keeps reaching the ears, the auditory receptors adapt to the sound and we do not hear it.

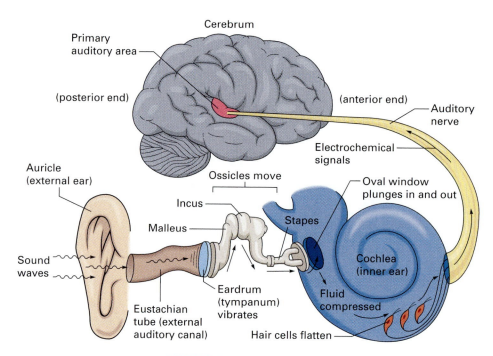

FIGURE 10-11 *Pathway of hearing*

PATHWAY OF EQUILIBRIUM

Movement of head ⟶ stimulates equilibrium receptors in the semi-circular and vestibule areas of the inner ear ⟶ vestibular nerve (part of the vestibulocochlea nerve) ⟶ cerebellum of the brain for interpretation.

LOUD NOISE AND HEARING LOSS

Your hearing is both sensitive and fragile. Loud noise heard for too long will damage your hearing. If the delicate hair cells in the organ of Corti in the inner ear become overstimulated, they will become damaged. Repeated exposure to the loud noise causes the loss to become permanent as more cells and their nerve receptors are destroyed.

The alarming increase of hearing loss in young people is most likely caused by loud music usually heard through headphones. The symptoms of hearing loss may be tinnitus (ringing in the ears) or difficulty in understanding what people are saying (they seem to be mumbling). Words with high-frequency sounds like "pill," "hill" and "fill" may sound alike.

Sound is measured in decibels. The scale runs from the faintest sound the human ear can hear, labeled 0dB, to the scream of a jet engine or a shotgun blast at over 165 dB. Exposure to more than 90 decibels for eight hours (busy city traffic noise) may be dangerous to your hearing. At 100 dB, the noise level of a chain saw, it take two hours to do the same damage to your hearing. *NOTE:* Noise heard long enough and loud enough over time will cause damage.

To protect your hearing, turn down the volume on the stereo, find a quiet place, and wear earplugs or ear muffs.

EAR DISORDERS

Otitis media is an infection of the middle ear. It usually causes earache. This disorder is often a complication of the common cold in children. Treatment with antibiotics will cure the infection. In some cases, there may be a build up of fluid or pus which can be relieved by a **myringotomy** (an opening made in the tympanic membrane). Tubes may be placed in the ear to allow fluids to drain off, especially in cases of chronic otitis media.

Otosclerosis is an inherited disorder in which the bone stapes of the middle ear first become sponge and then harden. This causes the stirrup or stapes to become fixed or immovable. Otosclerosis is a common cause of deafness in young adults. Stapedectomy, a total replacement of the stapes, is the treatment of choice.

Tinnitus is a sensation of ringing or buzzing that is perceived in the ear in the absence of an actual sound stimulus. It may be caused by impacted wax, otitis media, otosclerosis, loud noise, blockage of normal blood supply to the cochlea, or the effects of various drugs like the salicylates (painkillers).

Presbycusis is a condition which causes deafness due to the aging process. This can be helped with the use of hearing aids.

Meniere's disease is a condition which affects the semicircular canals of the inner ear, causing marked **vertigo** (dizziness). Vertigo can occur at any time and without warning, causing the patient to be very frightened. In addition, the vertigo is accompanied by nausea, vomiting, and a ringing sensation in the ears. Bed rest is sometimes necessary during an acute attack. Medication may be given to relieve vertigo and nausea. The patient should avoid any sudden movement, since it may precipitate an attack. The cause is unknown and the symptoms subside; however, an attack occurs without any warning.

Types of Hearing Loss

- *Conductive hearing loss* occurs when sounds to the inner ear are blocked by ear wax or there is fluid in the middle ear or abnormal bone growth.

- *Sensorineural damage* to parts of the inner ear of auditory nerve results in a partial or complete deafness. In cases of profound deafness, cochlear implants improve communication ability which leads to positive psychological and social changes. At the present time, children after the age of two and adults with profound deafness are candidates for cochlear implants.

THE NOSE

The human nose can detect about 10,000 different smells. Smell accounts for about 90% of what we think of as taste. Hold your nose and see if you can tell the difference between eating a piece of orange and a piece of pear. Odor molecules inhaled through the nose get warmed and moistened as they pass through the nasal cavity.

In the nasal cavity, Figure 10-12, there is a patch of tissue about the size of a postage

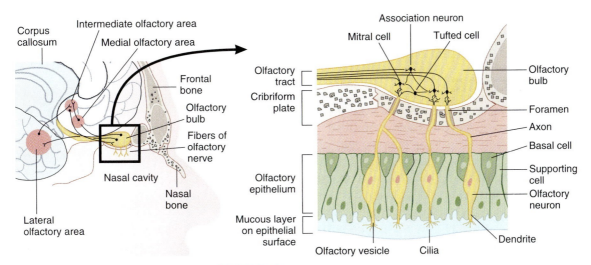

FIGURE 10-12 *The nasal cavity*

stamp called the olfactory epithelium, which has a plentiful supply of nerve cells with specialized receptors. The receptors send signals to the adjoining olfactory bulbs, an extension of the brain. The stimulus is transmitted by the olfactory nerve to the limbic system, thalamus, and frontal cortex. The limbic system generates our basic emotions such as affection, aggression, and fear. This relationship may explain why odors are tied to feelings. For example, we may associate the smell of something cooking usually with a good experience.

Scientists are starting to do research on how smells may affect learning, weight loss, aggression levels, and behavior.

DISORDERS OF THE NOSE

Rhinitis is an inflammation of the lining of the nose which may cause nasal congestion, nasal drainage, sneezing, or itching. The cause may be allergies, infection, or other factors such as fumes, odors, emotional changes, or drugs. Treatment includes eliminating the allergens, if possible, or reducing exposure to them. Some antihistamines are effective for short periods of time.

Nasal polyps are growths in the nasal cavity associated with rhinitis. In severe cases, surgery may be necessary to remove the polyps.

Deviated nasal septum is a condition in which there is a bend in the cartilage structure of the septum. Symptoms that result are a blockage in the airflow through one nostril, difficulty sleeping, headaches, loud breathing or snoring, dry nose, and nose bleeds. Treatment has been surgical correction. In June of 1996, a new product was introduced called Breathe Right. This nasal strip goes across the nose and provides temporary relief of breathing problems associated with a deviated nasal septum. This product improves breathing by reducing nasal airflow resistance. It can be effective in reducing snoring and in the temporary relief of nasal congestion.

A & P
CHALLENGE

THE TONGUE

The tongue is a mass of muscle tissue which has structures called papillae. Located on the papilla are the taste buds, which are stimulated by the flavors of foods. The receptors in the taste buds send stimuli through three cranial nerves to the cerebral cortex for interpretation.

CAREER PROFILES

THE SPECIAL SENSES

AUDIOLOGISTS

Audiologists assess and treat those with hearing and hearing related disorders. They use audiometers and other testing devices to measure the loudness at which a person begins to hear sounds, the ability to distinguish between sounds, and the extent of the hearing loss. Audiologists coordinate the results with medical and educational information to make a diagnosis and determine a course of treatment. Treatment may consist of cleaning the ear canal, fitting a hearing aid, auditory training, and instruction in speech or lip reading.

A master's degree is the standard credential in this field. Patience and compassion are critical traits to have since the client's progress may be very slow. Job outlook is higher than average because hearing loss is associated with the aging process.

OPTOMETRISTS

Over half the people in the United States wear glasses. Optometrists (Doctors of Optometry) provide most of the primary vision care people need.

Optometrists examine eyes to diagnose vision problems and eye disease. Optometrists use instruments and observations to examine eye health and to test patient's visual acuity, depth and color perception as well as their ability to focus and coordinate the eyes. They analyze test results and develop a treatment plan. Optometrists prescribe eyeglasses, contact lenses, and vision therapy. They prescribe drugs for other eye problems such as conjunctivitis, glaucoma, and corneal infection.

Optometrists differ from opthamologists. Opthamologists diagnose and treat eye diseases, perform surgery, and prescribe drugs. All states require optometrists to be licensed. Applicants must have a Doctor of Optometry from an accredited school and pass a licensing examination.

DISPENSING OPTICIANS

Dispensing opticians fit eyeglasses and contact lenses. Dispensing opticians help customers select appropriate frames, order the necessary opthalmic laboratory work, and adjust the finished eyeglasses. They examine written prescriptions to determine lens specification and measure the client's eyes. They prepare work orders which give the laboratory technicians information needed to grind and insert lenses.

Dispensing opticians keep records, work orders, and payments as well as track inventory and perform other administrative duties.

Employers generally hire individuals with no background in opticianry and then provide the required training. Mechanical drawing is particularly useful because training in this field usually includes instruction in optical mathematics, optical physics, and the use of precision measuring instruments and other machinery and tools. Formal training may be offered in community colleges. Job outlook is greater than average in response to rising demand for corrective lenses. Fashion also influences demand, encouraging people to buy more than one pair of eyeglasses.

● REVIEW QUESTIONS

Select the letter of the choice that best completes the statement.

1. The outer tough coat of the eye is the:
   a. retina
   b. sclera
   c. choroid
   d. lens

2. The clear anterior portion of the sclera is called:
   a. cornea
   b. lens
   c. pupil
   d. iris

3. The muscle that regulates how much light enters the eye is called:
   a. conjunction
   b. iris
   c. cornea
   c. lens

4. The posterior chamber of the eye is filled with fluid called:
   a. tears
   b. ciliary body
   c. vitreous humor
   d. aqueous humor

5. The area of the eye that contains the rods and cones is called:
   a. retina
   b. choroid
   c. sclera
   d. cornea

6. The tube that connects the throat to the ear is called:
   a. pinna
   b. eustachian
   c. cochlear
   d. auditory

7. Hardening of the bones of the middle ear is called:
   a. otitis media
   b. presbycusis
   c. otosclerosis
   d. presbyopia

8. Near sightedness is also known as:
   a. myopia
   b. hyperopia
   c. presbyopia
   d. strabismus

9. A clouding of the lens is called:
   a. myopia
   b. glaucoma
   c. hyperopia
   d. cataract

10. An infectious disease known as pink eye is also called:
    a. kernicterus
    b. otitis
    c. conjunctivitis
    d. strabismus

● LABELING

Identify the structures on the following figure and write and your answers in the spaces provided.

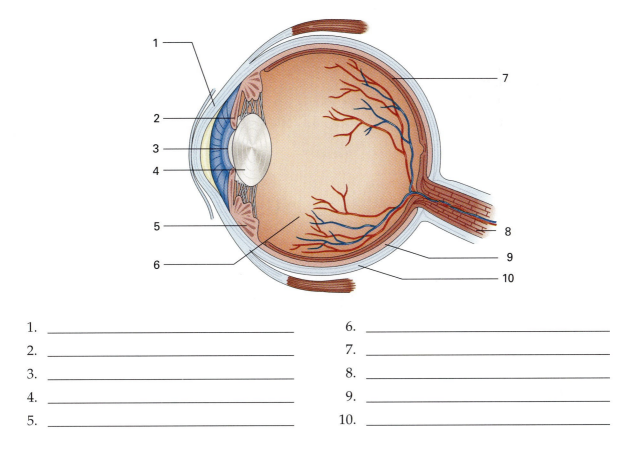

1. _____   6. _____
2. _____   7. _____
3. _____   8. _____
4. _____   9. _____
5. _____   10. _____

● APPLYING THEORY TO PRACTICE

1. You have heard that your eye works like a camera. Explain how you see and track the pathway of light from the cornea to the occipital lobe of the brain.

2. Explain to a friend how your outer ear catches a sound and where in the brain it is interpreted.

3. One of the most serious side effects of aging is sensory loss. Explain how the aging process affects vision and hearing in the elderly.

4. A patient comes to the doctor's office for treatment of glaucoma. She states, "I am so tired of taking these eyedrops. I don't want to use them anymore." How would you respond and what instructions would you give her?

5. The phrase "stop and smell the roses" means slow down and enjoy life. What conditions may interfere with your ability to smell the roses?

CHAPTER

11

Endocrine System

KEY WORDS

acromegaly
Addison's disease
adrenal glands
adrenalin
   (epinephrine)
adrenocorticotropic
   hormone (ACTH)
androgen
anterior pituitary
   lobe
Basal Metabolic Rate
   (BMR)
calcitonin
cretinism
Cushing's syndrome
diabetes insipidus
diabetes mellitus
dwarfism
endocrine gland
estrogen
exocrine gland
exophthalmos
follicle-stimulating
   hormone (FSH)
gigantism
glucagon

glucocorticoids
   (G-C^s)
goiter
gonads
growth hormone
   (GH)
hyperglycemia
hyperthyroidism
hypoglycemia
hypothyroidism
insulin
interstitial cell-stim-
   ulating hormone
   (ICSH)
islets of Langerhans
lactogenic hormone
   (LTH)
luteinizing hormone
   (LH)
melatonin
mineralocorticoids
   (M-C^s)
myxedema
negative feedback
norepinephrine
oxytocin

pancreas
parathormone
parathyroid gland
pineal gland
pituitary gland
polydypsia
polyphagia
polyuria
posterior pituitary
   lobe
progesterone
prolactin hormone
   (PR)
prostaglandin
somatotropin
testosterone
tetany
thymus
thyrotropin
thyroid gland
thyroid-stimulating
   hormone (TSH)
thyroxin (T$_4$)
triiodothyronine (T$_3$)
vasopressin

A&P
CHALLENGE

A gland is any organ that produces a secretion. **Endocrine glands**, Figure 11-1, are organized groups of tissues which use materials from the blood or lymph to make new compounds called hormones. Endocrine glands are also called ductless glands and glands of internal secretion; the hormones are secreted directly into the bloodstream as the blood circulates through the gland. The secretions are often transported to all areas of the body where they have a special influence on cells, tissues, and organs. There is another type of gland called an **exocrine gland**, in which the secretions from the gland must go through a

duct. This duct then carries the secretion to a body surface or organ. Exocrine glands include sweat, salivary, lacrimal, and pancreas. Their functions are included in chapters on the relevant body systems. See Figure 11-2.

One of the endocrine glands, the pancreas, can perform both as an exocrine gland and an endocrine gland. The pancreas produces pancreatic juices which go through a duct into the small intestines. The endocrine gland function is when a special group of cells known as **islets of Langerhans** secrete the hormone insulin directly into the bloodstream.

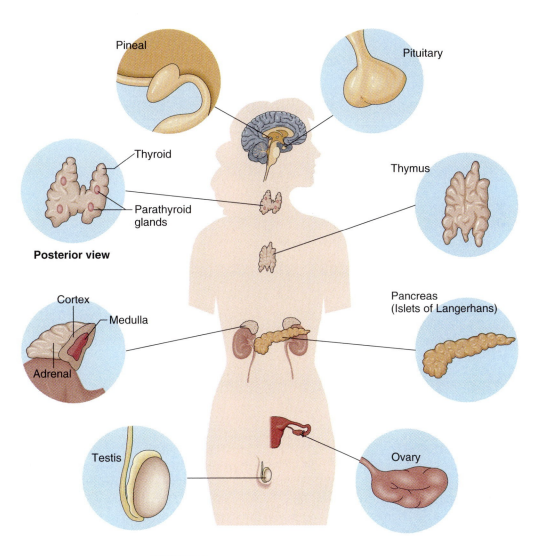

Pineal

Pituitary

Thyroid

Thymus

Parathyroid glands

Posterior view

Cortex

Medulla

Pancreas (Islets of Langerhans)

Adrenal

Testis

Ovary

FIGURE 11-1 *Locations of the endocrine glands*

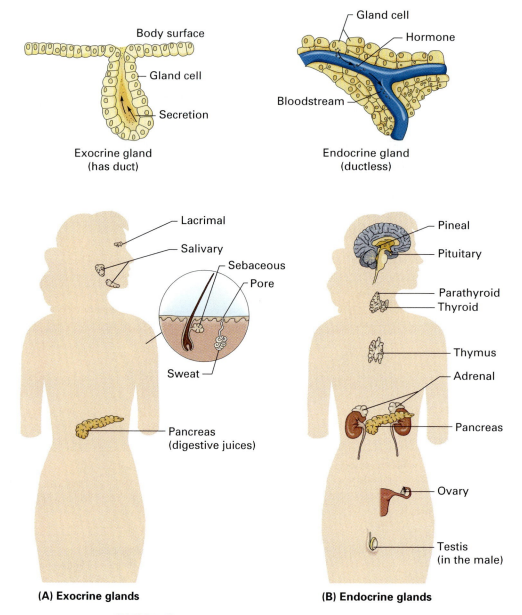

FIGURE II-2 *(a) Exocrine glands, (b) Endocrine glands*

FUNCTION OF THE ENDOCRINE SYSTEM

The major function of the endocrine system is to secrete hormones or chemical messengers which coordinate and direct the activities of target cells and target organs. See Table 11-1.

The major glands of the endocrine system include pituitary, pineal, thyroid, parathyroid, thymus, adrenals, pancreas, and the gonads (ovaries in the female and testes in the male).

Figure 11-1 shows the locations of the endocrine glands in the body. Each has specific functions to perform. Any disturbance in the functioning of these glands may cause changes in the appearance or functioning of the body.

TABLE II-I • *Endocrine Glands*

GLAND	LOCATION	HORMONE	PRINCIPAL EFFECTS
PITUITARY Anterior lobe	Undersurface of the brain in the sella turcica of the skull	Growth hormone (GH) Thyroid stimulating hormone (TSH) (Thyrotropin) Adrenocorticotropic hormone (ACTH) Melanocyte-stimulating hormone (MSH) Follicle-stimulating hormone (FSH) Luteinizing hormone (LH) Interstitial-cell stimulating hormone (ICSH)	Normal growth of body tissues Stimulates growth and activity of thyroid cells to produce thyroid hormone Stimulates the cortex of the adrenal gland Increases skin pigmentation Stimulates the maturity of the graafian follicle to rupture and to produce estrogen in the female. In the male it stimulates the development of the testes and the production of sperm. Causes the development of the corpus luteum, which then secretes progesterone in the female. ICSH in the male stimulates the interstitial cells of the testes to produce testosterone.
Posterior lobe		Prolactin (PR) Oxytocin Vasopressin or Antidiuretic hormone (ADH)	Develops breast tissue and stimulates secretion of milk from mammary glands Stimulates contraction of uterus, especially during childbirth; causes ejection of milk from mammary glands Acts on cells of kidney tubules to concentrate urine and conserve fluid in the body. Also acts to constrict blood vessels.
THYROID	Lower portion of anterior neck	Thyroxine (T_4) and Triiodothyronine (T_3) Thyrocalcitonin	Increases metabolism; influences both physical and mental activity; promotes normal growth and development Causes calcium to be stored in bones; reduces blood level of calcium
PARATHYROID	Posterior surface of thyroid gland	Parahormone	Regulates exchange of calcium between the bones and blood
ADRENAL Medulla	Superior surface of each kidney	Adrenaline (Epinephrine) Aldosterone (Mineral corticoid)	Increases heart rate, blood pressure, and flow of blood; decreases intestinal activity Controls electrolyte balances by regulating the reabsorption of sodium and the excretion of potassium
Cortex		Glucocorticoids Sex hormones (Androgens)	Affect the metabolism of protein, fat, and glucose, thereby increasing blood sugar Govern sex characteristics, especially those that are masculine
PANCREAS	Behind the stomach	Insulin Glucagon	Essential to the metabolism of carbohydrates; reduces the blood sugar level Stimulates the liver to release glycogen and converts it to glucose to increase blood sugar levels
THYMUS	Under the sternum	Thymosin	Reacts upon lymphoid tissue to produce T lymphocyte cells to develop immunity to certain disease
PINEAL BODY	Third ventricle in the brain	Melatonin	Controls onset of puberty
OVARIES	Female pelvis	Estrogen Progesterone	Promotes growth of primary and secondary sexual characteristics Develops excretory portion of mammary glands; aids in maintaining pregnancy
TESTES	Male scrotum	Testosterone	Develops primary and secondary sexual characteristics; stimulates maturation of sperm

HORMONAL CONTROL

The secretion of the hormones operates on a negative feedback system or under the control of the nervous system.

Negative Feedback

In **negative feedback** there is a drop in the level of the hormone, which triggers a chain reaction of responses to increase the amount of hormone in the blood. A description follows of how the negative feedback system functions as it relates to the thyroid gland:

1. The blood level of thyroxine (thyroid hormone) falls →

2. hypothalamus in the brain gets the message →

3. hypothalamus responds by sending a releasing hormone for TSH →

4. to the anterior pituitary gland to release TSH →

5. TSH stimulates the thyroid gland to produce thyroxine →

6. thyroxine blood level rises which in turn shuts off the releasing hormone for TSH.

Nervous Control

The nervous system controls the glands which are stimulated by nervous stimuli, as in the adrenal medulla where the gland is stimulated by the sympathetic nervous system. For example, when we become afraid, the adrenal medulla secretes adrenalin.

PITUITARY GLAND

The **pituitary gland** is a tiny structure having a diameter of about 10mm and a weight of approximately .5 grams, about the size of a grape. It is located at the base of the brain within the sella turcica, a small bony depression in the sphenoid bone of the skull, Figure 11-3. The pituitary gland is connected to the hypothalamus by a stalk called the infundibulum. The pituitary gland is divided into an anterior lobe and a posterior lobe, Figure 11-4.

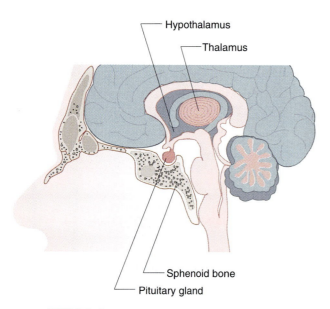

FIGURE II-3 *The pituitary gland in relation to the brain*

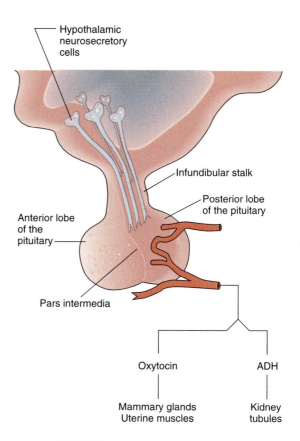

FIGURE II-4 *The pituitary gland*

Pituitary-Hypothalamus Interaction

The hormones of the anterior pituitary are controlled by the releasing chemicals or factors produced by the hypothalamus in the brain. As the pituitary hormones are needed by the body, the hypothalamus releases a specific releasing factor for each hormone. See Figure 11-4. For example, the thyroid-stimulating hormone (TSH) has a TSH releasing factor. In addition, when a sufficient amount of the hormone is released, a different releasing factor will inhibit the anterior pituitary from secreting TSH.

The hypothalamus is considered part of the nervous system. However, it produces two hormones: vasopressin, which converts to antidiuretic hormone (ADH), and oxytocin. These hormones are stored in the posterior lobe of the pituitary and are released into the blood stream in response to nerve impulses from the hypothalamus.

HORMONES OF THE PITUITARY GLAND

Anterior Pituitary Lobe

The **anterior pituitary lobe** secretes the following hormones:

1. **Growth hormone** (**GH**) (or **Somatotropin**) which is responsible for growth and development. This hormone also helps fat to be used for energy, saving glucose and helping to maintain blood sugar levels.

2. **Prolactin hormone** (**PR**) develops breast tissue and stimulates the production of milk after childbirth. The function in males is unknown.

3. **Thyroid-stimulating hormone** or **TSH** stimulates the growth and secretion of the thyroid gland.

4. **Adrenocorticotropic hormone** (**ACTH**) stimulates the growth and secretion of the adrenal cortex.

5. **Follicle-stimulating hormone** (**FSH**) stimulates the growth of the graafian follicle and the production of estrogen in females, and stimulates the production of sperm in the male.

6. **Luteinizing hormone** (**LH**) stimulates ovulation and the formation of the corpus luteum, which produces progesterone in females.

7. **Interstitial cell-stimulating hormone** (**ICSH**) is necessary for the production of testosterone by the interstitial cells of the testes in men.

Posterior Pituitary Lobe

The hormones produced by the hypothalamus are stored in the **posterior pituitary lobe**.

1. **Vasopressin** converts to antidiuretic hormone or ADH in the bloodstream. The name vasopressin may cause confusion since it causes little or no vasoconstriction. ADH maintains the water balance by increasing the absorption of water in the kidney tubules. Sometimes drugs called *diuretics* are used to inhibit the action of ADH. The result is an increase in urinary output and a decrease in blood volume, thus decreasing blood pressure.

2. **Oxytocin** is released during childbirth causing strong contractions of the uterus. It also causes strong contractions when a mother is breastfeeding. A synthetic form of oxytocin is called *pitocin* and is given to help start labor or make uterine contractions stronger.

The pituitary gland is known as the *master gland* because of its major influence on the body's activities. See Table 11-2. It is even more amazing when you consider the size of this incredible gland.

THYROID AND PARATHYROID GLANDS

The thyroid and parathyroid glands are located in the neck, close to the cricoid cartilage (or the "Adam's apple"). The thyroid regulates body metabolism. The parathyroid maintains the calcium-phosphorus balance.

TABLE II-2 • *Pituitary Hormones and Their Known Functions*

PITUITARY HORMONE	KNOWN FUNCTION
Anterior Lobe	
TSH — Thyroid-Stimulating Hormone (Thyrotropin)	Stimulates the growth and the secretion of the thyroid gland.
ACTH — Adrenocortiotrophic Hormone	Stimulates the growth and the secretion of the adrenal cortex.
FSH — Follicle-Stimulating Hormone	Stimulates growth of new graafian (ovarian) follicle and secretion of estrogen by follicle cells in the female and the production of sperm in the male.
LH — Luteinizing Hormone (female)	Stimulates ovulation and formation of the corpus luteum. Corpus luteum secretes progesterone.
ICSH — Interstitial Cell-Stimulating Hormone (male)	Stimulates testosterone secretion by the interstitial cells of the testes.
PR — Prolactin	Stimulates secretion of milk in females. Function in males is unknown.
GH — Growth Hormone (Somatotropin, STH)	Accelerates body growth and causes fat to be used for energy; this helps to maintain blood sugar.
Posterior Lobe	
VASOPRESSIN — (Antidiuretic Hormone ADH)	Maintains water balance by reducing urinary output. It acts on kidney tubules to reabsorb water into the blood more quickly. In large amounts, it causes constriction of arteries.
OXYTOCIN	Promotes milk ejection and causes contraction of the smooth muscles of the uterus.

THYROID GLAND

The **thyroid gland** is a butterfly-shaped mass of tissue located in the anterior part of the neck, Figure 11-5. It lies on either side of the larynx, over the trachea. Its general shape is that of the letter "H." It is about two inches long, with two lobes joined by strands of thyroid tissue called the isthmus. Coming from the isthmus is a finger-like lobe of tissue known as the intermediate lobe. This intermediate lobe projects upward toward the floor of the mouth, as far up as the hyoid bone. The thyroid gland has a rich blood supply. In fact, it has been estimated that about 4 to 5 liters

(some 8 1/2 to 10 1/2 pints) of blood pass through the gland every hour.

The thyroid gland secretes three hormones: thyroxine, triiodothyronine, and calcitonin. The first two are iodine-bearing derivatives of the amino acid, tyrosine. Triiodothyronine is five to ten times more active than thyroxine, but its activity is less prolonged. However, the two have the same effect. Both hormones are produced in the follicle cells of the thyroid gland. These cells are stimulated to secretory activity by a hormone from the anterior lobe of the pituitary gland. This thyroid-stimulating hormone (TSH) controls the production and

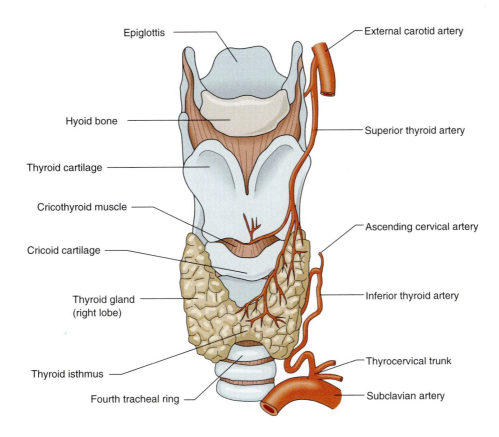

Epiglottis

External carotid artery

Hyoid bone

Superior thyroid artery

Thyroid cartilage

Cricothyroid muscle

Cricoid cartilage

Ascending cervical artery

Inferior thyroid artery

Thyroid gland
(right lobe)

Thyrocervical trunk

Thyroid isthmus

Subclavian artery

Fourth tracheal ring

FIGURE II-5 *Thyroid gland*

secretion of the thyroid hormone from the thyroid gland. The thyroid hormones contain iodine. Most of the iodine needed for their synthesis comes from the diet. Iodides are circulated to the thyroid gland, where they are "trapped." Here the iodides combine with the amino acid tyrosine to form the hormones **Triiodothyronine** (T_3) and **thyroxine** (T_4).

Under normal circumstances, the presence of these two hormones (T_3 and T_4) in the bloodstream serves to regulate the system. On the other hand, an excess would suppress TSH secretion. When the concentration of thyroid hormones is lowered in the bloodstream, the pituitary gland secretes more TSH. This, in turn, stimulates thyroid gland activity. (The consequences of hyposecretion and hypersecretion of the thyroid hormones is discussed later in this chapter.)

Thyroxine controls the rate of metabolism, heat production, and oxidation of all cells, with the possible exception of the brain and spleen cells. It can speed up or slow down the activities of the body as needed. In the liver, the two thyroid hormones affect the conversion of glycogen from sources other than sugar. It also helps to change glycogen into glucose, raising the glucose level of the blood.

To summarize, the functions of thyroxin are as follows:

1. Controls the rate of metabolism in the body; how cells use glucose and oxygen to produce heat and energy.

2. Stimulates protein synthesis and thus helps in tissue growth.

3. Stimulates the breakdown of liver glycogen.

Calcitonin

Calcitonin is another hormone produced and secreted by the thyroid gland. It controls the calcium ion concentration in the body by maintaining a proper calcium level in the bloodstream.

Calcium is an essential body mineral. Approximately 99% of the calcium in the body is stored in the bones. The rest is located in the blood and tissue fluids. Calcium is necessary for blood clotting, holding cells together, and neuromuscular functions. The constant level of calcium in the blood and tissues is maintained by the action of calcitonin and parathormone (produced by the parathyroid gland).

When blood calcium levels are higher than normal, calcitonin secretion is increased. Calcitonin lowers the calcium concentration in the blood and body fluids by decreasing the rate of the bone resorption or osteoclastic activity and by increasing the calcium absorption by bones or osteoblastic activity. Proper secretion of calcitonin into the blood stream prevents hypercalcemia, a harmful rise in the blood calcium level.

PARATHYROID GLANDS

The **parathyroid glands**, usually four in number, are tiny glands the size of grains of rice. These are attached to the posterior surface of the thyroid gland, and secrete the hormone **parathormone**. Parathormone, like calcitonin, also controls the concentration of calcium in the bloodstream. When the blood calcium level is lower than normal, parathormone secretion is increased.

Parathormone stimulates an increase in the number and size of specialized bone cells referred to as osteoclasts. Osteoclasts quickly invade hard bone tissue, digesting large amounts of the bony material containing calcium. As this process continues, calcium leaves the bone and is released into the bloodstream, increasing the calcium blood level.

Bone calcium is bonded to phosphorus in a compound called calcium phosphate ($CaPO_4$). When calcium is released into the bloodstream, phosphorus is released along with it. Parathormone stimulates the kidneys to excrete any excess phosphorus from the blood; at the same time, it inhibits calcium excretion from the kidneys. Consequently, the concentration of blood calcium rises.

Thus, parathormone and calcitonin of the thyroid have opposite, or antagonistic effects to one another (see Figure 11-6 for a summary of their actions). Parathormone, however, acts much more slowly than calcitonin. It may be hours before the effects of parathormone become apparent. In this manner, the secretion of parathormone and calcitonin serve as complementary processes controlling the level of calcium in the bloodstream.

THYMUS GLAND

The **thymus** gland is both an endocrine gland and lymphatic organ. It is located under the sternum, anterior and superior to the heart. Fairly large during childhood, it begins to disappear at puberty. Recent research has discovered that the thymus gland secretes a large number of hormones. The major hormone is thymosin which helps to stimulate the lymphoid cells that are responsible for the production of T cells, which fight certain diseases.

ADRENAL GLANDS

One of the two **adrenal glands** is located on top of each kidney, Figure 11-7. Each gland has two parts: the cortex and the medulla. Adrenocorticotrophic hormone (ACTH) from the pituitary glands stimulates the activity of the cortex of the adrenal gland. The hormones secreted by the adrenal cortex are known as corticoids. The corticoids are very effective as anti-inflammatory drugs.

The cortex secretes three groups of corticoids, each of which is of great importance:

1. **Mineralocorticoids** (**M-Cs**)—mainly aldosterone, affects the kidney tubules by speeding up the reabsorption of sodium into the blood circulation and increasing

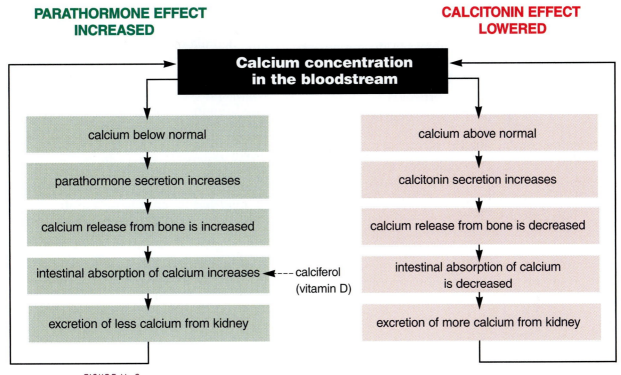

**PARATHORMONE EFFECT
INCREASED**

**CALCITONIN EFFECT
LOWERED**

**Calcium concentration
in the bloodstream**

PARATHORMONE EFFECT INCREASED	CALCITONIN EFFECT LOWERED
calcium below normal	calcium above normal
parathormone secretion increases	calcitonin secretion increases
calcium release from bone is increased	calcium release from bone is decreased
intestinal absorption of calcium increases ← calciferol (vitamin D)	intestinal absorption of calcium is decreased
excretion of less calcium from kidney	excretion of more calcium from kidney

FIGURE II-6 *Effects of parathormone and calcitonin on the level of calcium in the blood*

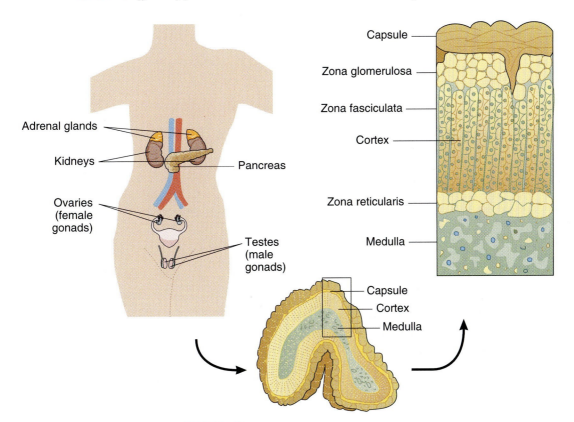

Adrenal glands

Kidneys

Pancreas

Ovaries
(female
gonads)

Testes
(male
gonads)

Capsule

Zona glomerulosa

Zona fasciculata

Cortex

Zona reticularis

Medulla

Capsule
Cortex
Medulla

FIGURE II-7 *Locations of adrenal and gonads*

the excretion of potassium from the blood. They also speed up the reabsorption of water by the kidneys. Aldosterone (M-C) is used in the treatment of Addison's Disease to replace deficient secretion of mineralocorticoids.

2. **Glucocorticoids** (**G-Cs**)—namely cortisone and cortisol, increase the amount of glucose in the blood. This is presumably done by: (1) conversion of the protein brought to the liver into glycogen, followed by (2) breakdown of the glycogen into glucose. These glucocorticoids also help the body resist the aggravations caused by various everyday stresses. In addition, these hormones seem to decrease edema in inflammation and reduce pain by inhibiting pain-causing **prostaglandin**.

3. Sex hormones are in both males and females. **Androgens** are male sex hormones which, together with similar hormones from the gonads, bring about masculine characteristics. Some estrogens are also present.

Medulla of the Adrenal Gland

The medulla of the adrenal gland secretes **epinephrine** and **norepinephrine**, Table 11-3. Epinephrine (generic name), or **Adrenalin** (trade), is a powerful cardiac stimulant. It functions by bringing about a release of more glucose from stored glycogen for muscle activity and increasing the force and rate of the heartbeat. This chemical activity increases cardiac output and venous return, and raises the systolic blood pressure. The adrenal medulla responds to the sympathetic nervous system. The hormones produced are referred to as the "fight or flight" hormones, since they prepare the body for an emergency situation.

GONADS

The **gonads**, or sex glands, include the ovaries in the female and the testes in the male. The ovary is responsible for producing the ova or egg and the hormones **estrogen** and **progesterone**. The testes are responsible for producing sperm and the hormone **testosterone**.

TABLE II-3 ● *Comparison of the Effects Between Epinephrine and Norepinephrine*

EPINEPHRINE	NOREPINEPHRINE
1. Bronchial relaxation	No effect
2. Dilation of iris	No effect
3. Excitation of central nervous system	No effect
4. Increased conversion of stored glycogen to glucose	Much less effect
5. Increased heart rate	Little effect
6. Increased cardiac output and venous return	Slight effect
7. Increased blood flow to muscles	Vasoconstriction in muscle
8. Increased myocardial strength	About the same
9. Increased basal metabolic rate (BMR)	Much less effect
10. Increased systolic blood pressure	Raises both systolic and diastolic blood pressure
11. Increased lipolytic effects; frees fatty acids from fat deposits	Slightly greater effects
12. Relaxation of uterine myometrial muscles	Pilomotor contraction

Female Hormones—Estrogen and Progesterone

Estrogen is produced by the graafian follicle cells of the ovary. It stimulates the development of the reproductive organs, including the breast, and secondary sex characteristics such as pubic and axillary hair.

Progesterone is produced by the cells of the corpus luteum of the ovary. Progesterone works with estrogen to build up the lining of the uterus for the fertilized egg. If no fertilization occurs, menstruation takes place. This cycle depends on the secretion of the anterior pituitary gland. (See Chapter 20.)

Male Hormone—Testosterone

Testosterone is produced by the interstitial cells of the testes and is responsible for the development of the male reproductive organs and secondary sex characteristics. Testosterone influences the growth of a beard and other body hair, deepening of the voice, increase in musculature, and the production of sperm. The secretion of the hormone depends on the pituitary gland. (See Chapter 20.)

A&P CHALLENGE

PANCREAS

The **pancreas** is located behind the stomach and functions as both an exocrine and endocrine gland. The exocrine portion secretes pancreatic juices which are excreted through a duct into the small intestines. There they become part of the digestive juices. The endocrine portion is involved in the production of insulin by the B cells of the islets of Langerhans on the pancreas.

The islet cells are distributed throughout the pancreas. These cells were named the **islets of Langerhans** after the doctor who discovered them, Figure 11-8. B cells produce **insulin** which: (1) promotes the utilization of glucose in the cells, necessary for maintenance of normal levels of blood glucose, (2) promotes fatty acid transport and fat deposition into cells, (3) promotes amino acid transport into cells, and (4) facilitates protein synthesis. Lack of insulin secretion by the island (islet) cells causes diabetes mellitus.

The A cells contained in the islets of Langerhans secrete the hormone **glucagon**. The action of glucagon may be antagonistic or opposite to that of insulin. Glucagon's function is to increase the level of glucose in the bloodstream. This is done by stimulating the conversion of liver glycogen to glucose. The control of glucagon secretion is achieved by negative feedback (refer to Negative Feedback, page 160.) Low glucose levels in the bloodstream stimulate the A cells to secrete glucagon, which quickly increases the glucose level in the bloodstream.

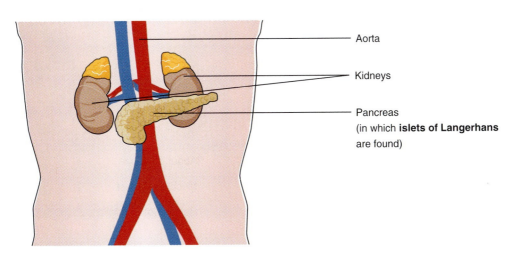

Aorta

Kidneys

Pancreas
(in which **islets of Langerhans** are found)

FIGURE 11-8 *Location of islets of Langerhans*

PINEAL GLAND

The pineal gland or body is a small pine-cone-shaped organ attached by a slim stalk to the roof of the third ventricle in the brain. The hormone produced by the pineal gland is called melatonin. The pineal gland is stimulated by a group of nerve cells called the suprachiasmatic nucleus (SCN), which are located in the brain over the pathway of fibers of the optic nerve. The amount of light entering the eye stimulates the SCN which then stimulates the pineal gland to release its hormone. The amount of light affects the amount of melatonin secreted. The darker it is, the more melatonin is produced; the lighter it is, the less melatonin is produced. There are no clear answers to the function of melatonin; however, melatonin causes body temperature to drop. For example, falling asleep is associated with lowered body temperature while waking up is associated with rising body temperature.

It is also thought that melatonin combines with a hypothalmic substance to prevent the early onset of puberty.

OTHER HORMONES PRODUCED IN THE BODY

Prostaglandins

In various tissues, throughout the body, hormones are secreted which are called prostaglandins. Their activity depends on which tissue secretes them. Some prostaglandins can cause constriction of the blood vessels; others may cause dilation. Prostaglandins can be used to induce labor and cause severe muscular contractions of the uterus. The exact nature and function of the prostaglandins are being extensively studied by scientists.

DISORDERS OF THE ENDOCRINE SYSTEM

Endocrine gland disturbances may be caused by several factors such as disease of the gland itself, infections in other parts of the body, autoimmune causes and dietary deficiencies. Most disturbances result from: (1) hyperactivity of the glands, causing oversecretion of hormones, or (2) hypoactivity of the gland, resulting in undersecretion of hormones. Health care workers most often see these patients in a doctor's office.

PITUITARY DISORDERS

Disturbances of the pituitary gland may produce a number of body changes. This gland is chiefly involved in the growth function. However, as the master gland, the pituitary indirectly influences other activities.

Hyperfunction of Pituitary

Hyperfunctioning of the pituitary gland (often due to a pituitary tumor) causes hypersecretion of the pituitary growth hormone. This can lead to two conditions: gigantism and acromegaly.

Gigantism. When this occurs during preadolescence it causes gigantism, an overgrowth of the long bones leading to excessive tallness.

Acromegaly. If hypersecretion of the growth hormone occurs during adulthood, acromegaly results. This is an overdevelopment of the bones of the face, hands and feet, Figure 11-9. In adults whose

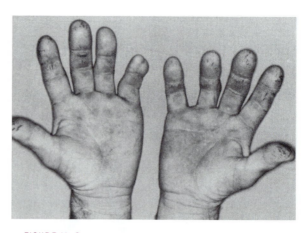

FIGURE 11-9 *Effects of acromegaly on fingers and hands (Armed Forces Institute of Pathology negative 72-14615)*

Sunshine Disorder

It is called "cabin fever" or "winter blues." It is the depression or anxiety many people feel during the dark days of winter. To feel better many people look for a winter vacation in the sunshine. Scientists have identified this "phenomena" and call it "Seasonal Affective Disorder" or SAD. Scientists Norman Rosenthal and his colleagues at the National Institute of Mental Health described SAD and the preliminary findings regarding a form of treatment with light was documented.

They conducted a study to observe how a group of people reacted to amounts of daylight. As daylight began decreasing during the fall, people started to develop symptoms of lethargy, anxiety, mood changes, appetite increases (especially a craving for carbohydrates), and a decrease in physical activity. As winter progressed and the days shortened, the symptoms increased. When spring arrived, the symptoms diminished; by the end of May almost everyone in the study group exhibited no symptoms at all.

During this study, the scientists found that they could reverse the symptoms by supplying light. They used two different kinds of light: the dimmer yellow light had no effect, but the brighter light (with a frequency spectrum more or less simulating the frequencies in sunlight) produced a marked change in mood in most of the patients who received this treatment.

Our bodies have evolved to respond to a "biological clock," being alert by daylight and sleepy as the sun fades into the night. A small cluster of brain cells called the *suprachiasmatic nucleus* (*SCN*) has been identified as the probable site for the biological clock in our bodies. One type of information has to do with the amount of light coming in through the eyes. **Note:** *Supra* means *over*; *chiasmatic* refers to *optic chiasma* which is the site where the fibers (nerve endings) from the retinas of the right and left eye cross. The SCN nerve cluster is located directly above a part of our vision system.

The SCN sends its message about the amount of light through the sympathetic nervous system to the pineal gland. The pineal gland secretes melatonin—the more light, the less secretion of melatonin; the less light the more melatonin is secreted. Light suppresses the secretion of melatonin.

For people affected by Seasonal Affective Disorder, the suggested treatment is bright light exposure for one-half to three hours, usually in the morning. In addition, prepare for the change in daylight hours by planning special activities for shorter days of winter. Expose yourself to as much bright light as possible. On sunny days go outside; on dark days use bright lights. Proper diagnosis is essential for proper treatment. If these symptoms develop, seek professional advice.

---

long bones have already matured, the growth hormone attacks the cartilaginous regions and the bony joints. Thus the chin protrudes, and the lips, nose, and extremities enlarge disproportionately. Lethargy and severe headaches frequently set in as well.

Treatment of acromegaly and gigantism is drug therapy (which inhibits GH), and radiation therapy.

Hypofunction of Pituitary

Dwarfism. Hypofunctioning of the pituitary gland during childhood leads to pituitary dwarfism. Growth of the long bones is abnormally decreased by an inadequate production of growth hormone. Despite the small size, however, the body of a dwarf is normally proportioned and intelligence is normal. Unfortunately, the physique remains juvenile and sexually immature. Treatment involves early diagnosis and injections of human growth hormone. The treatment period is five years or more.

Diabetes Insipidus

Another disorder caused by posterior lobe dysfunction is **diabetes insipidus**. In this condition, there is a drop in the amount of ADH, which causes an excessive loss of water and electrolytes. The affected person complains of excessive thirst (**polydypsia**).

THYROID DISORDERS

Since the thyroid gland controls metabolic activity, any disorder will affect other structures besides the gland itself. Persons at risk include those with other immune system problems, such as arthritis sufferers. Signs and symptoms of the disorders most frequently seen are discussed in this unit.

DIAGNOSTIC TESTS FOR THYROID

To diagnose thyroid function, a blood test is done; blood levels of TSH, T_3, and T_4 are checked to see if they are within normal limits.

A thyroid scan is another diagnostic tool which is used to determine the activity of the thyroid gland. The patient takes radioactive iodine; after the dye is taken, a scan is done to measure how the radioactive iodine is taken up by the thyroid gland. A large uptake indicates hyperthyroidism.

The radioactive iodine uptake test measures the activity of the thyroid gland. Dilute radioactive iodine is given orally. The amount which accumulates in the thyroid gland is calculated by use of a scan.

Hyperthyroidism

Hyperthyroidism is due to the overactivity of the thyroid gland. Too much thyroxin is secreted (hypersecretion), leading to enlargement of the gland. People with hyperthyroidism consume large quantities of food, but

nevertheless suffer a loss of body fat and weight. Symptoms include feeling too hot, fast growing and rougher fingernails, and weakened muscles. They may suffer from increased blood pressure and heartbeat, hand tremors, perspiration, and irritability. In addition, the liver releases excess glucose into the bloodstream, increasing the blood sugar level and causing a mild case of glycosuria. The most pronounced symptoms of hyperthyroidism include enlargement of the thyroid gland (**goiter**), bulging of the eyeballs (**exophthalmos**), dilation of the pupils, and wide-opened eyelids. In the United States, 70-80% of people who have hyperthyroidism have the type also known as Graves Disease.

The immediate cause of exophthalmos is not completely known, Figure 11-10. It is not directly caused by the hyperthyroidism, because removal of the thyroid does not always cause the eyeballs to return to their normal

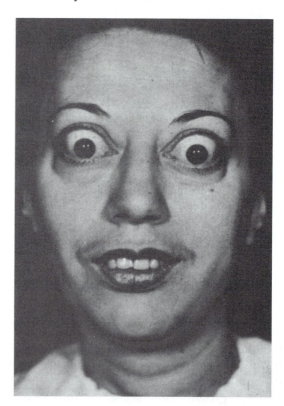

FIGURE 11-10 *Hyperthyroidism (reproduced with permission from S.L. Robbins and R.S. Cotran, Pathological Basis of Disease, Philadelphia: W.B. Sanders)*

state. Treatment of hyperthyroidism includes total or partial removal of the thyroid and administration of drugs like propylthiouracil and methylthiouracil to reduce the thyroxin secretion. The use of radioactive iodine to suppress the activity of the thyroid gland is another treatment for hyperthyroidism.

Hypothyroidism

Hypothyroidism is a condition in which the thyroid gland does not secrete sufficient thyroxin (hyposecretion). This is manifested by low T_3 or T_4 levels or increased TSH blood levels.

Adult hypothyroidism may occur because of iodine deficiency. A simple goiter may indicate this condition. Because iodized salt is commonly used in the United States, that is not the usual cause of a hypothyroid condition. The major cause is an inflammation of the thyroid which destroys the ability of the gland to make thyroxine. This inflammation is an autoimmune disease that attacks the body's own thyroid gland. Symptoms include dry and itchy skin, dry and brittle hair, constipation, and muscle cramps at night. If this condition goes untreated, a condition known as myxedema occurs.

Depending upon the time hypothyroidism strikes its victims, two different sets of disorders may occur: myxedema or cretinism.

Myxedema. The face becomes swollen, weight increases, and initiative and memory fails when a person experiences **myxedema**. Treatment is daily medication of thyroid hormone. It is important for the health care worker to be sure the patient understands the necessity of taking the medication. Follow-up tests to measure TSH blood levels are also important.

Cretinism. This disorder develops in early infancy or childhood. It is characterized by a lack of mental and physical growth, resulting in mental retardation and malformation (dwarfism or **cretinism**). The sexual development and physical growth of cretins do not proceed beyond that of seven or eight-year-old children.

In treating cretinism, thyroid hormones or thyroid extract may restore a degree of normal development if administered in time. In most cases, however, normal development cannot be completely restored once the affliction has set in.

PARATHYROID DISORDERS

The parathyroid glands regulate the use of calcium and phosphorus. Both of these minerals are involved in many of the body systems.

Hyperfunctioning of the parathyroid glands may cause an increase in the amount of blood calcium, thereby increasing the tendency for the calcium to crystallize in the kidneys as kidney stones. Excess amounts of calcium and phosphorus are withdrawn from the bones; this may lead to eventual deformity. So much calcium can be removed from the bones that they become honeycombed with cavities. Afflicted bones become so fragile that even walking can cause fractures.

Hypofunctioning of the parathyroid glands leads to a condition known as **tetany**. In this case, severely diminished calcium levels affect the normal function of nerves. Convulsive twitchings develop, and the afflicted person dies of spasms in the respiratory muscles. Treatment consists of administering vitamin D, calcium, and parathormone to restore a normal calcium balance.

ADRENAL DISORDERS

Hyperfunction of Adrenal

Cushing's syndrome results from the hypersecretion of the glucocorticoid hormones from the adrenal cortex, Figure 11-11. This hypersecretion may be caused by an adrenal cortical tumor or the prolonged use of prednisone. (Oddly enough, more women than men tend to develop this endocrine disorder.) Symptoms include high blood pressure, muscular weakness, obesity, poor healing of skin lesions, a tendency to bruise easily, hirsutism (excessive hair growth), menstrual disorders in women, and hyperglycemia. The most noticeable characteristics are a rounded "moon" face and a "buffalo hump" that develops from the redistribution of body fat. Therapy consists of surgical removal of the adrenal cortical tumor.

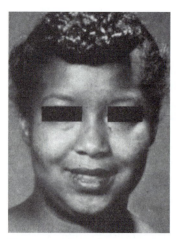

Preoperative   Postoperative (6 months later)

FIGURE II-II *Cushing's syndrome*

Hypofunction of Adrenal

Hypofunctioning of the adrenal cortex can also lead to **Addison's disease**. Persons with Addison's disease exhibit the following symptoms: excessive pigmentation prompting the characteristic "bronzing" of the skin, decreased levels of blood glucose, hypoglycemia, low blood pressure which falls further when standing, pronounced muscular weakness and fatigue, diarrhea, weight loss, vomiting, and a severe drop of sodium in the blood and tissue fluids, causing a serious imbalance of electrolytes.

The medical treatment of Addison's disease is focused on the replacement of the deficient hormones.

STEROID ABUSE IN SPORTS

Athletes of today have turned to the use of androgenic anabolic steroids to build bigger, stronger muscles and thus hope to achieve status in the world of sports.

The risks of taking steroids far outweigh any temporary improvement that an athlete may hope to gain. Effects on males who abuse steroids include liver changes, decrease in spleen production, atrophy of the testicles, breast enlargement and increased risk of cardiovascular disease. Effects on females include amenorrhea (loss of menstrual cycle), abnormal placement of body hair, baldness, and voice changes. In addition, both sexes complain of headaches, dizziness, hypertension, mood swings, and aggressiveness.

GONAD DISORDERS

Disturbances in the ovaries may consist of cysts and tumors, abnormal menstruation, and menopausal changes. Turner's Syndrome may occur in either the male or female; this is a chromosomal disorder. (See Chapter 20.)

PANCREATIC DISORDERS

Diabetes mellitus is a condition caused by decreased secretion of insulin from the islet cells of the pancreas or by the ineffective use of insulin. Insulin is necessary for the cells to use glucose. Carbohydrate metabolism in diabetes mellitus is disturbed which has an adverse effect on protein and fat metabolism.

Diabetes is divided into two types: insulin dependent (IDDM) or Type I and non-insulin dependent (NIDDM) or Type II. The insulin dependent type of the disease is also known as juvenile diabetes, since the onset is usually in children or young adults. The cause of Type I is thought to be an auto immune reaction which involves genetic and virus factors which destroys the Islets of Langerhans cells. Type I diabetics must take insulin and monitor daily blood glucose levels.

Symptoms of Type I or insulin dependent diabetes mellitus (IDDM):

- **polyuria**—excessive urination

- **polydypsia**—excessive thirst

- **polyphagia**—excessive hunger

- weight loss

- blurred vision

- possible diabetic coma

Insulin deficiency causes glucose to accumulate in the bloodstream, rather than be transported to the cells and converted into energy. Eventually the excess becomes too much for the kidneys to reabsorb, and the excess glucose is excreted in the urine. Excretion of excess glucose requires an accompanying excretion of large amounts of water. This occurs to insure that the sugar concentration does not rise too high. Diabetics are constantly thirsty because the lost water must be replaced.

Since sufficient glucose is not available for cellular oxidation in diabetes mellitus, the body starts to burn up protein and fats. The diabetic is constantly hungry and usually eats voraciously, but loses weight nonetheless.

When fats are utilized as a fuel source, they are rapidly but incompletely oxidized. One product of this abnormal rate of fat oxidation is ketone bodies. Ketone bodies are highly toxic; the type most commonly formed is acetoacetic acid. These ketone acids accumulate in the blood, promoting the development of acidosis, giving the breath and urine an odor of "sweet" acetone. If acidosis is severe, diabetic coma and death may result. Prolonged diabetes leads to atherosclerosis, heart disease, and kidney damage. Therapy consists of daily insulin injections and a controlled diet.

Patient education is critical in the treatment of diabetes. The insulin dependent diabetic must be educated in the signs of **hypoglycemia** (low blood sugar; insulin shock) and **hyperglycemia** (high blood sugar; diabetic coma), as illustrated in Table 11-4.

TABLE 11-4 • *Signs of Hypoglycemia and Hyperglycemia*

	HYPOGLYCEMIA (↓ BLOOD SUGAR)	HYPERGLYCEMIA (↑ BLOOD SUGAR)
Onset	Sudden	Slow
Reason	Too much insulin Too much exercise Not enough food	Not enough insulin Not enough exercise Too much food
Skin	Pale, moist to wet Sweating	Flushed, dry, hot No Sweating
Symptoms	Nervous, trembling, confusion, irritable	Drowsy, lethargic, weak, lapses into unconsciousness
Breath	Normal odor	Fruity odor
Respiration	Normal to rapid	Kussmaul breathing (air hunger)
Glycosuria	Little to none	High amount
Ketonuria	None	Present
Blood Sugar	Low-below 80	High-above 150
Treatment	Rapid response; give sugar in form of soft drink or orange juice Glucagon (IM); Glucose 50% IV	Slow response IV fluids Regular insulin

Characteristics and symptoms of Type II or non-insulin dependent diabetes (NIDDM):

- gradual onset
- most common in adults over age fifty-five
- feelings of tiredness or illness
- frequent urination, especially at night
- unusual thirst
- frequent infections and slow healing of sores

Non-insulin dependent or Type II diabetes makes up ninety to ninety-five percent of diabetics. It is usually a familial disease which occurs later in life. In this condition, insulin is secreted but in lowered amounts. The treatment focus is on diet, weight reduction, and medication. Oral hypoglycemic agents are given which stimulate the pancreatic cells to produce more insulin or increase the effectiveness of the insulin that is produced.

Treatment of Diabetes Mellitus

Patients with diabetes can lead normal, productive lives if they follow their treatment. Diabetics need instruction on how to use the glucose monitoring system, how to inject insulin, exercise and its effects on the blood sugar, and how to use their calculated diet and the food exchange listings.

Diabetes is widely recognized as one of the leading causes of death and disability in the United States. Diabetes is associated with long-term complications that affect almost every part of the body. It can cause blindness, heart disease, strokes, kidney failure, amputations, and nerve damage.

Diabetics should wear a medic-alert bracelet and carry an identification card which states they are diabetic.

Tests for Diabetes Mellitus

The diagnostic tests to determine the presence of glucose are done on urine and blood samples. The most common test done is a finger prick to obtain a blood sample that is then measured in a *glucometer* (glucose monitor). This test may be done by the patient at home. The normal blood sugar is 80 to 120 mg of glucose per 100 ml of blood.

Another blood test for diabetes is glycosylated hemoglobin (HbA1c). The glucose exposed to hemoglobin attaches itself to the protein in a way that reflects the average blood glucose concentration for the preceding two to three months. The test is done every three months.

Urine may also be tested by using a specifically coded dipstick. A urine sample is obtained, then the tape is dipped into the urine and compared with the special coding bar that is found on the outside of the dipstick container.

MEDICAL HIGHLIGHT: RESEARCH

Diabetes

There are about fourteen million Americans who have diabetes mellitus, a serious lifelong disorder that is yet incurable. About one-half of these people do not know they have the disease and are not under medical care. Researchers in the past fifteen years have made advances in managing diabetes and treating its complications. Major advances include:

- New forms of purified insulin such as human insulin produced through genetic engineering.
- Development of better ways for patients to monitor blood glucose levels at home.
- Development of external and implantable insulin pumps which deliver appropriate amounts of insulin and replace daily injections.

- The use of laser treatment for diabetic eye disease, reducing the risk of blindness.
- Successful transplantation of kidneys in diabetics with kidney failure.
- Better ways of managing diabetic pregnancies and improving chances of a successful outcome.
- Development of new drugs to treat NIDDM and better ways to manage this type through weight control.
- Proof that intensive management of blood glucose levels reduces and may prevent development of microvascular complications of diabetes, such as peripheral vascular disease.
- Firm evidence that antihypertensive drugs called ACE-inhibitors prevent or delay kidney failure in people with diabetes.

- In the future, insulin may be administered through nasal sprays or taken in the form of a pill.
- Devices to read blood glucose levels without having to prick a finger to get the blood sample are also being developed.

Researchers continue to look for the exact cause of diabetes and methods to prevent and cure diabetes mellitus. Some genetic markers for IDDM have been identified and it is now possible to screen relatives of people with IDDM to see if they are at risk for diabetes. Studies are now under way using drugs that stop the immune system from attacking the beta cells, to try to prevent IDDM from developing in people who are at high risk for the IDDM type of diabetes.

CAREER PROFILE

RADIOLOGIC TECHNOLOGISTS

Medical uses of radiation go far beyond the diagnosis of broken bones by x-ray. Radiation is used to produce images of the interior of the body and to treat cancer. The term "diagnostic imaging" does not only involve x-ray technique but includes ultrasound and magnetic resonance scans.

Radiographers produce x-ray films for use in diagnosing disease. They prepare the patients for procedures by explaining the process, positioning the patient, being certain to prevent unnecessary radiation exposure, and taking the picture. Experienced radiographers may perform more complex imaging tests such as fluoroscopy, operate computerized tomography scanners, and use magnetic resonance machines.

Radiation therapy technologists prepare cancer patients for treatment and administer prescribed doses of ionizing radiation to specific body parts. They check for radiation side effects.

Sonographers project non-ionizing, high frequency sound waves into specific areas of the patient's body; the equipment then collects the reflected echoes to form an image.

Education for these positions is offered in hospitals, colleges, and vocation-technical institutes. Course of study includes class and clinical practice. The Joint Review Committee on Education in Radiologic Technology accredits most formal training programs in this field. Since January 1995, thirty-one states require radiographers to be licensed and twenty-six require radiation therapists to be licensed. The job outlook in this field is expected to grow faster than average.

● REVIEW QUESTIONS

Select the letter of the choice that best completes the statement.

1. The master gland is known as:
   a. pituitary
   b. thyroid
   c. adrenal
   d. ovary

2. The hormone which is necessary to govern metabolism is:
   a. FSH
   b. MSH
   c. TSH
   d. ACTH

3. The hormones that affect neuromuscular functioning, blood clotting, and holding the cells together are:
   a. thyroxine and calcitonin
   b. thyroxine and parathormone
   c. calcitonin and thymosin
   d. calcitonin and parathormone

4. The gland that governs the production of antibodies is the:
   a. thymus
   b. thyroid
   c. parathyroid
   d. pituitary

5. The hormone that is responsible for stimulating ovulation is:
   a. TSH
   b. ICSH
   c. FSH
   d. LTH

6. The hormone that prepares us to fight or flee is:
   a. aldosterone
   b. epinephrine
   c. cortisol
   d. corticoid

7. The secretions of the ovaries are:
   a. estrogen and LTH
   b. estrogen and LH
   c. progesterone and LTH
   d. progesterone and estrogen

8. A decrease in the production of insulin causes:
   a. diabetes mellitus
   b. diabetes insipidus
   c. cretinism
   d. exophthalmos

9. A hypofunction of the thyroid gland causes:
    a. exophthalmos
    b. glycosuria
    c. cretinism
    d. Graves disease

10. An over secretion of the adrenal cortex is known as:
    a. myxedema
    b. Cushing's syndrome
    c. Addison's disease
    d. dwarfism

● COMPLETION

Complete the following chart.

GLAND	HORMONE	NORMAL FUNCTION	DISORDERS
Pituitary			
Pineal			
Thyroid			
Parathyroid			
Thymus			
Adrenals			
Gonads			
Pancreas			

● MATCHING

Match each term in Column I with its correct description in Column II.

Column I	Column II
_____ 1. ACTH	a. master gland of the endocrine system
_____ 2. adrenals	b. any gland of internal secretion
_____ 3. cortisone	c. a hormone secreted by adrenals
_____ 4. gonad	d. regulates use of calcium
_____ 5. endocrine	e. the secretion of any endocrine gland
_____ 6. hormone	f. helps body meet emergencies
_____ 7. insulin	g. sex gland
_____ 8. parathyroid	h. regulates body metabolism
_____ 9. pituitary	i. one of the hormones secreted by pituitary gland
_____ 10. thyroid	j. a hormone which regulates carbohydrates and metabolism
	k. hypofunction of endocrine glands

● APPLYING THEORY TO PRACTICE

1. You have a thermostat in your house which regulates the heat or the air conditioner. When a certain temperature is reached, it automatically shuts off. This principle applies also to negative feedback in hormonal control. Explain how this functions in relation to the thyroid gland.

2. A patient comes to the doctor's office and tells the doctor she is experiencing leg cramping, which she has heard has to do with calcium. Explain to the patient how calcium is affected by the action of the thyroid gland and parathyroid.

3. When you arrive at your office in the health maintenance organization, a patient calls out to you. He is near hysteria; he tells you he is experiencing heart palpitations and feels he is "jumping out of his skin." You check the records and note this patient has been on thyroid medication. Explain to the patient what you think may be the cause of his symptoms and what action should be taken.

4. Your brother wants to be a football player. He is 5'7"; he heard "steroids" could help him. Explain the action of steroids and why they should not be used.

5. Remember a time when you were frightened; think about it. How did your body react?

6. Diabetes mellitus affects one in ten Americans. You have to do a presentation to the class. Explain diabetes: its causes, treatments, signs of insulin shock (hypoglycemia), diabetic coma (hyperglycemia), diet, and the research currently being conducted.

CHAPTER

12

Blood

KEY WORDS

abscess	fibrin	pathogenic
agranulocyte	fibrinogen	pernicious anemia
albumin	gamma globulin	phagocytosis
anemia	globin	plasma
antibody	globulin	polycythemia
anticoagulant	granulocyte	polymorphonuclear
antigen	hematoma	leukocyte
antiprothrombin	heme	prothrombin
(heparin)	hemoglobin	pus
antithromboplastin	hemolysis	pyrexia
aplastic anemia	hemophilia	Rh factor
B-lymphocyte	inflammation	RHO Gam
basophil	iron-deficiency	sedimentation rate
clotting time	anemia	septicemia
coagulation	leukemia	sickle cell anemia
Cooley's anemia	leukocyte	T-lymphocyte
diapedesis	leukocytosis	thrombin
edema	leukopenia	thrombocyte
embolism	lymphocyte	thrombocytopenia
eosinophil	macrophage	thromboplastin
erythrocyte	monocyte	thrombosis
erythroblastosis	myeloblast	thrombus
fetalis	neutrophil	universal donor
erythropoiesis	oxyhemoglobin	universal recipient

The average adult has eight to ten pints of blood in his or her body. Loss of more than two pints at any one time leads to a serious condition.

FUNCTION OF BLOOD

Blood is the transporting fluid of the body. It carries nutrients from the digestive tract to the cells, oxygen from the lungs to the cells, waste products from the cells to the various organs of excretion, and hormones from secreting cells to other parts of the body. It aids in the distribution of heat formed in the more active tissues (such as the skeletal muscles) to all parts of the body. Blood also helps to regulate the acid-base balance and to protect against infection. Consequently, it is a vital fluid to our life and health. See Table 12-1.

BLOOD COMPOSITION

Blood is made up of these major components:

- **Plasma**, the liquid portion of blood without its cellular elements. Serum is the name given to plasma after a blood clot is formed. Serum=plasma−(fibrinogen+prothrombin).

- *Cellular elements* which include *erythrocytes*, or red blood cells (RBC's), *leukocytes*, or white blood cells (WBC's), and *thrombocytes* (*platelets*), Figure 12-1.

BLOOD PLASMA

Plasma is a straw colored, complex liquid, comprising about 55% of the blood volume and containing the following seven substances in solution:

1. *Water*—Water makes up about 92% of the total volume of plasma. This percentage is maintained by the kidneys and by water intake and output.

2. *Blood proteins*—There is a protein found in *red blood cells* known as *hemoglobin*, which comprises about two-thirds of the blood proteins.

TABLE 12-1 • *Summary of the Various Functions of Blood*

FUNCTION	EFFECT ON BODY
Nutritive	Transporting nutrient molecules (glucose, amino acids, fatty acids, and glycerol) from the small intestine or storage sites to the tissues.
Respiratory	Transporting oxygen from the lungs to the tissues and carbon dioxide from the tissue to the lungs.
Excretory	Transporting waste products (lactic acid, urea, and creatinine) from the cells to the excretory organs.
Regulatory	Transporting hormones and other chemical substances that control the proper functioning of many organs.
	Circulating excess heat to the body surfaces and to the lungs, through which it is lost (controls body temperature).
	Maintains water balance and a constant environment for tissue cells.
Protective	Circulating antibodies and defensive cells throughout the body to combat infection and disease.

3. *Plasma proteins*—These three proteins are the most abundant of those found in plasma: fibrinogen, serum albumin, and serum globulin.

   a. **Fibrinogen** is necessary for blood clotting. Without fibrinogen, the slightest cut or wound would bleed profusely. It is synthesized in the liver.

   b. **Albumin** is the most abundant of all the plasma proteins. Another product of the liver, albumin helps to maintain the blood's osmotic pressure and volume. It provides the "pulse pressure" needed to hold and pull water from the tissue fluid back into the blood vessels. Normally, plasma proteins do

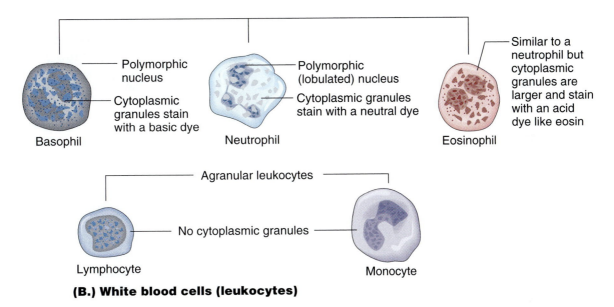

(A.) Red blood cells (erythrocytes)

Front view

Side view — Biconcave on both sides

Basophil — Polymorphic nucleus / Cytoplasmic granules stain with a basic dye

Neutrophil — Polymorphic (lobulated) nucleus / Cytoplasmic granules stain with a neutral dye

Eosinophil — Similar to a neutrophil but cytoplasmic granules are larger and stain with an acid dye like eosin

Agranular leukocytes

Lymphocyte — No cytoplasmic granules — Monocyte

(B.) White blood cells (leukocytes)

FIGURE 12-1 *Cellular elements of the blood*

not pass through the capillary walls, since their molecules are relatively large. They are colloidal substances; they can give up, or take up, water-soluble substances thus regulating the osmotic pressure within the blood vessels.

c. **Globulin** is formed not only in the liver, but also in the lymphatic system (discussed in Chapter 15). **Gamma globulin** has been fractionated (separated) from globulin. This portion helps in the synthesis of antibodies, which destroy or render harmless various disease-causing organisms. **Prothrombin** is yet another globulin, formed continually in the liver, which helps blood to coagulate. Vitamin K is necessary in aiding the process of prothrombin synthesis.

4. *Nutrients*—Nutrient molecules are absorbed from the digestive tract. Glucose, fatty acids, cholesterol, and amino acids are dissolved in the blood plasma.

5. *Electrolytes*—The most abundant electrolytes are sodium chloride and potassium. These come from foods and chemical processes occurring in the body.

6. *Hormones, vitamins, and enzymes*—These three substances are found in very small amounts in the blood plasma. They generally help the body to control its chemical reactions.

7. *Metabolic waste products*—All of the body's cells are actively engaged in chemical reactions to maintain homeostasis. As a result of this, waste products are formed and subsequently carried by the plasma to the various excretory organs.

RED BLOOD CELLS

Red blood cells (RBC's), or erythrocytes, are biconcave, disc-shaped cells. They are caved in on both sides, with a thin center and thicker margins. When viewed from above, they appear to have a doughnut shape, see Figure 12-1.

Hemoglobin

Erythrocytes contain a red pigment(coloring agent) called hemoglobin, which provides its characteristic color. Hemoglobin is composed of a protein molecule called globin and an iron compound called heme. A single blood cell contains several million molecules of hemoglobin. Hemoglobin is vital to the function of the red blood cell, helping it to transport oxygen to the tissues and some carbon dioxide away from the tissues. Normal hemoglobin count for men is 14-18 gm and for women is 12-16 gm per 100cc.

Function

In the capillaries of the lung, erythrocytes pick up oxygen from the inspired air. The oxygen chemically combines with the hemoglobin, forming the compound oxyhemoglobin. The oxyhemoglobin-laden erythrocytes circulate to the capillaries of tissues. Here oxygen is released to the tissues. The carbon dioxide that is formed is picked up by the plasma as a bicarbonate; and it is known as carbaminohemoglobin. The red blood cells circulate back to the lungs to give up the carbon dioxide and absorb more oxygen. Arteries carry blood away from the heart and veins carry blood towards the

heart, but there are exceptions. Blood cells that travel in the arteries (except for pulmonary arteries) carry oxyhemoglobin, which gives blood its bright red color. Blood cells in the veins (except for pulmonary veins) contain carbaminohemoglobin, which is responsible for the dark, crimson-blue color characteristic of venous blood.

Carbon monoxide (CO) poisoning is a serious and sometimes fatal condition. Carbon monoxide is an odorless gas present in the exhaust of gasoline engines. Carbon monoxide rapidly combines with hemoglobin; and binds at the same site on the hemoglobin molecule as oxygen and crowds it out. The cells are deprived of their oxygen supply. Symptoms which may occur are headache, dizziness, drowsiness, and unconsciousness. Death may occur in severe cases of carbon monoxide poisoning. It is important to remember that carbon monoxide gas is odorless. Carbon monoxide is also present in the flue gases of furnaces and gas or oil-fired space heaters. Damaged or improperly-installed furnaces and heaters, as well as plugged or defective chimneys and vents can bring carbon monoxide into the home. Always be certain to allow for proper ventilation of home and work areas. NEVER allow a car to run in an unventilated garage. Commercial carbon monoxide detectors are now available for home use.

Erythropoiesis

Erythropoiesis, or the manufacture of red blood cells, occurs in the red bone marrow of essentially all bones, until adolescence. (In the fetus, red blood cells are also produced by the spleen and liver.) As one grows older, the red marrow of the long bones is replaced by fat marrow; erythrocytes are thereafter formed only in the short and flat bones.

Erythrocytes come from stem cells in the red bone marrow called hemocytosblasts. (See Figure 12-1.) As the hemocytoblast matures into an erythrocyte, it loses its nucleus and cytoplasmic organelles. The hemocytoblast also becomes smaller, gains hemoglobin, develops a biconcave shape, and enters into the bloodstream. To aid in erythropoiesis, vitamin B_{12}, folic acid, copper, cobalt, iron, and proteins are needed.

Since erythrocytes are enucleated (contain no nucleus), they only live about 120 days. Destruction occurs as the cells age, rendering them more vulnerable to rupturing. They are broken down by the spleen and liver. Hemoglobin breaks down into globin and heme; the iron content of heme is used to make new red blood cells. The normal count of red blood cells ranges from 4.5 to 6.2 million/µl venous blood for men and 4.2 to 5.4 million/µl venous blood for women.

Hemolysis

A rupture or bursting of the red blood cell (erythrocyte) is called **hemolysis**. This sometimes occurs as a result of a blood transfusion reaction or other disease processes.

WHITE BLOOD CELLS

White blood cells (WBC's) are known as **leukocytes**. They are larger than the erythrocytes, ranging from one and one quarter to two times their diameter. They are granular or agranular, translucent, and ameboid in shape. Leukocytes are manufactured in both red bone marrow and in lymphatic tissue.

Types of Leukocytes

Leukocytes are classified into two major groups of cells: the **granulocytes** (**granular leukocytes**) and the **agranulocytes** (**agranular leukocytes**). This classification is due to the presence of cytoplasmic granules, nuclear structure, and reactions to stains like Wright's stain. Granulocytes are synthesized in red bone marrow from cells called **myeloblasts**. Granulocytes are destroyed as they age and as a result of participating in bacterial destruction. The life-span of white blood cells is variable, but most granulocytes live only a few days.

There are three types of granulocytes: neutrophils, eosinophils, and basophils.

Neutrophils, also called **polymorphonuclear leukocytes**, phagocytize bacteria with lysosomal enzymes. (**Phagocytosis** is a process that surrounds, engulfs and digests harmful bacteria.) **Eosinophils** phagocytize the remains of antibody-antigen reactions. They also increase in great numbers in allergic conditions, malaria, and in worm infestations. **Basophils** perform phagocytosis, and their count increases during chronic inflammation and during the healing from an infection. Basophils produce *histamine*, a vasodilator, and *heparin*, an anticoagulant.

Agranulocytes are divided into lymphocytes and monocytes. **Lymphocytes** are further subdivided into **B-lymphocytes**, which are synthesized in the bone marrow, and **T-lymphocytes** from the thymus gland. Still others are formed by the lymph nodes and spleen. Their life-span ranges from a few days to several years. They basically help the body by synthesizing and releasing antibody molecules and by protecting against the formation of cancer cells.

Monocytes are formed in bone marrow and the spleen. They assist in phagocytosis, and are able to leave the bloodstream to attach themselves to tissues; here they become tissue **macrophages**, or histiocytes. During an inflammation, histiocytes help to wall off and isolate the infected area.

The aforementioned types of leukocytes (basophils, neutrophils, eosinophils, and monocytes) which can perform phagocytosis are called phagocytes. Unlike erythrocytes, they can move through the intercellular spaces of the capillary wall into neighboring tissue. This process is known as **diapedesis**.

A normal leukocyte count averages from 3,200 to 9,800/µl.

To summarize, leukocytes help protect the body against infection and injury. This is achieved through: (1) phagocytosis and destruction of bacteria, (2) synthesis of antibody molecules, (3) "cleaning up" of cellular remnants at the site of inflammation, and (4) the walling off of the infected area. See Tables 12-2 and 12-3.

TABLE 12-2 • *The Different Types of Leukocytes and Their Sizes*

MAJOR TYPES OF LEUKOCYTES	SPECIFIC KINDS OF LEUKOCYTES	SIZE
Granulocytes 60-70%	Neutrophils	9-12 mu
	Eosinophils	10-14 mu
	Basophils	8-10 mu
Agranulocytes Lymphocytes 20-30%	Small	7-10 mu
	Large	up to 20 mu
Monocyte 5-8%	Mononuclear	9-12 mu
	Transitional	9-12 mu

TABLE 12-3 • *Characteristics and Functions of the Leukocytes*

LEUKOCYTE	WHERE FORMED	TYPE OF NUCLEUS	CYTOPLASM	FUNCTION
Agranular leukocytes 1. Lymphocyte	Lymph glands and nodes, bone marrow, spleen	One large, spherical nucleus; may be indented Sharply defined and stains dark blue	Cytoplasm stains a pale blue and contains scattered violet granules	Helps to form antibodies at a site of inflammation; protects against cancer
2. Monocyte (macrophage)	Lymph glands and nodes, bone marrow, spleen	One lobulated or horseshoe-shaped nucleus that stains blue	Abundant cytoplasm that stains a gray-blue	Phagocytosis of cellular debris and foreign particles
Granular leukocytes 1. Neutrophil	Formed in bone marrow from neutrophilic myelocytes	Lobulated: contains 1 to 5 or more lobes, stains deep blue	Cytoplasm has a pink tinge with very fine granules.	Displays marked phagocytosis toward bacteria during infections and inflammations. Contributes to pus formation.
2. Eosinophil	Formed in bone marrow from eosinophilic myelocytes	Irregularly shaped with 2 lobes, stains blue, but less deeply than neutrophils	Cytoplasm has a sky-blue tinge with many coarse, uniform, round or oval bright-red granules.	Marked increase during parasitic, worm infections and allergic attacks.
3. Basophil (mast cell)	Formed in bone marrow from basophilic myelocytes	Centrally located, slightly lobulated nucleus, stains a light purple and hidden by granules	Cytoplasm has a mauve color with many large deep-purple granules.	Phagocytosis; releases heparin and histamine and promotes the inflammatory response.

INFLAMMATION

If living tissue is damaged in any way, the body usually responds to the damage by either neutralizing or eliminating the cause of the damage. When this happens, the damaged body part goes through an inflammation process. Inflammation occurs when tissues are subjected to chemical or physical trauma (cut or heat). Invasion by pathogenic (disease-causing) microorganisms like bacteria, fungi, protozoa, and viruses also can cause inflammation.

The characteristic symptoms of inflammation are redness, local heat, swelling, and pain. This is due to irritation by bacterial toxins, to increased blood flow, to congestion of blood vessels, and to the collection of blood plasma in the surrounding tissues (edema). Histamine released from the basophil and other chemical substances increase blood flow to the injured area as well as increasing capillary permeability. Thus, large amounts of blood plasma and fibrinogen enter the damaged area. The damaged area is walled off as a result of the clotting action of fibrinogen on the damaged tissue and macrophage action.

Neutrophils move very quickly to the damaged area. The neutrophils move through the capillary walls by diapedesis and begin phagocytosis of the pathogenic microorganisms. Macrophages also participate in phagocytosis.

In most inflammations, a cream-colored liquid called pus forms. Pus is a combination of dead tissue, dead and living bacteria, dead leukocytes, and blood plasma. If the damaged area is below the epidermis, an abscess (pus-filled cavity) forms. If it is on the skin or a mucosal surface, it is called an ulcer. In many inflammations, chemical substances called pyrogens are formed, which are circulated to the hypothalamus. In the hypothalamus, the pyrogens affect the temperature-control center, which raises the body's temperature causing fever or pyrexia.

In inflammation, there is an increased production of neutrophils by bone marrow. If the white blood cell count exceeds 10,000 cells/µl, a condition called leukocytosis exists. Following healing, the leukocyte count returns to normal. Sometimes, a decrease in the number of white blood cells occurs. This is called leukopenia. Leukopenia can be caused by taking marrow-depressant drugs, by pathologic conditions, or by radiation.

THROMBOCYTES (BLOOD PLATELETS)

Thrombocytes are the smallest of the solid components of blood. They are ovoid-shaped structures, synthesized from the larger megakaryocytes in red bone marrow. Thrombocytes are not cells but fragments of the megakaryocytes cytoplasm, see Figure 12-1.

The normal blood platelet count ranges from 250,000 to 450,000 per cubic millimeter of blood. Platelets function in the initiation of the blood-clotting process. When a blood vessel is damaged, as in a cut or wound, the vessel's collagen fibers come into contact with the platelets. The platelets are then stimulated to produce sticky projecting structures, allowing them to stick to the collagen fibers. This reaction occurs countless times, creating a "platelet plug" to stop the bleeding. The platelets secrete a chemical called *serotin* which causes the blood vessel to spasm and narrow and a decrease in blood loss until the clot forms. Subsequently, the blood clotting process follows to "harden" the platelet plug. Old platelets eventually disintegrate in the bone marrow.

Coagulation

Blood clotting or coagulation is a complicated and essential process which depends in large part on thrombocytes. When a cut or other injury ruptures a blood vessel, clotting must occur to stop the bleeding.

Although the exact details of this process are not clear, there is a general agreement that the following reaction occurs. Whenever a blood vessel or tissue is injured, platelets and injured tissue release thromboplastin. An injury to a blood vessel makes the lining rough; as blood platelets flow over the roughened area, they disintegrate, releasing thromboplastin.

Thromboplastin is a complex substance that can only cause coagulation if calcium ions and prothrombin are present. Prothrombin is a plasma protein synthesized in the liver.

The thromboplastin and calcium ions act as enzymes in a reaction that converts prothrombin into thrombin. This reaction occurs only in the presence of bleeding, because normally there is no thrombin in the blood plasma.

In the next stage of coagulation, the thrombin just formed acts as an enzyme, changing fibrinogen (a plasma protein) into fibrin. These gel-like fibrin threads layer themselves over the cut, creating a fine, meshlike network. This fibrin network entraps the red blood cells, platelets, and plasma, creating a blood clot. At first, *serum* (a pale yellow fluid) oozes out of the cut. As the serum slowly dries, a crust (scab) forms over the fibrin threads, completing the common clotting process.

In order for coagulation to occur successfully, two anticoagulants (substances preventing coagulation) must be neutralized. These are called antithromboplastin and antiprothrombin (heparin); they are neutralized by thromboplastin.

Prothrombin is dependent on vitamin K. Vitamin K is manufactured in the body by a type of bacteria found in the intestines. See Table 12-4 for a summary of the coagulation process. It is important to note that prothrombin and fibrinogen are plasma proteins which are manufactured in the liver; therefore serious liver disease may interfere with the blood clotting process.

Clotting Time. The time it takes for blood to clot is known as its clotting time. The clotting time for humans is from five to fifteen minutes. This information is quite useful prior to surgery.

TABLE 12-4 • *Blood Clotting Process*

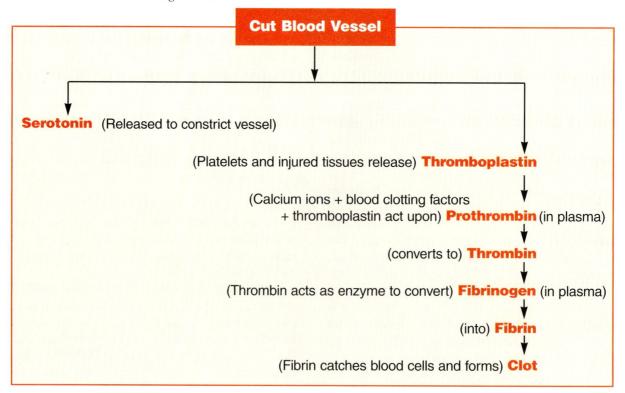

Cut Blood Vessel

Serotonin (Released to constrict vessel)

(Platelets and injured tissues release) **Thromboplastin**

(Calcium ions + blood clotting factors + thromboplastin act upon) **Prothrombin** (in plasma)

(converts to) **Thrombin**

(Thrombin acts as enzyme to convert) **Fibrinogen** (in plasma)

(into) **Fibrin**

(Fibrin catches blood cells and forms) **Clot**

BLOOD TYPES

There are four major groups, or types of blood: A, B, AB, and O. Blood type is inherited from one's parents. It is determined by the presence—or absence—of the blood protein called agglutinogen or **antigen**, on the surface of the *red blood cell*. People with type A blood have the A antigen on their red blood cells; type B blood has the type B antigen; type AB has both A and B antigen; and type O has *neither* of the antigens.

There is a protein present in the *plasma* known as agglutinin or **antibody**. An individual with type A blood has *b* antibodies in the blood plasma. Type B blood possesses *a* antibodies; type O contains *both a* and *b* antibodies; and type AB contains *no* antibodies.

Knowledge of one's correct type is important in cases of blood transfusions and surgery. A test known as type and cross match is done before receiving a blood transfusion. This determines the blood type of both recipient and donor. Antibodies react with the antigens of the same type, causing the red blood cells to clump together. The clumping of blood, a process known as agglulation, clogs up the blood vessels, impeding circulation, thus causing death.

By way of example, if a person with type A blood needs a transfusion, he *must receive only type A blood*. Should he receive type B, the B antigens of the type B blood would clump with the b antibodies of the person's type A blood. This would prove fatal! In an emergency, persons with type A blood can receive both types A and O blood. How is this possible? Because the red blood cells of type O contain no A or B antigens. Therefore they may not clump with the b antibodies of type A nor the a antibodies of type B. Thus blood type O can be donated to all four blood types, for which reason it is known as the **universal donor**. This is only done in an emergency situation.

Conversely, type AB, having no antibodies in its plasma, can receive all four blood types. The reason is that, lacking antibodies, AB cannot agglutinate the red blood cells of any donor. It is thus called the **universal recipient**. This is only done in emergency situations. Blood should always be given to same type to avoid serious reactions. Table 12-5 provides a summary of pertinent facts about blood types.

Rh FACTOR

Human red blood cells, in addition to containing antigens A and B, also contain the Rh antigen. We know it as the **Rh factor** since it was found in the Rhesus monkey. The Rh factor is found on the surface of red blood cells.

TABLE 12-5 ● *Blood Types*

BLOOD TYPE	PERCENT OF US POPULATION	ANTIGEN ON RED BLOOD CELLS	ANTIBODY IN PLASMA	CAN RECEIVE	CAN DONATE TO
A	41%	A	b	A or O only	A or AB only
B	12%	B	a	B or O only	B or AB only
AB	3%	A and B	none	A, B, AB, O (universal recipient)	AB only
O	44%	None	a and b	O only	A, B, AB, O (universal donor)

People possessing the Rh factor are said to be Rh positive (Rh+). Those without the Rh factor are Rh negative (Rh-).

About 85% of North Americans are Rh positive and 15% are Rh negative. Neither Rh negative nor Rh positive blood contains antibodies, or agglutinins in its plasma. However, if an Rh negative individual receives a transfusion of Rh positive blood, he or she will develop antibodies to it. The antibodies take two weeks to develop. Generally there is no problem with the first transfusion. But, if a second transfusion of Rh positive blood is given, the accumulated Rh antibodies will clump with the Rh antigen (agglutinogen) of the blood being received. So, both blood type and Rh factor must be taken into account for safe and successful transfusions.

The same problem arises when an Rh negative mother is pregnant with an Rh positive fetus. The mother's blood can develop anti-Rh antibodies to the fetus' Rh antigens. The first-born child will normally suffer no harmful effects. However, subsequent pregnancies will be affected, because the mother's accumulated anti-Rh antibodies will clump the baby's red blood cells. If the condition is left untreated, the baby will usually be born with the condition known as **erythroblastosis fetalis** (hemolytic disease of newborn). This condition is rare today because of the use of the drug **RHO Gam**, which is special preparation of immune globulin. RHO Gam is given to the Rh negative (Rh-) mother within seventy-two hours after delivery. (Some doctors also give this drug during the last trimester of pregnancy.) The antibodies in the RHO Gam will destroy any Rh positive (Rh+) cells of the baby's which may have entered the mother's bloodstream; therefore, the mother's immune system will not be stimulated to produce antibodies.

A&P CHALLENGE BLOOD NORMS

Tests have been devised to use physiological blood norms in diagnosing and following the course of certain diseases. Some of these norms are listed in Table 12-6.

Patients who are taking anticoagulant medications to prolong the clotting time of their blood must have prothrombin time (PT) and a partial thromboplastin test (PTT) done frequently. The dosage of their medication is based on their clotting times.

Sedimentation rate is the time required for erythrocytes to settle to the bottom of an upright tube at room temperature. It indicates whether disease is present and is very valuable in observing the progression of inflammatory conditions.

VENIPUNCTURE BY SYRINGE PROCEDURE

The purpose of this procedure is to obtain venous blood acceptable for laboratory testing when it is required by the physician. The following supplies are required to properly perform this procedure:

- gloves
- safety glasses and mask
- a syringe
- a disposable 21 or 22 gauge needle for the syringe

TABLE 12-6 • *Blood Tests*

TEST	NORMAL RANGE
Bleeding time	1 to 3 minutes
Coagulation time	5 to 15 minutes
Hemoglobin count	Men: 14 to 18 gm/dl Women: 12-16 gm/dl
Platelet count	150,000 to 350,000/mm^3
Prothrombin time (quick)	9.5 to 11 seconds
Sedimentation rate (Westergren) in first hour	Men: 0 to 10 mm/hour Women: 0 to 20 mm/hour
Red blood cell count	Men: 4.5 to 6.2 million/µl Women: 4.2 to 5.4 million/µl
White blood cell count	3,200 to 9,800/µl
Cholesterol level	below 200 mg/dl

- evacuated tube(s) or special collection tube(s)
- a tourniquet
- a 70% isopropyl alcohol swab
- gauze or cotton balls
- adhesive bandage or tape
- sharps container

Procedure Steps

1. Position and identify the patient. Ask the patient's name and verify it with the computer label or identification number.

2. If a fasting specimen is required, verify that the patient has not had anything to eat or drink.

3. Wash hands.

4. Put on gloves, goggles, and mask if there is a potential for blood splatter.

5. Open the sterile needle and syringe packages, attaching the needle if necessary.

6. Prevent the plunger from sticking by pulling it halfway out and pushing it all the way in one time.

7. Select the proper tube(s) to transfer the blood to after collection.

8. Find the vein and apply the tourniquet, Figure 12-2a.

9. Ask the patient to close the hand. The patient must not be allowed to pump the hand. Pumping of the hand will change the values of the laboratory tests being collected. Place the patient's arm in a downward position if possible.

10. Select a vein, noting the location and direction of the vein.

11. Clean the venipuncture site with a 70% isopropyl alcohol swab in a circular motion from the center outward, Figure 12-2b.

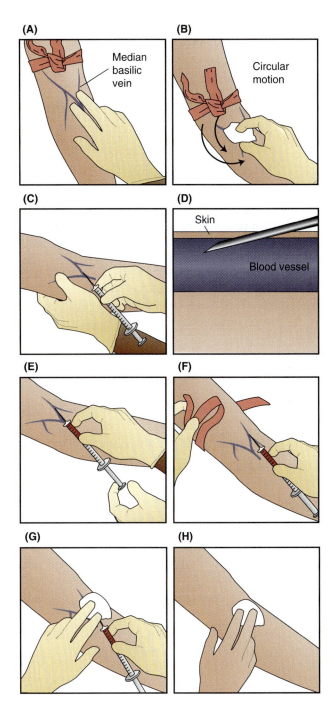

FIGURE 12-2 *(a) Find vein and apply tourniquet, (b) Apply alcohol and allow to air dry, (c) Draw skin taut and insert needle, (d) Needle entering the blood vessel, (e) Withdraw blood slowly, (f) Release tourniquet, (g) Apply sterile pad before withdrawing needle, (h) Have patient apply pressure and flex the arm at elbow until clot forms.*

12. Do not touch the venipuncture site.

13. Draw the patient's skin taut with your thumb. Place the thumb 1 to 2″ below the puncture site, Figure 12-2c.

14. With the bevel up, line up the needle with the vein and perform the venipuncture, (Figure 12-2d).

15. Do not enter at the exact location at which the vein is felt. Enter the vein approximately ¼″ below the vein location. The bevel of the needle must enter the skin at the point where the vein was palpated. Push the needle into the skin. A sensation of resistance will be followed by easy penetration as the vein is entered. This is known as feeling the "pop." Once this point is reached, stop and do not move.

16. Take the opposite hand and pull on the plunger of the syringe. Pull gently and only as fast as the syringe will fill with blood. Pulling too hard or fast will cause temporary collapse of the vein. If the vein does collapse, stop pulling on the plunger and let the vein refill with blood, Figure 12-2e.

17. Pull the plunger back until the desired amount of blood has been obtained.

18. Ask the patient to open the hand.

19. Release the tourniquet, Figure 12-2f.

20. Lightly place a sterile gauze square or cotton ball above the venipuncture site.

21. Remove the needle from the arm, Figure 12-2g.

22. Apply pressure to the site for three to five minutes. The patient may assist if able by elevating the arm above heart level, Figure 12-2h.

23. Eject blood into appropriate tube(s). Puncture the stopper of the evacuated tube with the syringe needle and allow the blood to enter the tube until the flow stops. Mix if any anticoagulant is present.

24. Immediately discard the syringe and needle in the appropriate containers; e.g., needle to sharps container.

25. Discard the gauze and other waste in biohazard containers.

26. Label all tubes before leaving the examination room.

27. Apply an adhesive bandage.

28. Remove and discard gloves, goggles, and mask in a biohazard container.

29. Wash hands.

30. Document procedure.

VENIPUNCTURE BY EVACUATED TUBE SYSTEM

The purpose of this procedure is to obtain venous blood acceptable for laboratory testing when it is required by the physician. The venous blood is collected by evacuated tubes; the volume of blood collected is dependent on the size of the tube used and the test requirements. The following supplies are required to properly perform this procedure:

- gloves
- goggles and a mask
- an evacuated tube holder
- a tourniquet
- a 70% isopropyl alcohol swab
- a 20, 21, or 22 gauge disposable needle for evacuated system
- evacuated tube(s) or special collection tube(s)
- gauze or cotton balls
- adhesive bandage or tape
- sharps container

Procedure Steps

1. Position and identify the patient. Ask the patient's name and verify it with the computer label or identification number.

2. If a fasting specimen is required, verify that the patient has not had anything to eat or drink.

3. Wash hands.

4. Put on gloves, and goggles and mask if there is a potential for blood splatter.

5. Assemble equipment.

6. Break the needle seal. Thread the appropriate needle into the holder using the needle sheath as a wrench.

7. Before using, tap all tubes that contain additives to ensure that all the additive is dislodged from the stopper and wall of the tube.

8. Insert the tube into the holder until the needle slightly enters the stopper. Avoid pushing the needle beyond the recessed guideline, because a loss of vacuum may result. If the tube retracts slightly, leave it in the retracted position to avoid prematurely puncturing the rubber stopper.

9. Apply the tourniquet.

10. Ask the patient to close the hand. The patient must not be allowed to pump the hand. Pumping the hand will change the values of the laboratory tests being drawn. If possible, place the patient's arm in a downward position.

11. Select a vein, noting the location and direction of the vein.

12. Clean the venipuncture site with a 70% isopropyl alcohol swab.

13. Do not touch the venipuncture site.

14. Draw the patient's skin taut with your thumb. Place the thumb 1 to 2" below the puncture site, Figure 12-3.

15. With the bevel up, line up the needle with the vein and puncture the vein. Remove your hand from drawing the skin taut. Grasp the flange of the evacuated tube holder and push the tube forward until the butt end of the needle punctures the stopper. Do not change hands while performing the venipuncture. The hand performing the venipuncture is the hand that holds the evacuated tube holder. The opposite hand manipulates the tubes.

16. Fill the tube until the vacuum is exhausted and blood flow into the tube ceases.

This will assure the proper blood to anticoagulant ratio.

17. When the blood flow ceases, remove the tube from the holder. While securely grasping the evacuated tube holder with one hand, use the other hand to change the tubes. The shutoff valve recovers the point, stopping the flow of blood until the next tube of blood is inserted.

18. After drawing, immediately mix each tube that contains an additive. Gently inverting the tube five to ten times provides adequate mixing without causing hemolysis.

19. Ask the patient to open the hand.

20. Release the tourniquet.

21. Lightly place a sterile gauze square or cotton ball above the venipuncture site.

22. Remove the needle from the arm. Be certain the last tube drawn has been removed from the holder before removing

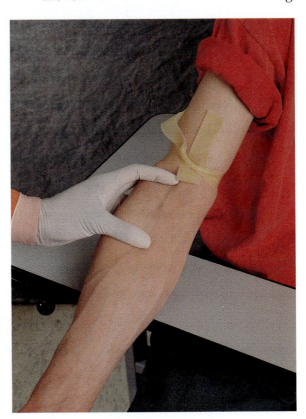

FIGURE 12-3 *Pull the skin taut to prevent vein roll.*

the needle. This prevents blood dripping off the tip of the needle.

23. Apply pressure to the site for three to five minutes. The patient may assist if able by elevating the arm above heart level to reduce blood flow.

24. Label all tubes at the patient's side before leaving the examination room.

25. Apply an adhesive bandage.

26. Remove and discard gloves, goggles, and mask in a biohazard container.

27. Wash hands.

28. Document procedure.

DISORDERS OF THE BLOOD

Anemia is a deficiency in the number and/or percentage of red blood cells and the amount of hemoglobin in the blood. Anemia results from a large or chronic loss of blood (hemorrhage) which decreases the number of erythrocytes. Extreme erythrocyte destruction and malformation of the hemoglobin of red blood cells also causes this condition. Since there is always some hemoglobin deficiency, there is never enough oxygen transported to the cells of cellular oxidation. Consequently, not enough energy is being released. Anemia is characterized by varying degrees of dyspnea, pallor, palpitation, and fatigue.

Iron-deficiency anemia is a condition that often exists in women, children, and adolescents. It is caused by a deficiency of adequate amounts of iron in the diet. This leads to insufficient hemoglobin synthesis in the red blood cells. The condition is easily alleviated by ingestion of iron supplements and green, leafy vegetables that contain the mineral iron.

Pernicious anemia is a form of anemia caused by a deficiency of Vitamin B_{12} and/or lack of the intrinsic factor. The intrinsic factor produced by the stomach mucosa is necessary for the absorption and utilization of Vitamin B_{12}. Vitamin B_{12} and folic acid are necessary for the development of mature red blood cells. Symptoms such as dyspnea, pallor, and fatigue are present as well as specific neurologic changes. Foods that contain Vitamin B_{12} are animal proteins such as liver and organ meats. Treatment for pernicious anemia involves injections of Vitamin B_{12}.

Aplastic anemia is a disease caused by the suppression of the bone marrow chemical agents, certain drugs, or radiation therapy. In this condition, bone marrow does not produce enough red blood cells and white blood cells. Treatment consists of removal of the toxic substances or discontinuing the drugs and radia-

MEDICAL HIGHLIGHT: TECHNOLOGY

Uses for Newborn's Umbilical or Cord Blood

The blood found in the umbilical cord contains the same immunity-producing stem cells found in the bone marrow and is far easier to transplant. While bone marrow transplants require an almost exact match, cord blood stem cells are too young and the brand new donor has not yet developed antibodies that turn against the recipient. At this time, these transplants are highly experimental and have been used mainly in children. Proponents of this treatment say it will give a new chance for life to people with some forms of leukemia, anemia, Hodgkin's disease, and other conditions.

MEDICAL HIGHLIGHT: TREATMENT

Drug Treatment for Sickle Cell Anemia

One of the most severe problems related to sickle cell anemia is that the rigid sickle red blood cells clog the blood vessels, causing vaso-occlusion and painful episodes. Daily administration of the drug *hydroxyurea* reduced the painful episodes by about 50%. However, this drug may not be appropriate for some patients with sickle cell anemia. It is a cytotoxic agent and has the potential to cause life threatening *cytopenia* (a decrease in the number of cells). Hydroxyurea is a treatment, not a cure, and positive results will only occur as long as the patient takes the prescribed dose. The FDA has not given its full approval for the drug at this time; however, the results were so promising after the initial trials that doctors were permitted to prescribe hydroxyurea for patients with sickle cell anemia.

tion. In severe conditions, a bone marrow transplant may be performed.

Sickle cell anemia is a chronic blood disease inherited from both parents. The disease causes red blood cells to form in the abnormal crescent shape. These cells carry less oxygen and break easily, causing anemia. The sickling trait, a less serious disease, occurs with inheritance from only one parent. Sickle cell anemia occurs almost exclusively among Blacks. Treatment of sickle cell anemia consists of the affected person receiving blood transfusions when necessary. Drug therapy and bone marrow transplants are being considered as treatment.

Cooley's anemia, also known as thalassemia major, is a blood disease caused by a defect in hemoglobin formation. It affects people of Mediterranean descent.

Polycythemia is a condition in which too many red blood cells are formed. This may be a temporary condition which occurs at high altitudes because there is less oxygen present. The disease polycythemia vera, cause unknown, is a condition of too many red blood cells. The increase in the number of red blood cells causes a thickening of the blood with possible blood clot formation. Treatment for this condition is phlebotomy—removal of approximately one pint of blood or drug therapy.

Embolism is a condition where an embolus is carried by the bloodstream until it reaches an artery too small for passage. An embolus is a substance foreign to the bloodstream. It may be air, a blood clot, cancer cells, fat, bacterial clumps, a needle or even a bullet that was lodged in tissue and breaks free.

Thrombosis is the formation of a blood clot in a blood vessel. The blood clot formed is called a **thrombus**. It is caused by unusually slow blood circulation, changes in the blood or blood vessel walls, immobility, or a decrease in mobility.

Hematoma is a localized clotted mass of blood found in an organ, tissue, or space. It is caused by an injury, like a blow, that can cause a blood vessel to rupture.

Hemophilia is a hereditary disease in which the blood clots slowly or abnormally. This causes prolonged bleeding with even minor cuts and bumps. Although sex-linked hemophilia occurs mostly in males, it is transmitted genetically by females to their sons. The person with hemophilia may be treated with the missing clotting factor. The hemophiliac is taught to avoid trauma, if possible, and report promptly any bleeding, no matter how slight.

Thrombocytopenia is a blood disease in which there is a decrease in the number of platelets (thrombocytes). In this condition, blood will not clot properly.

Leukemia is a cancerous or malignant condition in which there is a great increase in the number of white blood cells. The overabundant immature leukocytes replace the erythrocytes, thus interfering with the transport of oxygen to the tissues. They can also hinder the synthesis of new red blood cells from bone marrow. The acute form of the disease, which develops quickly and runs its course rapidly, occurs most often in children and young adults. Treatment today consists of drug therapy, bone marrow transplants, and radiation therapy which has given people with leukemia remissions which may last for several years.

Septicemia describes the presence of pathogenic (disease producing) organisms or toxins in the blood.

CAREER PROFILES

CLINICAL LABORATORY TECHNOLOGISTS AND TECHNICIANS

Clinical laboratory testing plays a critical role in the detection, diagnosis, and treatment of disease. Clinical laboratory technologists and technicians, also known as medical technologists or technicians, perform most of these tests. Clinical laboratory personnel obtain, examine, and analyze body fluids, tissues, and cells. They look for microorganisms, match blood for transfusions, and test for drug levels in the blood to see how a patient is responding to treatment. The complexity of tests performed, the level of judgment required, and the amount of responsibility workers assume depend largely on the amount of education and experience they have.

Medical technologists generally have a bachelor's degree in medical technology which includes specialized courses devoted to knowledge and skills used in the clinical laboratory. As of September 1, 1997, the Clinical Laboratory Improvement Act (CLIA) will require technologists who perform certain highly complex tests to have at least an associate's degree. Medical technicians generally have an associate's degree from a community college or a certificate from a hospital, or vocational technical school.

Clinical laboratory personnel work in either hospitals or independent laboratories. Employment is expected to grow about as fast as the average employment rate.

● REVIEW QUESTIONS

Select the letter of the choice that best completes the statement.

1. Blood of the universal donor is:
   a. type B
   b. type A
   c. type AB
   d. type O

2. Blood of the universal recipient is:
   a. type B
   b. type A
   c. type AB
   d. type O

3. Negative Rh blood is found in:
   a. 5% of the population
   b. 10% of the population
   c. 15% of the population
   d. 20% of the population

4. The blood type found in the largest percent of the population is:
   a. type O
   b. type A
   c. type AB
   d. type B

5. The prothrombin in the blood-clotting process is dependent upon:
   a. vitamin A
   b. vitamin K
   c. vitamin P
   d. vitamin D

6. Which of the following is not a blood cell?
   a. erythrocyte
   b. leukocyte
   c. osteocyte
   d. monocyte

7. Erythrocytes contain all but one of the following elements:
   a. Rh factor
   b. leukocytes
   c. hemoglobin
   d. globin and heme

8. What characteristic is not true of normal thrombocytes?
   a. They average 4500 for each cubic millimeter of blood
   b. They are also called platelets
   c. They are plate-shaped cells
   d. They initiate the blood-clotting process

9. The normal leukocyte cell:
   a. can only be produced in the lymphatic tissue
   b. goes to the infection site to engulf and destroy microorganisms
   c. is too large to move through the intracellular spaces of the capillary wall
   d. exists in numbers which amount to an average of 12,000 cells per cubic millimeter of blood

10. The blood-clotting process:
   a. requires a normal platelet count which is 5000 to 9000 for each cubic millimeter of blood
   b. is delayed by the rupture of platelets which produces thromboplastin
   c. occurs in less time with persons having type O blood
   d. requires Vitamin K of the synthesis of prothrombin

● COMPLETION

Briefly answer the following questions.

1. Name the three major types of blood cells.

2. What name is given to the straw-colored liquid portion of the blood?

3. What five proteins are contained in the blood and what are their functions?

4. Describe the process of blood clot formation.

● APPLYING THEORY TO PRACTICE

1. You hear that your friend has been in a car accident and needs a blood transfusion; you want to donate blood. You friend has type O+ blood and you have A+ blood. Can your blood be given to your friend? Explain the reason for your answer.

2. Why is blood considered the "gift of life?"

3. A patient comes to the doctor's office. She is pregnant and states she is Rh negative and her husband is Rh positive. She has heard that there may be a problem with the baby. Explain to her about the Rh factor and how this situation is taken care of today.

4. In the hospital you are caring for a six-year-old girl with leukemia. The mother asks what she did that caused the disease. What will your response be?

5. You are employed as a medical technologist. A patient comes to the lab and requires a complete blood count and sedimentation rate. The patient asks you to explain these tests and what they are for.

CHAPTER

13

Heart

KEY WORDS

angina pectoris
angioplasty (balloon surgery)
aorta
aortic semilunar valve
apex
arrhythmia
ascites
atrial fibrillation
atrioventricular bundle (bundle of His)
atrioventricular node (AV)
atrium
bicuspid valve (mitral)
bradycardia
cardiac arrest
cardiopulmonary circulation
cardiopulmonary resuscitation (CPR)

cardiotonics
conduction defect
congestive heart failure
coronary by-pass
defibrillator
deoxygenated
diuretics
dyspnea
edema
electrocardiogram (ECG or EKG)
endocardium
endocarditis
fibrillation
heart block
heart failure
left ventricle
lubb dupp
mitral valve prolapse
murmur
myocardial infarction

myocarditis
myocardium
oxygenated
palpitations
pericarditis
pericardium
pulmonary artery
pulmonary semi-lunar valve
pulmonary veins
Purkinje fibers
rheumatic heart disease
right ventricle
septum
sinoatrial node (SA) (pacemaker)
systemic curation
stethoscope
tachycardia
tricuspid valve
vena cava

The circulatory system is the longest system of the body. If one were to lay all of the blood vessels in a single human body end to end, they would stretch one fourth the way from earth to the moon, a distance of some 60,000 miles.[1]

FUNCTIONS OF THE CIRCULATORY SYSTEM

1. The heart is the pump necessary to circulate blood to all parts of the body.

2. Arteries, veins, and capillaries are the structures that take blood from the heart to the cells and return blood from the cells back to the heart.

3. Blood carries oxygen and nutrients to the cells and carries the waste products away.

4. The lymph system (see Chapter 15) returns excess fluid from the tissues to the general circulation. The lymph nodes produce lymphocytes and filter out pathogenic bacteria.

COMPONENTS OF THE CIRCULATORY SYSTEM

The organs of the circulatory system include the heart, arteries, veins, and capillaries. The blood and lymphatic system are part of the circulatory system.

The heart is the muscular pump which is responsible for circulating the blood throughout the body.

MAJOR BLOOD CIRCUITS

Blood leaves the heart through arteries and returns by veins. The blood uses two circulation routes:

1. The general (or systemic) circulation carries blood throughout the body, Figure 13-1.

2. The **cardiopulmonary circulation** carries blood from the heart to the lungs and back, Figure 13-2.

CHANGES IN THE COMPOSITION OF CIRCULATING BLOOD

The major substances added to and removed from the blood as it circulates through organs along the various sites of the

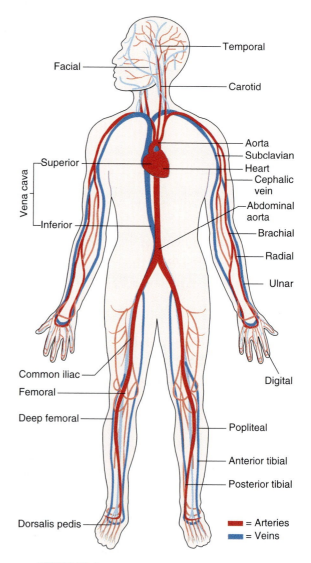

FIGURE 13-1 *General or systemic circulation*

---

[1] I. Sherman and V. Sherman, *Biology: A Human Approach* (New York: Oxford University Press, 1979).

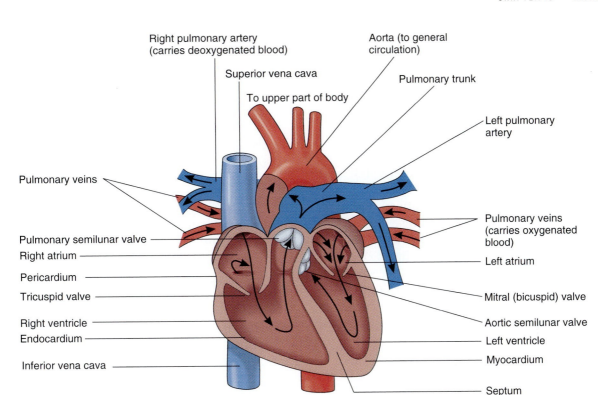

Right pulmonary artery
(carries deoxygenated blood)

Aorta (to general
circulation)

Superior vena cava

Pulmonary trunk

To upper part of body

Left pulmonary
artery

Pulmonary veins

Pulmonary veins
(carries oxygenated
blood)

Pulmonary semilunar valve

Right atrium

Left atrium

Pericardium

Tricuspid valve

Mitral (bicuspid) valve

Right ventricle

Aortic semilunar valve

Endocardium

Left ventricle

Myocardium

Inferior vena cava

Septum

FIGURE 13-2 *Schematic of heart pulmonary circulation*

circulatory system are outlined in Table 13-1. (This table includes only the major changes in the blood as it passes through certain specialized organs or structures.)

THE HEART

The blood's circulatory system is extremely efficient. The main organ responsible for this efficiency is the heart, a tough, simply-constructed muscle about the size of a closed fist.

The adult human heart is about 5" long and 3.5" wide, weighing less than one pound (12-13 oz). The importance of a healthy, well-functioning heart is obvious: to circulate life-sustaining blood throughout the body. When the heart stops beating, life stops as well! To explain further, if the blood flow to the brain ceases for five seconds or more, the subject loses consciousness. After fifteen to twenty seconds, the muscles twitch convulsively; after six to nine minutes without blood flow, the brain cells are irreversibly damaged.

TABLE 13-1 • *Changes in the Composition of the Blood*

ORGANS	BLOOD LOSES	BLOOD GAINS
Digestive glands	Raw materials needed to make digestive juices and enzymes	Carbon dioxide
Kidneys	Water, urea, and mineral salts	Carbon dioxide
Liver	Excess glucose, amino acids, and worn-out red blood cells	Released glucose, urea, and plasma proteins
Lungs	Carbon dioxide and water	Oxygen
Muscles	Glucose and oxygen	Lactic acid and carbon dioxide
Small intestinal villi	Oxygen	End products of digestion (glucose) and amino acids)

The heart is located in the thoracic cavity. This places the heart between the lungs, behind the sternum, in front of the thoracic vertebrae and above the diaphragm. Although the heart is centrally located, its axis of symmetry is not along the midline. The heart's **apex** (conical tip) lies on the diaphragm and points to the left of the body. It is at the apex where the heartbeat is most easily felt and heard through the **stethoscope**.

Try this simple demonstration: place the disk or bowl of a stethoscope over the heart's apex. This is the area between the fifth and sixth ribs, along an imaginary line extending from the middle of the left clavicle. Since the heartbeat is felt and heard so easily at the apex, this gives rise to the popular but incorrect notion that the heart is located on the left side of the body.

Knowledge of the correct position of the heart can make all the difference in the treatment of **cardiac arrest**. During such a medical emergency, the combination of manual heart compression and artificial respiration can save a life. This life-saving technique is known as **cardiopulmonary resuscitation** (CPR) and should be performed only by those specifically trained in CPR.

STRUCTURE OF THE HEART

The heart is a hollow, muscular, double pump which circulates the blood through the blood vessel to all parts of the body. At rest, the heart pumps two ounces of blood with each beat, five quarts per minute, seventy-five gallons per hour. The heart contracts about seventy-two times per minute, or about 100,000 times each day.

Surrounding the heart is a double layer of fibrous tissue called the **pericardium**, Figure 13-3. Between these two pericardial layers is a

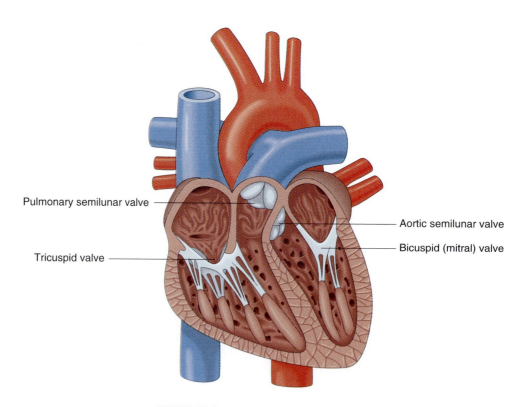

Pulmonary semilunar valve

Tricuspid valve

Aortic semilunar valve

Bicuspid (mitral) valve

FIGURE 13-3 *The heart and its valves*

space filled with a lubricating fluid called peri-cardial fluid. This fluid prevents the two layers from rubbing against each other and creating friction. The thin inner layer covering the heart is the visceral or serous pericardium. The tough outer membrane is the parietal or fibrous pericardium.

Cardiac muscle tissue, or **myocardium**, makes up the major portion of the heart. On the inner lining lies a smooth tissue called the **endocardium**. The endocardium covers the heart valves and lines the blood vessels providing smooth transit for the flowing blood.

A frontal view of the human heart reveals a thick, muscular wall separating it into a right half and a left half. This partition, known as the **septum**, completely separates the blood in the right half from that in the left half. See Figure 13-2.

Structures leading to and from the heart are:

- Superior **vena cava** and inferior vena cava—the large veinous blood vessels which bring **deoxygenated** blood (which has lesser amounts of oxygen) to the right atrium from all parts of the body.

- **Coronary sinus**—from the heart muscle to the right atrium.

- **Pulmonary artery**—takes blood away from the right ventricle to the lungs for oxygen.

- **Pulmonary veins**—bring **oxygenated** blood from the lungs to the left atrium.

- **Aorta**—takes blood away from the left ventricle to the rest of the body.

Chambers and Valves

The human heart is separated into right and left halves by the septum. In turn, each half is divided into two parts, thus creating four chambers. The two upper chambers are called the right atrium and the left atrium (pl. atria). The **atrium** may be referred to as the auricle. The lower chambers are the **right ventricle** and the **left ventricle**, Figure 13-4.

The heart has four valves which permit the blood to flow in one direction only. These valves open and close during the contraction of the heart, preventing the blood from flowing backwards, Figure 13-3.

Atrioventricular valves are located between the atria and the ventricles.

- The **tricuspid valve** is positioned between the right atrium and the right ventricle. Its name comes from the fact that there are three points, or cusps, of attachment. It allows blood to flow from the right atrium into the right ventricle, but not in the opposite direction.

- The **bicuspid** or **mitral valve** is located between the left atrium and the left ventricle. Blood flows from the left atrium into the left ventricle, while backflow from the left ventricle to the left atrium is prevented.

Semi-lunar valves are located where blood will leave the heart:

- The **pulmonary semilunar valve** is found at the orifice (opening) of the pulmonary artery. It lets blood travel from the right ventricle into the pulmonary artery, and then into the lungs.

- The **aortic semilunar valve** is at the orifice of the aorta. This valve permits the blood to pass from the left ventricle into the aorta, but not backwards into the left ventricle. See Figure 13-3.

Physiology of the Heart

The structure of the heart allows it to function as a double pump. (Think of the heart as having a right side and a left side.) Two major functions occur each time the heart beats:

- *Right heart*—Blood (deoxygenated) flows into the heart from the superior and inferior vena cava to the right atrium to the tricuspid valve to the right ventricle through the pulmonary semilunar valves to the pulmonary artery, which takes blood to the lungs for oxygen.

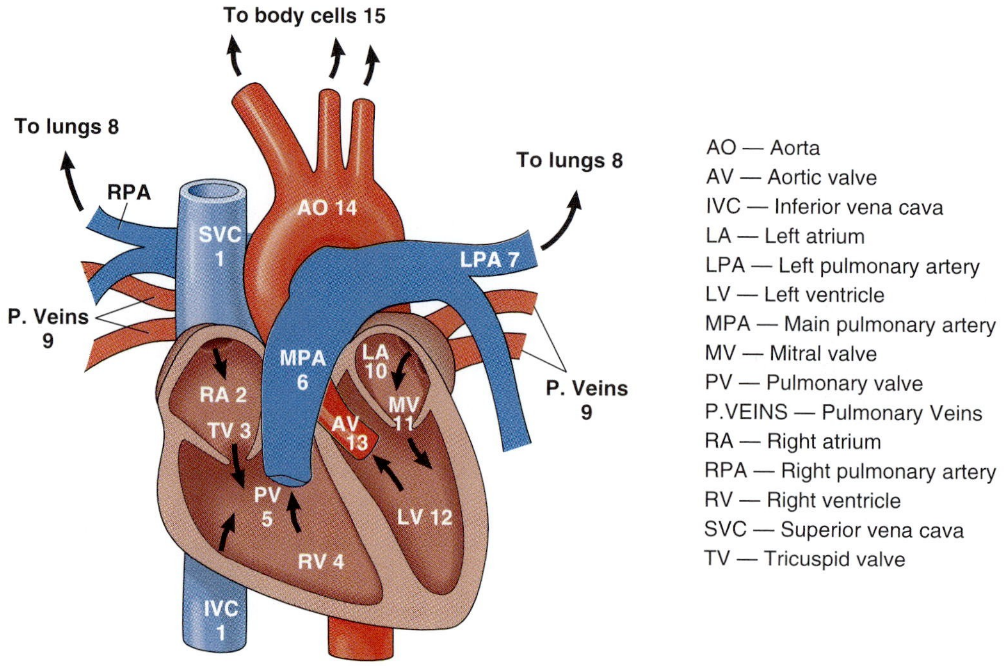

1. Blood reaches heart through superior vena cava (SVA) and inferior vena cava (IVC)
2. To right atruim
3. To tricuspid valve
4. To right ventricle
5. To pulmonary valve (semi-lunar)
6. To main pulmonary artery
7. To left pulmonary artery and right pulmonary artery

8. To lungs—blood receives O_2
9. From lungs to pulmonary veins
10. To left atrium
11. To mitral (bicuspid) valve
12. To left ventricle
13. To aortic valve (semi-lunar valve)
14. To aorta (largest artery in the body)
15. Blood with oxygen then goes to all cells of the body

FIGURE 13-4 *Normal heart*

● *Left heart*—Blood (oxygenated) flows into the heart from the lungs by the pulmonary veins to the left atrium through the bicuspid valve (mitral) to the left ventricle to the aorta to general circulation.

It is sometimes hard to imagine this idea of two pumping actions occurring at the same time. Each time the ventricles contract, blood leaves the right ventricle to go to the lungs, and blood leaves the left ventricle to go to the aorta.

Blood Supply to the Heart

The heart receives its blood supply from the coronary artery, which branches into right

and left coronary arteries. (Further discussion on this subject can be found in Chapter 14.)

Heart Sounds

The physician listens at specific locations on the chest wall to hear how the heart is functioning. During the cardiac cycle, the valves make a sound when they close. These are referred to as the lubb dupp sounds. The lubb sound is heard first and is made by the valves (tricuspid and bicuspid) closing between the atria and ventricles. The physician refers to it as the S_1 sound. It is heard loudest at the apex of the heart.

The dupp sound is heard second and is shorter and higher pitched. It is caused by the semilunar valves in the aorta and the pulmonary artery closing. The physician refers to it as the S_2 sound. Certain conditions can cause changes in the action of the heart valves.

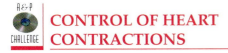

CONTROL OF HEART CONTRACTIONS

A heart removed from the body will continue to beat rhythmically, which shows that heartbeat generates in the heart muscle itself. The heart rate is also affected by the endocrine and nervous system. The myocardium contracts rhythmically in order to perform its duty as a forceful pump.

Control of heart muscle contractions is found within a group of conducting cells located at the opening of the superior vena cava into the right atrium. These cells are known as the **sinoatrial (SA) node**, or **pacemaker**. The SA node sends out an electrical impulse that begins and regulates the heart. The impulse spreads out over the atria, making them contract or depolarize. This causes blood to flow downward from the upper atrial chamber to the atrioventricular openings. The electrical impulse eventually reaches the **atrioventricular (AV) node**, which is another conducting cell group located between the atria and ventricle.

From the AV node, the electrical impulse is carried to conducting fibers in the septum. These conducting fibers are known as the **atrioventricular bundle** or the bundle of His. It divides into a right and left branch: each branch then subdivides into a fine network of branches spreading throughout the ventricles called the Purkinje network. The electrical impulse shoots along the **Purkinje fibers** to the ventricles causing them to contract. The heart then rests briefly (repolarizes). See Figure 13-5.

The combined action of the SA and AV nodes is instrumental in the cardiac cycle. The cardiac cycle comprises one complete heartbeat, with both atrial and ventricular contractions.

1. The SA node stimulates the contraction of both atria. Blood flows from the atria into the ventricles through the open tricuspid and mitral valves. At the same time, the ventricles are relaxed, allowing them to fill with the blood. At this point, since the semilunar valves are closed, the blood cannot enter the pulmonary artery or aorta.

2. The AV node stimulates the contraction of both ventricles so that the blood in the ventricles is pumped into the pulmonary artery and the aorta through the semilunar valves which are now open. At this point the atria are relaxed and the tricuspid and mitral valves closed.

3. The ventricles relax; the semilunar valves are closed to prevent the blood flowing back into the ventricles. The heart rests briefly (repolarization). The cycle begins again with the signal from the SA node.

This action of the heart is known as the cardiac cycle and represents one heart beat. Each cardiac cycle takes 0.8 seconds. The average person's heart rate is between seventy-two to seventy-five beats per minute.

Electrocardiogram (ECG or EKG)

The ECG or EKG is a device used to record the electrical activity of the heart that causes the contraction (systole) and the relaxation (diastole) of the atria and ventricles during the cardiac cycle, Figure 13-5.

The baseline, or isoelectric line, of the ECG is the flat line that separates the various waves. It is present when there is no current flowing in the heart. The waves are either deflecting upward, known as *positive deflection*, or deflecting downward, known as *negative deflection*. The P, QRS, and T waves recorded during the ECG represent the depolarization (contraction) and repolarization (relaxation) of the myocardial cells. The P wave represents atrial depolarization; QRS represents ventricular depolarization; and the T wave represents ventricular repolarization.

By observing the size, shape, and location of each wave, the physician can analyze and

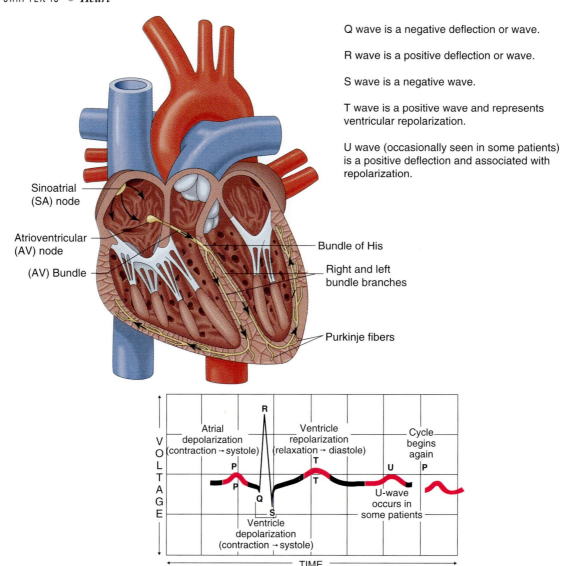

Q wave is a negative deflection or wave.

R wave is a positive deflection or wave.

S wave is a negative wave.

T wave is a positive wave and represents ventricular repolarization.

U wave (occasionally seen in some patients) is a positive deflection and associated with repolarization.

Sinoatrial (SA) node

Atrioventricular (AV) node

(AV) Bundle

Bundle of His

Right and left bundle branches

Purkinje fibers

VOLTAGE

Atrial depolarization (contraction → systole)

Ventricle repolarization (relaxation → diastole)

Cycle begins again

R

P
P

T
T

U
P

Q

S

Ventricle depolarization (contraction → systole)

U-wave occurs in some patients

TIME

FIGURE 13-5 *Cardiac cycle and ECG reading*

interpret the conduction of electricity through the cardiac cells, the heart's rate, the heart's rhythm, and the general health of the heart.

TWELVE-LEAD ELECTROCARDIOGRAM, SINGLE CHANNEL

The purpose of performing a twelve-lead electrocardiogram is to:

- obtain an accurate, graphic, artifact-free reading of the electrical activity of a patient's heart

- identify arrhythmias
- estimate damage caused by MI
- assess effects of cardiac medication
- determine whether electrolyte imbalance is present
- identify cardia ischemia
- determine the effects of hypertension or disorders of the heart

The procedure requires the following supplies in order to be performed successfully:

- examination or ECG table with a pillow and a sheet or blanket

- a patient gown
- single channel electrocardiograph with patient cable wires
- electrolyte (gel, lotion, paste, or presaturated pads)
- ECG tracing paper
- metal electrodes (sensors)
- rubber straps
- gauze squares
- mounting form

Procedure Steps

1. Perform tracing in a quiet, warm, and comfortable room away from electrical equipment that may cause artifacts. The patient will be less apprehensive in a quiet atmosphere. Alternating current (AC) interference is minimized when ECG is performed away from electrical equipment.

2. Wash hands, gather equipment, identify the patient, and explain the procedure to the patient. Following these universal steps minimizes transmissions of micro-organisms and reassures patient.

3. Have the patient remove clothing from the waist up and uncover lower legs; socks can be kept on. Provide a sheet or blanket for privacy and warmth. Place the patient in supine position on the examination table with arms and legs supported. Pillows may be used under the knees and head. All four limbs and chest must be uncovered for proper electrode placement.

4. Explain that the procedure is painless and why it is necessary not to move or talk during the procedure. Patient cooperation ensures good quality tracing.

5. Place the electrocardiograph with the power cord pointing away from the patient. Do not allow the cable to go underneath the table. This helps reduce AC interference.

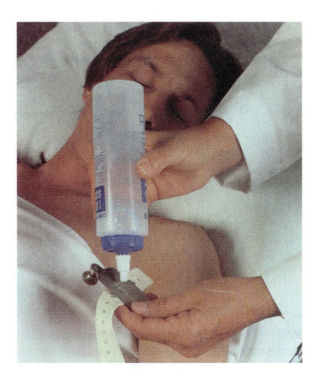

FIGURE 13-6 *The rubber strap is attached to the metal electrode and a small amount of electrolyte gel is placed on the side of the electrode applied to the patient's skin.*

6. Apply the limb electrodes by first connecting the rubber straps to the tabs on the electrodes. Apply a pea-size dab of electrolyte to the electrode; either paste or gel can be used, Figure 13-6. Apply the electrodes to the fleshy parts of the four limbs. Rub the electrolyte into the patient's skin. Lead connectors of the electrodes should be pointing toward the feet. Pull the rubber strap around the limb until it just meets, then pull tighter one more hole and secure, Figures 13-7 and 13-8. A more stable connection with the lead wires is possible when the lead connectors point to the feet. Electrolyte rubbed into the patient's skin helps ensure a good contact between the electrode and the skin. Straps applied too

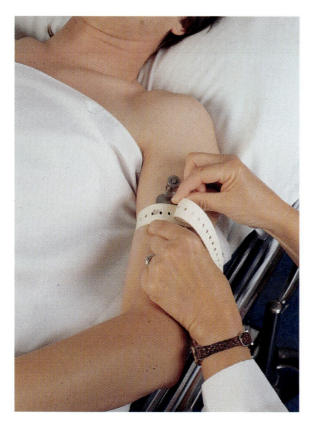

FIGURE 13-7 *Application of rubber strap and electrode to patient's upper arm. Placing an electrode on the upper arm minimizes somatic tremor.*

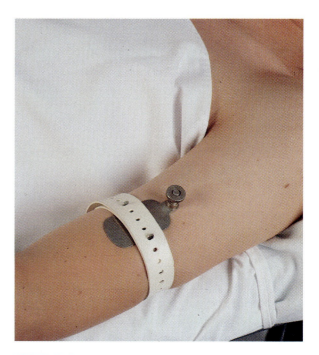

FIGURE 13-8 *The electrode is held in place on the upper arm by the rubber strap. Pull the strap around until the holes line up with the protrusions on the electrode with no tension. Then, pull the strap one hole tighter and secure.*

tightly or too loosely can cause artifacts. By applying electrodes to the fleshy part of the limbs, artifacts are minimized.

7. If using a Welch cup chest electrode, apply electrolyte to positions V_1 through V_6, rub the edge of each cup in the electrolyte, and secure it in position by squeezing the bulb end of the cup to create suction on the skin of the chest wall, Figure 13-9.

8. Tightly connect the lead wires to the electrodes. Be sure to connect the correct lead wires to the correct electrodes. The lead wires are labeled with abbreviations (RA, LA, RL, LL, and V or C). The lead wires should follow the patient's body contour. Following body contour minimizes artifacts, Figure 13-10.

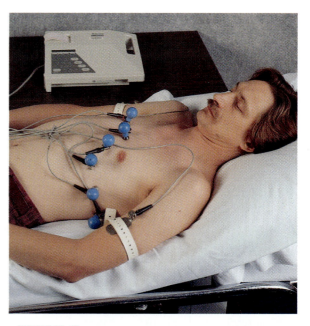

FIGURE 13-9 *An electrocardiograph showing all six chest leads applied simultaneously using Welch electrodes.*

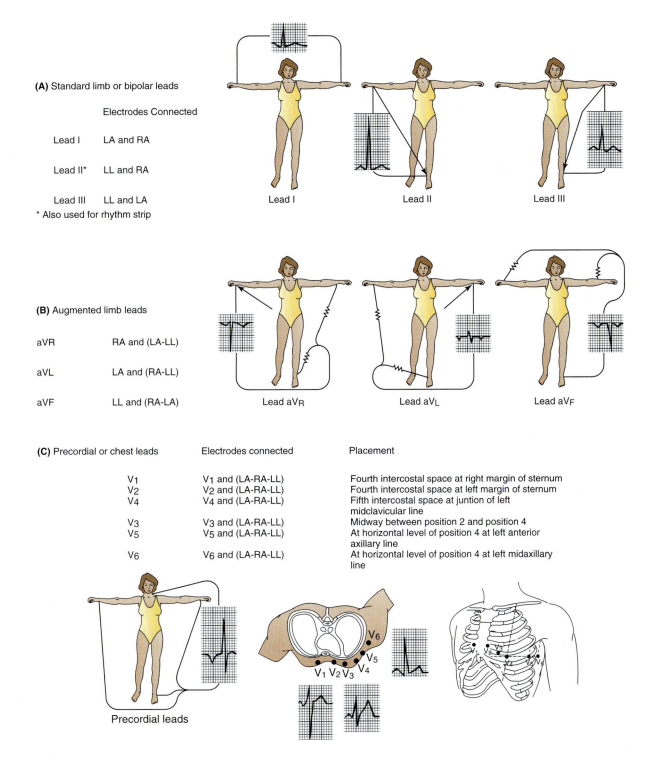

(A) Standard limb or bipolar leads

Electrodes Connected

Lead I   LA and RA

Lead II*   LL and RA

Lead III   LL and LA

* Also used for rhythm strip

Lead I   Lead II   Lead III

(B) Augmented limb leads

aVR   RA and (LA-LL)

aVL   LA and (RA-LL)

aVF   LL and (RA-LA)

Lead aV$_R$ Lead aV$_L$ Lead aV$_F$

(C) Precordial or chest leads   Electrodes connected   Placement

V$_1$	V$_1$ and (LA-RA-LL)	Fourth intercostal space at right margin of sternum
V$_2$	V$_2$ and (LA-RA-LL)	Fourth intercostal space at left margin of sternum
V$_4$	V$_4$ and (LA-RA-LL)	Fifth intercostal space at juntion of left midclavicular line
V$_3$	V$_3$ and (LA-RA-LL)	Midway between position 2 and position 4
V$_5$	V$_5$ and (LA-RA-LL)	At horizontal level of position 4 at left anterior axillary line
V$_6$	V$_6$ and (LA-RA-LL)	At horizontal level of position 4 at left midaxillary line

Precordial leads

FIGURE 13-10 *Lead types, connections, and placement: (a) Standard limb or bipolar leads, (b) Augmented limb leads, and (c) Precordial or chest leads*

9. The patient cable is supported either on the table or the patient's abdomen. Plug the patient cable into the electrocardiograph.

10. Turn instrument to ON.

11. The lead selector switch should be on STD (standard). Center the stylus. The record switch should be on Run (25 mm/sec). Check the standardization for the instrument by quickly pressing the standardization button. The standardization mark should be 10 mm or ten small squares high. If it is more or less than this, adjust the instrument appropriately. Standardization ensures a dependable and accurate tracing.

12. Center the stylus and run about 4 to 5" of each lead I, II, and III by placing the record switch on Run (25 m/sec) and turning the lead selector switch appropriately.

    • While recording be sure the stylus and recording are near the center of the paper. If not, use the position control knob to move up or down to adjust as needed. None of the waves should fall off the graph paper.

    • Watch for artifacts and correct if present.

    • Determine if a change in standard or stylus position is needed by observing the amplitude of the R wave.

13. Continue with leads aVR, aVL, aVF, and record about 4 to 5" of each lead by turning the lead selector to the appropriate position.

14. Record 6 to 8" each of the V leads by turning the lead selector control to the appropriate position.

15. Place another standardization at the end of the tracing by putting the lead selector on STD and depressing the button. Run the tracing through the instrument and turn the machine to OFF. Remove the tracing from the instrument and immediately label with patient's name, date, and time of day. Sign your initials. Unplug the power cord.

16. Disconnect the lead wires and remove the rubber straps and electrodes from the patient. Cleanse or wipe patient's skin to remove paste or gel electrolyte.

17. Assist patient as needed.

18. Provide physician with uncut tracing.

19. Clean and return equipment per OSHA guidelines.

20. Wash hands.

21. Document procedure.

22. Cut and mount the tracing remembering to handle carefully. Label appropriately and place in patient's record.

A & P CHALLENGE — DISEASES OF THE HEART

One of the leading causes of death is cardiovascular disease. Some of the common symptoms of heart disease are:

• **Arrhythmia** or dysrhythmia—the term used to discuss any change or deviation from the normal rate or rhythm of the heart.

• **Bradycardia**—the term used for slow heart rate (less than sixty beats per minute).

• **Tachycardia**—the term used for rapid heart rate (more than 100 beats per minute).

• **Murmurs**—indicate some defects in the valves of the heart. When valves fail to close properly, a gurgling or hissing sound will occur. Cardiac murmurs may be classified according to which valve is affected or according to the heart's cardiac cycle. If the murmur occurs when the heart is contracting it is called a systolic murmur. If the heart is at rest it is called a diastolic murmur. A surgical procedure can be done to replace the defective valve.

- **Mitral valve prolapse**—a condition in which the valve between the left atria and the left ventricle closes imperfectly. Symptoms are thought to occur because of a response to stress. These symptoms include fatigue, **palpitations** (heart feels like it is racing), headache, chest pain, and anxiety. Exercise, restricting sugar and caffeine intake, adequate fluid intake, and relaxation techniques help to alleviate symptoms.

Infectious Diseases of the Heart

A bacteria or virus is usually the cause of infectious diseases of the heart. These conditions may be treated with antibiotic therapy.

- **Pericarditis** is an inflammation of the outer membrane covering the heart. The symptoms are pain in the chest area overlying the heart, cough, **dyspnea** (difficulty in breathing), rapid pulse, and fever.

- **Myocarditis** is an inflammation of the heart muscle. The symptoms may be the same as the pericarditis.

- **Endocarditis** is an inflammation of the membrane that lines the heart and covers the valves. This causes the formation of rough spots in the endocardium, which may lead to the development of a fatal blood clot (thrombus).

- **Rheumatic heart disease** may be a result of a person having frequent strep throat infections during childhood; these infections may lead to rheumatic fever. The antibodies which form to protect the child from the strep throat or rheumatic fever may also attack the lining of the heart, especially the bicuspid or mitral valve. The valve becomes inflamed and may be scarred, which leads to narrowing of the valve. The mitral valve is then unable to close properly which interferes with the blood flow from the left atrium to the left ventricle. It is most important that children who have streptococcal infections are treated with antibiotic therapy.

Coronary Artery Disease

The coronary artery supplies the heart muscle, or the myocardium, with its blood supply.

- **Angina pectoris** is the severe chest pain which arises when the heart does not receive enough oxygen. It is not a disease in itself, but a symptom of an underlying problem with the coronary circulation. The chest pain radiates from the precordial area to the left shoulder, down the arm along the ulnar nerve. Victims often experience a feeling of impending death. Angina pectoris occurs quite suddenly; it may be brought on by stress or physical exhaustion. It may be treated with the drug nitroglycerine which helps to dilate the coronary arteries to permit blood flow to the heart.

- **Myocardial infarction**, commonly known as an "MI" or "heart attack," is caused by a lack of blood supply to the heart muscle, the myocardium. This may be due to blocking of the coronary artery by a blood clot, narrowing of the coronary artery as a result of arteriosclerosis (a loss of elasticity and thickening of the wall), or atherosclerosis (caused by plaque build up in the arterial walls), Figure 13-11. The heart muscle becomes damaged due to lack of blood supply. The amount of tissue affected depends on how much of the heart area is deprived of blood. Symptoms are crushing, severe chest pain radiating to the left shoulder, arm, neck, and jaw. Patients may also complain of nausea, increased perspiration, fatigue, and dyspnea. Mortality is highest when treatment is delayed; therefore, immediate medical care is critical. Treatment consists of bed rest, oxygen, and medications. Morphine or demerol is given to alleviate the pain, drugs such as tPA are used to dissolve the blood clot, and **cardiotonic** drugs such as digitalis are used to slow and strengthen the heartbeat. Anticoagulant therapy is used to prevent further clots from forming. Angioplasty and bypass surgery may also be necessary.

Cross sections through a coronary artery
undergoing progressive atherosclerosis
and arteriosclerosis

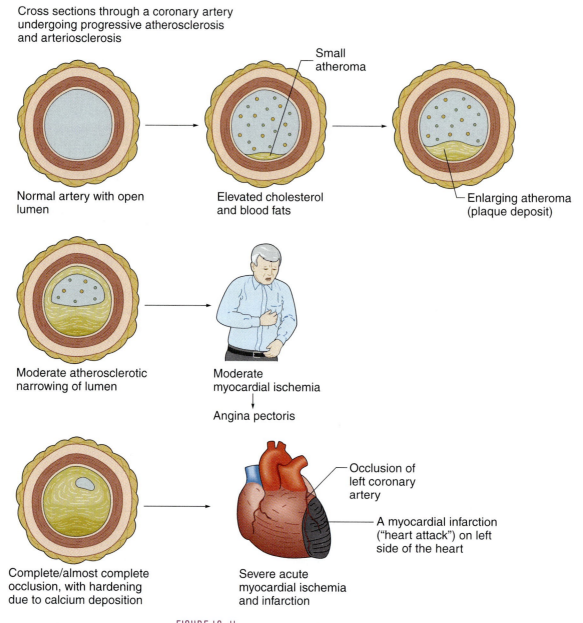

Small
atheroma

Normal artery with open
lumen

Elevated cholesterol
and blood fats

Enlarging atheroma
(plaque deposit)

Moderate atherosclerotic
narrowing of lumen

Moderate
myocardial ischemia

Angina pectoris

Occlusion of
left coronary
artery

A myocardial infarction
("heart attack") on left
side of the heart

Complete/almost complete
occlusion, with hardening
due to calcium deposition

Severe acute
myocardial ischemia
and infarction

FIGURE 13-11 *Progressive atherosclerosis*

Prevention of Heart Disease

The National Institute of Health has stated that the following lifestyle changes would reduce the risk of heart attacks. These include not smoking, regular exercise, maintaining ideal weight, estrogen replacement therapy for post-menopausal women, reduction of blood cholesterol levels, and maintaining normal blood pressure. In the blood there are two types of blood cholesterol: high density lipoprotein (HDL) and low density lipoprotein (LDL). The HDL type helps to remove a portion of the cholesterol plaque deposited by a related LDL. The benefits of increasing the HDL ratio to the LDL ratio are significant; medication and diet help to increase HDL.

Heart Failure

Heart failure occurs when the ventricles of the heart are unable to contract effectively and blood pools in the heart. Different symptoms can arise depending on which ventricle fails to beat properly. If the left ventricle fails, dyspnea occurs. If the right ventricle fails, engorgement of organs with venous blood occurs, as well as **edema** (excessive fluid in tissues) and **ascites** (abnormal accumulation of serous fluid in the abdominal cavity). Other symptoms may include lung congestion and coughing.

Congestive Heart Failure

Congestive heart failure is similar to heart failure, but in addition there is edema of the lower extremities. Blood backs up into the lung vessels, and fluid extends into the air passages. Treatment consists of cardiotonics (drugs used to slow and strengthen the heart beat, such as digoxin) and **diuretics** (drugs which reduce the amount of fluid in the body).

Rhythm/Conduction Defects

A **conduction**, or rhythm, **defect** is said to occur when the conduction system of the heart is affected.

- **Heart block** is the interruption of the AV node message from the SA.

- The interruption can occur in varying degrees. The abnormal patterns are seen on an electrocardiograph. *First degree block* is characterized by a momentary delay at the AV node before the impulse is transmitted to the ventricles. *Second degree block* can be of two forms. One occurs in cycles of delayed impulses until the SA node fails to conduct to the AV node, then returns to near normal. A second form is characterized by a pattern of only every second, third, or fourth impulse being conducted to the ventricles. This causes a decrease in heart output and usually progresses to the

third degree. *Third degree block* in known as "complete heart block." There is no impulse carried over from the pacemaker. Since the heart is essential to life, there is a built-in safety factor. The atria continue to beat seventy-two beats per minute while the ventricles contract independently at about half the atrial rate, adequate to sustain life by resulting in a severe decrease in cardiac output. Conduction defects may be treated by medications and/or the use of an *artificial pacemaker*.

- *Premature contractions* is an arrhythmia disorder which occurs when an area of the heart known as an ectopic (abnormal place) pacemaker (not the SA node) sparks and stimulates a contraction of the myocardium. There are three types identified by the area of their location: atrial, ventricular, or AV junctional. *Premature atrial contractions (PACs)* cause the atria to contract ahead of the anticipated time. *Premature junctional contractions (PJCs)* have the ectopic pacemaker focused at the junction of the AV node and the bundle of His. Usually, PACs and PJCs are of no clinical significance and are usually caused by stress, nicotine, caffeine, or fatigue. *Premature ventricular contractions (PVCs)* originate in the ventricles and cause contractions ahead of the next anticipated beat. They can be benign or deadly (ventricular fibrillation). If frequent (five to six per minute) or in pairs, they may require immediate intervention in order to decrease the irritability of the cardiac muscle and maintain cardiac output.

- In **fibrillation**, the rhythm breaks down and muscle fibers contract at random without coordination. This results in ineffective heart action and is a life-threatening condition. An electrical device called a **defibrillator** is used to discharge a strong electrical current through the patient's heart through electrode paddles held against the bare chest wall. The shock interferes with the uncoordinated action and attempts to shock the SA node to resume its control.

TYPES OF HEART SURGERY

- **Angioplasty**—a procedure to help open clogged vessels. This may also be referred to as **balloon surgery**. A small deflated balloon is able to be threaded into the coronary artery; when it reaches the blocked area the balloon is inflated. The balloon is then opened and closed a few times, until the blockage is pushed against the arterial wall and the area is unblocked. The balloon is then deflated and removed, Figure 13-12.

- **Coronary by-pass**—in this type of surgery a detour or by-pass is provided to allow the blood supply to go around the blocked area of the coronary artery. A healthy blood vessel, usually a vein from the leg, is used for this purpose. The vein is inserted before the blocked area and provides another route for the blood supply to the myocardium.

HEART TRANSPLANTS

A heart transplant is needed in cases where the individual's own heart can no longer function properly. This happens when someone has suffered repeated heart attacks and there is irreparable damage to the heart muscle, valves, or blood vessels leading to and from the heart. Occasionally, a baby or young child might need a heart transplant because of a congenital (present at birth) heart defect.

There are always problems that follow even the most "successful" of heart transplants, however. The problem is one of histocompatibility (matching of tissue type) and organ rejection. Heart transplants that occur between two unrelated people must be monitored carefully. When the heart from the donor is placed into the recipient's body, the recipient's body chemically recognizes the donated heart as a "foreign tissue." Thus, the recipient's immune system starts to reject the transplanted heart.

Medical science has counteracted the rejection by developing chemicals called immunosuppressants. These drugs suppress the recipient's immune system so it will not form antibodies to reject the donated heart. Unfortunately the effect of these chemicals is not permanent. Also, suppressing the recipient's immune system indefinitely is not medically wise be-

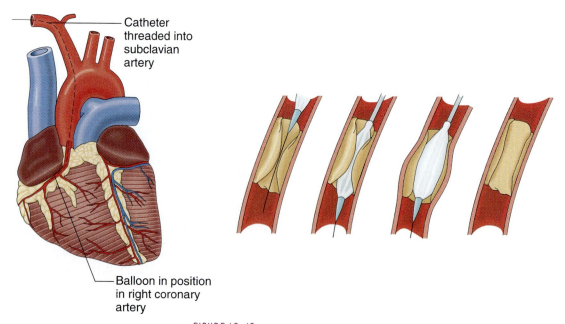

Catheter threaded into subclavian artery

Balloon in position in right coronary artery

FIGURE 13-12 *Balloon angioplasty*

cause he or she will be more susceptible to disease and infection. Often times a heart transplant patient dies not from problems arising from the donated heart but from a case of pneumonia! So the science and technology of heart transplants is still in its formative stages. However, a heart transplant can perhaps prolong the life and maybe even improve the quality of life for an individual with a chronic heart problem.

ARTIFICIAL HEART

The artificial heart was used for the first time on December 3, 1982. The use of the heart has not been as successful as scientists had hoped it would be. Scientists continue to do the necessary research to perfect an artificial heart.

MEDICAL HIGHLIGHT: TECHNOLOGY
Pacemakers, Implantable Difibrillators, and Stent Devices

Pacemakers

The most commonly used artificial pacemaker is the demand pacemaker which monitors the heart's activity and takes control only when the heart rate falls below a programmed minimum—usually sixty beats per minute, Figure 13-13. Today, newer types of pacemakers actually monitor a number of physical changes in the body which indicates an increase or decrease in activity. If the heart's own pacing system fails to respond, these rate-responsive pacemakers slowly raise or lower the heartbeat to the appropriate level, from sixty to perhaps 150 beats per minute.

Today's modern pacemakers are shielded from stray electromagnetic forces and people who use pacemakers no longer have to avoid microwave ovens. However, there is some evidence that the use of cellular phones, especially digital ones, can change the pace of pacemakers or speed up people's pulses when used near the heart-regulating devices. Medtronics, Inc., the world's largest developer and manufacturer of pacemakers, recommends that people keep cell phones at least six inches away from pacemakers.

Implantable Defibrillators

A defibrillator is a device that can shock the heart back to a regular rhythm. The im-

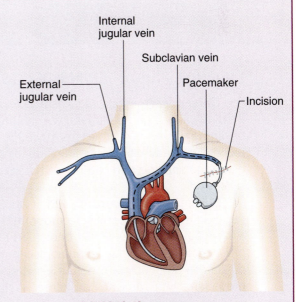

FIGURE 13-13 *A pacemaker*

plantable defibrillator protects patients at risk from severe ventricular tachycardia, a life-threatening arrhythmia. Mediation and pacemakers are the most common treatment for arrhythmias, but for a small proportion of patients the implantable defibrillator can save their lives. In May of 1996, the Food and Drug Administration also gave approval for the defibrillator to be used on patients who may have had at least one heart attack in the past but who are now without symptoms other than irregular heart rhythms picked up on an EKG. The defibrillator is implanted in the skin of the chest or abdomen and usually needs only one electrode to be routed to the heart through a vein. Through that electrode the tiny computer aboard the defibrillator constantly monitors the heartbeat. If it detects a minor arrhythmia, it activates a built-in conventional pacemaker to reestablish the heart rhythm. If that fails, it delivers a small defibrillating electrical jolt to the heart. The electrical jolt may be startling and a bit uncomfortable; however, the minor annoyance is acceptable to most patients since they realize that a potentially life-threatening heartbeat irregularity has been detected and corrected.

Angioplasty-Palmaz-Schatz Stent

This stent device is a tiny, expandable, stainless steel tube which holds arteries open following angioplasty. Following angioplasty, the coronary artery blockage can return within a matter of months if new plaque deposits develop or clot formation occurs.

CAREER PROFILES

CARDIOVASCULAR TECHNOLOGISTS AND TECHNICIANS

Cardiovascular technologists and *technicians* assist physicians in diagnosing and treating cardiac and peripheral vascular disease. Cardiovascular technicians may also be known as EKG technicians because they take electrocardiograms. More skilled technicians may also do Holter monitor and stress testing. Cardiovascular technologists who specialize in cardiac catheterization procedures are called *cardiology technologists*.

Education to prepare a technician for EKG, Holter, and stress testing usually requires a one year certificate program. Training for cardiology technologists involves a two year program which is dedicated to core courses and clinical practice. The job prospects for cardiology technologists are excellent. However, cardiovascular technologists' job prospects are not as good since nurses and others may be trained to do procedures such as EKG and stress testing.

● REVIEW QUESTIONS

Select the letter of the choice that best completes the statement.

1. The organs of the circulatory system include the:
   a. heart, blood vessels and liver
   b. heart, blood vessels and lungs
   c. heart, blood vessels and lymph
   d. heart, blood vessels and kidneys

2. The outer layer of the heart is called the:
   a. myocardium
   b. endocardium
   c. pericardium
   d. pleural lining

3. The muscle layer of the heart is called the:
   a. myocardium
   b. endocardium
   c. pericardium
   d. pleural lining

4. The valve between the right atrium and the right ventricle is called the:
   a. tricuspid valve
   b. aortic semilunar valve
   c. bicuspid valve
   d. pulmonary semilunar valve

5. The blood vessel that brings blood to the right atrium is called the:
   a. pulmonary vein
   b. aorta
   c. pulmonary artery
   d. vena cava

6. The pacemaker of the heart is the:
   a. SA node
   b. AV node
   c. Bundle branches
   d. Purkinje fibers

7. The heart contracts in this fashion:
   a. bundle branches, AV node, SA node
   b. AV node, bundle branches, SA node
   c. SA node, AV node, bundle branches
   d. bundle branches, SA node, AV node

8. The device used to measure the electrical activity of the heart is called an:
   a. EEG
   b. MRI
   c. EKG
   d. EMG

9. A heart rate below sixty is called:
   a. bradycardia
   b. tachycardia
   c. arrhythmia
   d. murmur

10. An inflammation of the inner layer of the heart is called:
    a. pericarditis
    b. myocarditis
    c. endocarditis
    d. phlebitis

11. The term "heart attack" is another name for:
    a. rheumatic heart disease
    b. myocardial infarction
    c. heart block
    d. congestive heart failure

12. The treatment for a heart attack may include all but:
    a. angioplasty
    b. antibiotics
    c. coronary by-pass
    d. anticoagulants

13. Another name for stationary blood clot is a:
    a. embolus
    b. stenosis
    c. thrombus
    d. thrombosis

14. The treatment for heart block may include:
    a. coronary by pass
    b. anticoagulants
    c. insertion of a pacemaker
    d. angioplasty

15. The circulation that carries blood from the heart to lungs and back to heart is the:
    a. coronary
    b. fetal
    c. cardiopulmonary
    d. portal

● LABELING

Locate and label the various structures of the heart. Also include valves, vessels, and nodes. Trace blood from right atrium to aorta.

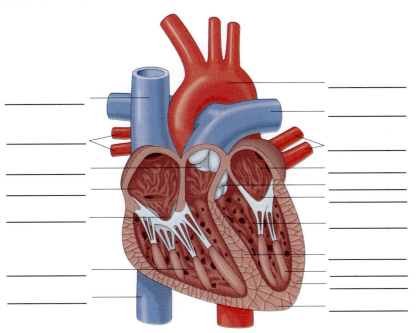

● MATCHING

Match each term in Column I with its correct description or function in Column II.

Column I	Column II
_____ 1. pulmonary artery	a. vein that carries freshly oxygenated blood from the lung to the heart
_____ 2. lymphatic system	
_____ 3. pulmonary vein	b. circulation route that carries blood to and from the heart and lungs
_____ 4. septum	
_____ 5. pulmonary circulation	c. divides the heart into right and left sides
	d. artery that carries deoxygenated blood from the heart to the lung
_____ 6. left ventricle	
_____ 7. general circulation	e. system that consists of lymph and tissue fluid derived from the blood
_____ 8. right ventricle	
_____ 9. aorta	f. blood from the pulmonary vein that re-enters the heart through the left atrium
	g. artery that carries blood with nourishment, oxygen and other materials from the heart to all parts of the body
	h. ventricle from which the aorta receives blood
	i. circulation that carries blood throughout the body
	j. ventricle from which the pulmonary artery leaves the heart

● APPLYING THEORY TO PRACTICE

1. Pretend you are a blood cell that has just arrived in the right atrium. Trace the journey you will take to get to the aorta.

2. A child has chronic strep throat. If this condition is not treated, what heart disease can occur? Describe what happens in the heart. How can this be prevented?

3. When a person has a heart attack, what happens to the cardiac muscle? Describe the types of surgery which can be done to treat this condition. Describe the feelings of the patient and the family.

4. A fifty-year-old female patient comes into the doctor's office and states, "People in my family all start to die at fifty from heart disease." What guidelines can you give her to help prevent the disease?

5. Many poems and songs are written about love and the heart. Why do you think there is a connection? Compare your answer with at least two classmates' answers.

CHAPTER 14

Circulation and Blood Vessels

KEY WORDS

aneurysm
aphasia
artery
arteriole
arteriosclerosis
atherosclerosis
blood pressure
brachial artery
capillary
cerebral hemorrhage
cerebral vascular
    accident (CVA)
claudication
common carotid
    artery
congenital heart
    defects
coronary artery
coronary
    circulation

coronary sinus
cyanosis
dorsalis pedis
    artery
diastolic blood
    pressure
dysphasia
ductus arteriosus
embolism
fetal circulation
foramen ovale
gangrene
hemiplegia
hepatic vein
hemorrhoids
hypertension
hypotension
peripheral vascular
    disease

phlebitis
portal circulation
portal vein
pulse
radial artery
stroke
systolic blood
    pressure
temporal artery
transient ischemic
    attacks (TIA)
tunica adventitia
    (externa)
tunica intima
tunica media
valves
varicose veins
vein
venule

The blood vessels circulate the blood through two major circulatory systems:

1. *cardiopulmonary circulation*—blood from the heart to the lungs and back to the heart.
2. *systemic circulation*—blood from the heart to the tissues and cells and back to the heart.

Specialized systemic routes are:

1. *coronary circulation*—brings blood to the myocardium.
2. *portal circulation*—takes blood from the organs of digestion to the liver through the portal vein.
3. *fetal circulation*—only occurs in the pregnant female. The fetus obtains oxygen and nutrients from the mother's blood.

CARDIOPULMONARY CIRCULATION

Cardiopulmonary circulation takes deoxygenated blood from the heart to the lungs where carbon dioxide is exchanged for oxygen.

The oxygenated blood returns to the heart. As stated in Chapter 13, blood enters the right atrium, which contracts, forcing the blood through the tricuspid valve into the right ventricle.

The right ventricle contracts to push the blood through the pulmonary valve into the pulmonary trunk. The pulmonary trunk bifurcates (divides in two). It branches into the right pulmonary artery, bringing blood to the right lung, and into the left pulmonary artery, bringing blood to the left lung, Figure 14-1.

Inside the lungs, the pulmonary arteries branch into countless small arteries called **arterioles**. The arterioles connect to dense beds of capillaries lying in the alveoli lung tissue. Here, gaseous exchange takes place: carbon dioxide leaves the red blood cells and is discharged into the air in the alveoli, to be excreted from the lungs. Oxygen from air in the alveoli combines with hemoglobin in the red blood cells. From these capillaries the blood travels into small veins or **venules**.

Venules from the right and left lung form large pulmonary veins. These veins carry oxy-

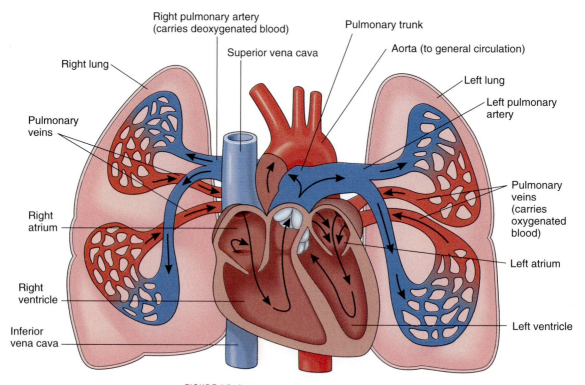

FIGURE 14-1 *Cardiopulmonary circulation*

genated blood from the lungs back to the heart and into the left atrium.

The left atrium contracts, sending the blood through the bicuspid, or mitral valve, into the left ventricle. This chamber, then, acts as a pump for newly oxygenated blood. When the left ventricle contracts, it sends oxygenated blood through the aortic semilunar valve, then into the aorta.

The function of the general (systemic) circulation is fourfold: it circulates nutrients, oxygen, water, and secretions to the tissues and back to the heart; it carries products such as carbon dioxide and other dissolved wastes away from the tissues; it helps equalize body temperature; it aids in protecting the body from harmful bacteria.

PATH OF SYSTEMIC/GENERAL CIRCULATION

The **aorta** is the largest artery in the body. The first branch of the aorta is the coronary artery which takes blood to the myocardium (cardial muscle). As the aorta emerges (ascending aorta) from the anterior (upper) portion of the heart, it forms an arch. This arch is known as the aortic arch. Three branches come from this arch: the brachiocephalic, the left common carotid and the left subclavian arteries, Figure 14-2. These arteries and their branches carry blood to the arms, neck and head.

From the aortic arch, the aorta descends along the mid-dorsal wall of the thorax and abdomen. Many arteries branch off from the

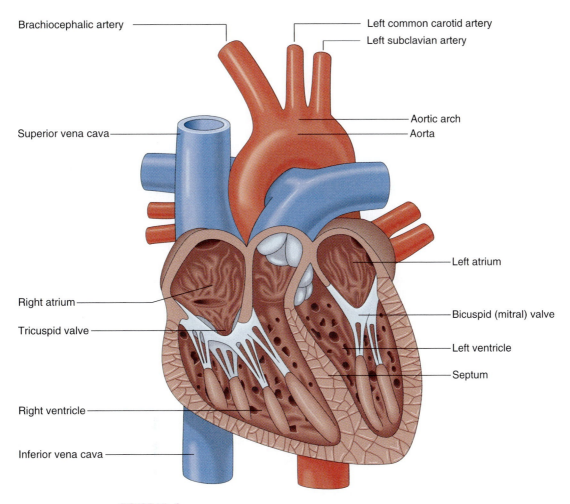

FIGURE 14-2 *Blood flow into, around, and out of the heart*

descending aorta, carrying oxygenated blood throughout the body.

As the descending aorta proceeds posteriorly, it sends off additional branches to the body wall, stomach, intestines, liver, pancreas, spleen, kidneys, reproductive organs, urinary bladder, legs, and so forth. Each of these arteries subdivides into still smaller arteries, then into arterioles, and finally into numerous capillaries embedded in the tissues. This is where hormones, nutrients, oxygen and other materials are transferred from the blood into the tissue.

In turn, metabolic waste products, such as carbon dioxide and nitrogenous wastes, are picked up by the blood. Hormones secreted by specialized tissues, and nutrients from the small intestines and liver, are also absorbed by the blood. Blood then runs from the capillaries first into tiny veins, through increasingly larger veins, and finally into one (or more) of the veins which exit from the organ. Eventually it empties into one of two largest veins in the body. See Figure 14-2.

Deoxygenated venous blood, returning from the lower parts of the body, empties into the interior vena cava. Venous blood from the upper body parts (arms, neck, and head) passes into the superior vena cava. Both the inferior and superior vena cava empty their deoxygenated blood into the right atrium.

Coronary Circulation

The **coronary circulation** brings oxygenated blood to the heart muscle. It has two branches: the left and right coronary arteries. These branches come off from the aorta just above the heart. The branches encircle the heart muscle with many tiny branches going to all parts of the heart muscle. Blood returns to the right atrium by a pocket or trough in the wall of the right atrium, the **coronary sinus** into which the coronary veins empty.

Portal Circulation

The **portal circulation** is a branch of the general circulation. Veins from the pancreas, stomach, small intestine, colon, and spleen empty their blood into the **portal vein** which goes to the liver, see Figure 14-3.

CAREER PROFILES

REGISTERED NURSES (R.N.'S)

Registered nurses are typically concerned with the "whole person," providing for the physical, mental, and emotional needs of their patients. They observe, assess, and record symptoms, reactions, and progress; they also assist physicians during treatments and examinations, administer medications, and assist in convalescence and rehabilitation. R.N.'s develop nursing care plans, instruct patients and their families in proper care, and help individuals and groups improve and maintain their health.

Registered nurses work in hospitals, the home, offices, nursing homes, public health services, and industries. At the advanced level, they work as nurse practitioners, clinical nurse specialists, nurse anesthetists, and nurse mid-wives.

In all states, students must graduate from an accredited school of nursing and pass a national licensing examination in order to become an R.N. There are three major educational paths to nursing: Associate degree programs (ADN) take two years, Bachelor of Science in Nursing (BSN) takes four years, and Diploma programs given in hospitals last two to three years.

Employment outlook is expected to be above average in the coming years. Job outlook is best for the nurse with a BSN.

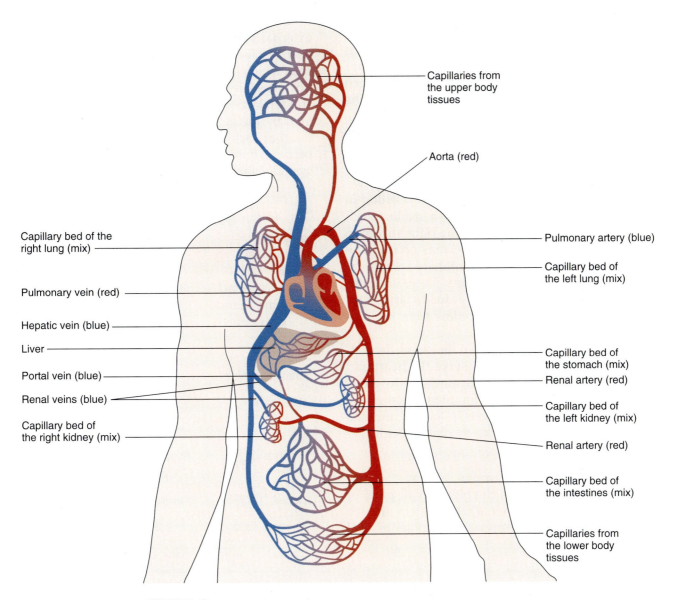

Capillaries from
the upper body
tissues

Aorta (red)

Capillary bed of the
right lung (mix)

Pulmonary vein (red)

Hepatic vein (blue)

Liver

Portal vein (blue)

Renal veins (blue)

Capillary bed of
the right kidney (mix)

Pulmonary artery (blue)

Capillary bed of
the left lung (mix)

Capillary bed of
the stomach (mix)

Renal artery (red)

Capillary bed of
the left kidney (mix)

Renal artery (red)

Capillary bed of
the intestines (mix)

Capillaries from
the lower body
tissues

FIGURE 14-3 *The systemic, pulmonary, renal, and portal blood circuits*

It is very important that venous blood makes a detour through the liver before returning to the heart. After meals, blood reaching the liver contains a higher than normal concentration of glucose. The liver removes the excess glucose, converting it to glycogen. In the event of vigorous exercise, work or prolonged periods without nourishment, glycogen reserves will be changed back into glucose for energy. This detour insures that the blood's glucose concentration is kept within a relatively narrow range.

The liver also detoxifies (neutralizes) drugs and toxins, breaks down hormones no longer useful to the body, and produces urea during the catabolism of amino acids. The liver also removes worn-out red blood cells from circulation.

Deoxygenated venous blood leaves the liver through the **hepatic vein**, which carries it to the inferior vena cava. From the inferior vena cava, blood enters the right atrium.

Fetal Circulation

Fetal circulation occurs in the fetus (unborn baby). Instead of using its own lungs and digestive system, the fetus obtains oxygen and nutrients from the mother's blood. The fetal and maternal blood do not mix. The exchange of gases, food, and waste takes place in the structure known as the placenta, located in the pregnant uterus.

In fetal circulation, blood may follow two paths: in the fetal heart there is an opening in the septum called the foramen ovale which permits blood to flow from the right atrium to the left atrium, and/or blood may go from the right ventricle to the pulmonary semilunar valve to the pulmonary artery. There is another fetal structure called the ductus arteriosus which allows the blood to flow from the pulmonary artery to the aorta.

In a fetus the purpose of the blood circulating through the heart is to give the heart and blood vessels oxygen and nutrients to grow. When birth occurs, the foramen ovale closes and the ductus arteriosus collapses and the normal cardiopulmonary circulation begins.

BLOOD VESSELS

The heart pumps the blood to all parts of the body through a remarkable system of three types of blood vessels: arteries, capillaries, and veins.

ARTERIES

Arteries carry oxygenated blood away from the heart to the capillaries. (There is one exception—the pulmonary arteries—which carry deoxygenated blood from the heart to the lungs). The arteries transport blood under very high pressure; they are elastic, muscular and thick-walled. The thickness of the arteries makes them the strongest of the three types of blood vessels. Table 14-1 lists the principal arteries and the areas they serve. See also Figure 14-4.

As seen in Figure 14-5, page 226 , the arterial walls are composed of three layers. The outer layer is called the **tunica adventitia** or **externa**. This layer is composed of fibrous connective tissue with bundles of smooth muscle cells which lends great elasticity to the arteries. This elasticity allows the arteries to withstand sudden large increases in internal pressure, created by the large volume of blood forced into them at each heart contraction. When arteries become hardened, as in arteriosclerosis, the systolic blood pressure increases greatly.

TABLE 14-1 • *Principal Arteries*

PRINCIPAL ARTERIES	AREA SERVED
Common carotid	head and face
Internal carotid	brain
External carotid	face (*pulse point*)
Vertebral	spinal column and brain
Brachiocephalic	right arm, head and shoulder
Subclavian	shoulder
Axillary	axilla area
Brachial	upper arm and elbow area (*pulse point*)
Radial	arm, wrist (*pulse point*)
Thoracic aorta	chest cavity
Celiac	liver, spleen, stomach and pancreas
splenic	spleen
hepatic	liver
Superior mesenteric	small intestines and colon
Renal	kidney
Common iliac	lower abdominal area
Internal iliac	pelvis and bladder
External iliac	groin and lower leg
Femoral	groin (*pulse point*)
Popliteal	knee area (*pulse point*)
Anterior tibialis	anterior lower leg
Posterior tibialis	posterior lower leg
Dorsalis pedis	ankle (*pulse point*)

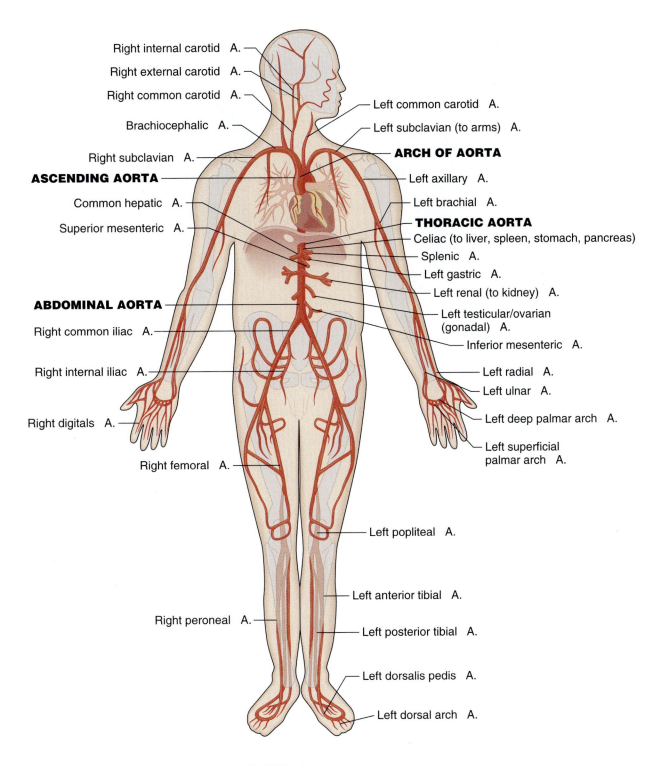

Right internal carotid A.
Right external carotid A.
Right common carotid A.
Brachiocephalic A.
Right subclavian A.
ASCENDING AORTA
Common hepatic A.
Superior mesenteric A.
ABDOMINAL AORTA
Right common iliac A.
Right internal iliac A.
Right digitals A.
Right femoral A.
Right peroneal A.

Left common carotid A.
Left subclavian (to arms) A.
ARCH OF AORTA
Left axillary A.
Left brachial A.
THORACIC AORTA
Celiac (to liver, spleen, stomach, pancreas)
Splenic A.
Left gastric A.
Left renal (to kidney) A.
Left testicular/ovarian
(gonadal) A.
Inferior mesenteric A.
Left radial A.
Left ulnar A.
Left deep palmar arch A.
Left superficial
palmar arch A.
Left popliteal A.
Left anterior tibial A.
Left posterior tibial A.
Left dorsalis pedis A.
Left dorsal arch A.

FIGURE 14-4 *Arterial distribution*

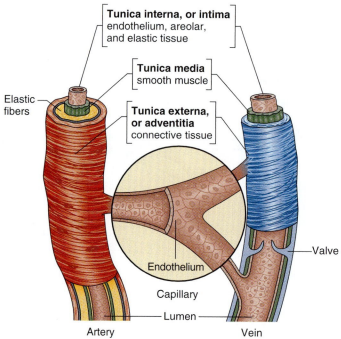

Tunica interna, or intima
endothelium, areolar,
and elastic tissue

Tunica media
smooth muscle

Tunica externa,
or adventitia
connective tissue

Elastic
fibers

Endothelium

Capillary

Lumen

Valve

Artery

Vein

(A) Types of blood vessels and their general structure

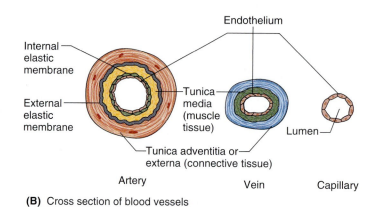

Endothelium

Internal
elastic
membrane

External
elastic
membrane

Tunica
media
(muscle
tissue)

Tunica adventitia or
externa (connective tissue)

Lumen

Artery

Vein

Capillary

(B) Cross section of blood vessels

FIGURE 14-5 *Different types of blood vessels and their cross-sectional views*

The **tunica media** is the middle arterial layer. It is composed of muscle cells arranged in a circular pattern. This layer controls the artery's diameter by dilation and constriction, which regulates the flow of blood through the artery. This keeps the blood flow steady and even and reduces the heart's work.

An inner layer (**tunica intima**) consists of three smaller layers: endothelium, areolar, and elastic tissue. The endothelium gives the artery a smooth lining which allows for the free flow of blood. See Figure 14-5.

The aorta leads away from the heart and branches into smaller arteries. These smaller arteries, in turn, branch into arterioles, which still have some smooth muscle in the walls and are also resistant vessels. Arterioles give rise to the capillaries, Figure 14-6.

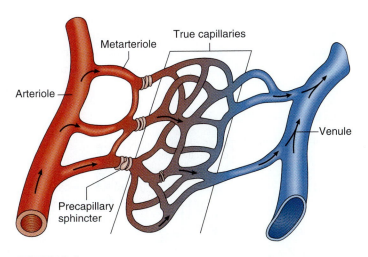

FIGURE 14-6 *Capillary bed connecting an arteriole with a venule*

CAPILLARIES

Capillaries are the smallest blood vessels which can only be seen through a compound microscope. Capillaries connect the arterioles with venules. Capillaries are branches of the finest arteriole divisions, known as metarterioles. The metarterioles have lost most of their connective tissue and muscle layers. Eventually, the last traces of these two tissues disappear and there remains only a simple endothelial cell layer. This endothelial cell layer constitutes the capillaries.

The capillary walls are extremely thin to allow for the selective permeability of various cells and substances. Nutrient molecules and oxygen pass out of the capillaries and into the surrounding cells and tissues. Metabolic waste products like carbon dioxide and nitrogenous wastes pass back from the cells and tissues into the bloodstream for excretion at their proper sites (i.e. lungs and kidneys).

Tiny openings in the capillary walls allow white blood cells to leave the bloodstream and enter the tissue spaces to help destroy invading bacteria. In the capillaries, some of the plasma diffuses out of the bloodstream and into the tissue spaces. This fluid is called interstitial fluid and is returned to the bloodstream in the form of lymph via the lymphatic vessels.

Sometimes, the diameter of red blood cells exceeds that of the capillaries: they become compressed and distorted as they flow through the capillary.

Blood flow through the capillaries can be controlled, despite the fact that muscle cells do not line the capillary walls. This is achieved by the action of small muscular bands called precapillary sphincters.

Although capillaries are ultimately responsible for transporting blood to all tissues, not all capillaries are open simultaneously. This system allows for regulation of blood flow to so-called "active" tissues. In the human brain, for instance, most of the capillaries remain open. However, in a resting muscle, only 1/20 to 1/50 of the capillaries transport blood to the muscle cells. Compare this to an actively contracting muscle where as many as 190 capillaries per square millimeter are open. If the same muscle is not active, there may be as few as five capillaries open per square millimeter.

VEINS

The **veins** carry deoxygenated blood away from the capillaries to the heart. The smallest vein is hardly larger than a capillary, but it contains a muscular layer which is not present within capillaries. Table 14-2 lists the principal veins and the areas they serve. See also Figure 14-7.

The veins are composed of three layers: the tunica externa, tunica media, and tunica intima. Veins are considerably less elastic and muscular than arteries. The walls of the veins

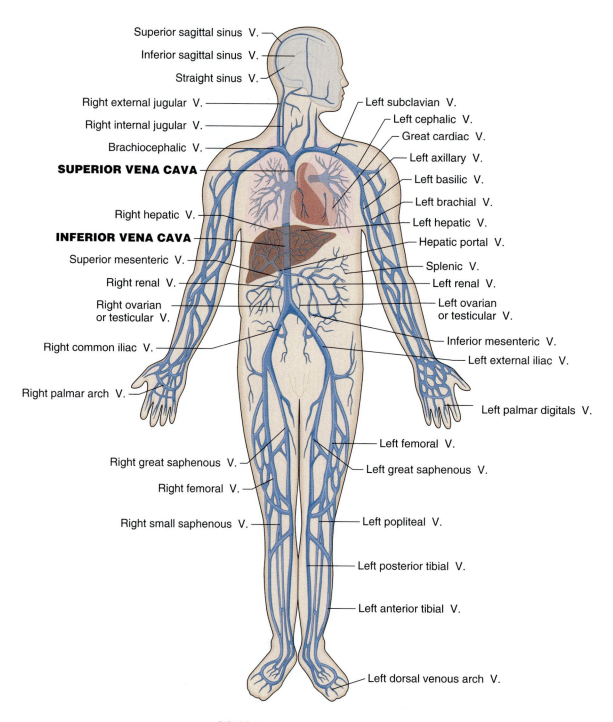

Superior sagittal sinus V.
Inferior sagittal sinus V.
Straight sinus V.
Right external jugular V.
Right internal jugular V.
Brachiocephalic V.
SUPERIOR VENA CAVA
Right hepatic V.
INFERIOR VENA CAVA
Superior mesenteric V.
Right renal V.
Right ovarian or testicular V.
Right common iliac V.
Right palmar arch V.
Right great saphenous V.
Right femoral V.
Right small saphenous V.

Left subclavian V.
Left cephalic V.
Great cardiac V.
Left axillary V.
Left basilic V.
Left brachial V.
Left hepatic V.
Hepatic portal V.
Splenic V.
Left renal V.
Left ovarian or testicular V.
Inferior mesenteric V.
Left external iliac V.
Left palmar digitals V.
Left femoral V.
Left great saphenous V.
Left popliteal V.
Left posterior tibial V.
Left anterior tibial V.
Left dorsal venous arch V.

FIGURE 14-7 *Venous distribution*

TABLE 14-2 • *Principal Veins*

PRINCIPAL VEINS	AREA(S) SERVED
External jugular	face
Internal jugular	head and neck
Subclavian	shoulder and upper limbs
Brachiocephalic	right side of head and shoulder
Left cephalic	shoulder and axillary
Axillary	axilla area
Brachial	upper arm
Radial	lower arm and wrist
Superior vena cava	upper part of body
Inferior vena cava	lower part of body and abdominal area
Hepatic	liver
Renal	kidney
Hepatic portal	organs of digestion
Splenic	spleen
Superior mesenteric	small intestine and colon
Common iliac internal iliac	lower abdominal and pelvis, bladder, and reproductive organs
external iliac	lower limbs
Great saphenous	upper leg
Femoral	upper leg and groin area
Popliteal	knee
Posterior tibialis	posterior leg
Dorsal venous arch	foot

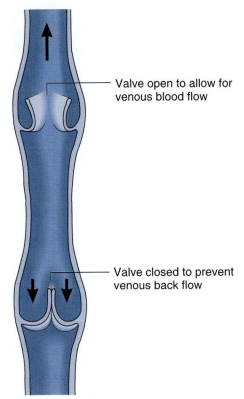

Valve open to allow for venous blood flow

Valve closed to prevent venous back flow

FIGURE 14-8 *Valves in the veins*

are much thinner than those of the arteries since they do not have to withstand such high internal pressures. This is because pressure from the heart's contraction is greatly diminished by the time the blood reaches the veins for its return journey. Thus the thinner walled veins can collapse easily when not filled with blood. Finally, veins have **valves** along their length. These valves allow blood to flow only in one direction, towards the heart. This prevents reflux (backflow) of blood toward the capillaries, Figure 14-8. Valves are found in abundance in veins where there is a greater chance of reflux. There are many valves in the lower extremities where blood has to oppose the force of gravity.

Eventually, all the venules converge to make up larger veins, which ultimately form the body's largest veins, the vena cavae. Venous blood from the upper part of the body returns to the right atrium via the superior vena cava; blood from the lower body parts is conducted to the heart via the inferior vena cava.

VENOUS RETURN

In addition to valves, the skeletal muscles contract to help push the blood along its path.

CAREER PROFILES

NURSING AIDES AND PSYCHIATRIC AIDES

Nursing aides and psychiatric aides help care for physically or mentally ill, injured, disabled, or infirm individuals confined to hospitals, nursing, or residential care facilities.

Nursing aides work under the supervision of nursing and medical staff. They answer call bells, deliver messages, serve meals, make beds, and help patients to eat, dress, and bathe. Aides may also provide skin care, take vital signs, and assist patients in and out of bed. They observe patients' physical, mental, and emotional states and report any changes to the nursing or medical staff. Nursing aides employed in nursing homes are often the principal caregiver, having far more contact with the residents than other staff members.

Psychiatric aides care for the mentally impaired and work under a health care team. In addition to helping patients with the activities of daily living, they socialize with the patients and lead them in educational and recreational activities. Because they have the closest contact with the patients, psychiatric aides have a great deal of influence on patients' outlook and treatment.

Most states require a nursing aide to have training. Nursing aides employed in the nursing homes must complete a minimum of seventy-five hours of mandatory training and pass a competency examination within four months of employment. Aides who complete the course are placed on the State Registry of Nursing Aides.

In response to the aging population, job outlook is good and is expected to grow faster than the average.

LICENSED PRACTICAL NURSES

Licensed practical nurses (L.P.N.'s) or Licensed Vocational Nurses (L.V.N.'s) (as they are called in Texas and California) care for the sick, injured, convalescing, and handicapped under the direction of a physician or registered nurse.

Most L.P.N.'s provide basic bedside care. They take vital signs, treat bedsores, prepare and give injections, and administer some treatments. They collect laboratory specimens, observe patients, and report any adverse reactions. They help patients with activities of daily living, keep them comfortable, and care for their emotional needs. In states where the law allows, they may administer prescribed medicines.

L.P.N.'s in nursing homes also evaluate residents' needs, develop care plans, and supervise nursing aides.

All states require L.P.N.'s to graduate from an accredited practical nursing program and pass a national licensing examination.

Job outlook for the practical nurse is good and is expected to increase faster than the average over the next few years.

In the abdominal and thoracic cavity, pressure changes occur when you breathe; this also helps to bring the venous blood back to the heart. Think about sitting for a long period of time, especially on a car ride. Think how sleepy you start to get. The reason may be that blood isn't getting back to the heart for oxygen. To reduce the drowsiness, you may stop the car, pull over, and get out and walk around for a while. This will improve circulation and the drowsiness should pass.

BLOOD PRESSURE

When the heart pumps blood into the arteries, the surge of blood filling the vessels creates pressure against their walls. The pressure measured at the moment of contraction is the **systolic blood pressure**. The lessened force of the blood (measured when the ventricles are relaxed) is called **diastolic pressure**. The pressure in arteries that are closest to the heart is greatest and gradually decreases as the blood travels further away from the heart.

The average systolic pressure in an adult is 120 mm/Hg. The average diastolic pressure in an adult is 80 mm/Hg. The blood pressure is recorded as 120/80. **Pulse pressure**, a term associated with blood pressure, is the difference between the systolic and diastolic; if blood pressure is 120/80, the pulse pressure is 40.

PULSE

If you touch certain areas (pulse points) of the body, such as the radial artery at the wrist, you will feel alternating, beating throbs. These throbs represent your body's pulse. A **pulse** is the alternating expansion and contraction of an artery as blood flows through it. The pulse rate usually is the same as the heart rate.

Try this simple demonstration: place your fingertips (except for the thumb that has its own pulse point) over an artery which is near the surface of the skin and over a bone. There are seven locations where you can conveniently feel your pulse. (See Figure 14-9.)

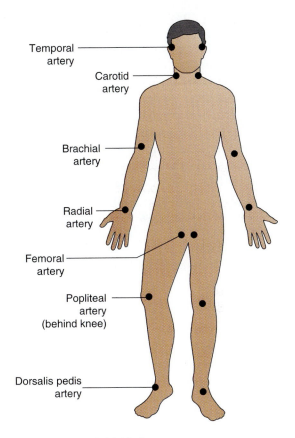

FIGURE 14-9 *Pulse points*

1. **Brachial artery**—located at the crook of the elbow, along the inner border of the biceps muscle.

2. **Common carotid artery**—found in the neck, along the front margin of the sternocleidomastoid muscle, near the lower edge of the thyroid cartilage.

3. **Femoral artery**—in the inguinal or groin area.

4. **Dorsalis pedis artery**—on the anterior surface of the foot, below the ankle joint.

5. **Popliteal artery**—behind the knee. May be hard to palpate.

6. **Radial artery**—at the wrist, on the same side as the thumb.

7. **Temporal artery**—slightly above the outer edge of the eye.

CONGENITAL HEART DEFECTS

Congenital heart defects occur when there is a malformation of the heart during fetal development. In addition to malformation, other conditions may exist because of the unique structure of the fetal heart. As mentioned in fetal circulation, when the baby is born the lungs begin to function, the foramen ovale closes, and the ductus arteriosus collapses. If this does not occur, proper oxygenation will not occur. The most common symptom of heart disease is cyanosis, which is a bluish discoloration to the skin and mucous membrane. Microscopic surgery today can be used to correct many congenital heart defects.

DISORDERS OF BLOOD VESSELS

Aneurysm is the ballooning out of an artery, accompanied by a thinning arterial wall, caused by a weakening of the blood vessel (almost like having a bubble on a tire). The aneurysm pulsates with each systolic beat. The symptoms are pain and pressure, however sometimes there are no symptoms. The most common aneurysm site is in the aorta.

Arteriosclerosis is the disease which occurs when the arterial walls thicken because of a loss of elasticity as aging occurs. Atherosclerosis is the disease which occurs when deposits of fatty substances form along the walls of the arteries. Exercise and low fat diet are recommended to prevent this disease. In both arteriosclerosis and atherosclerosis there is a narrowing of the blood vessel opening. This interferes with the blood supply to the body parts and causes hypertension. Symptoms develop where the circulation is impaired (numbness and tingling of the lower extremities or loss of memory indicates interference with circulation). See Figure 14-10.

Gangrene is death of body tissue due to an insufficient blood supply caused by disease or injury.

Phlebitis is an inflammation of the lining of a vein, accompanied by clotting of blood in the vein. Symptoms include edema (swelling) of the affected area, pain and redness along the length of the vein.

Embolism is a traveling blood clot. A pulmonary embolism is a blood clot in the lungs.

Varicose veins are the swollen veins which result from a slowing down of blood flow back to the heart. Blood backs up in the veins if the muscles do not massage them. The weight of the stagnant blood distends the valves; the continued pooling of blood then causes distention and inelasticity of the vein walls. This condition develops due to hereditary weakness in vein structure. In addition the human posture, prolonged periods of standing, and physical exertion can cause valves in the superficial leg veins to enlarge and weaken. Age and pregnancy are other factors responsible for varicose veins.

Hemorrhoids are varicose veins in the walls of the lower rectum and the tissues around the anus.

Cerebral hemorrhage refers to bleeding from blood vessels within the brain. It can be caused by arteriosclerosis, disease, or injury, such as a blow to the head.

Peripheral vascular disease is caused by blockage of the arteries, usually in the legs. Symptoms are pain or cramping in the legs or buttocks while walking. This pain is called claudication. As the condition worsens, symptoms may include pain in the toes or feet while at rest, numbness, paleness, and cyanosis in the foot or leg. The condition must be treated or amputation may be necessary. Treatments include medication to reduce cholesterol, improved and/or modified diet, and other treatments to improve circulation.

Hypertension or high blood pressure is frequently called the "silent killer" since there are usually no symptoms of the disease. This condition leads to strokes, heart attacks, and kidney failure. Most people discover that they have the condition during a routine physical. Hypertension means that blood pressure is 140/90 or higher. According to the July 1995 journal *Hypertension*, one in five Americans has hypertension. Incidence of hypertension is higher in black Americans and post-menopausal women. Risk factors for hypertension

AFFECTED SITE   **COMPLICATION**

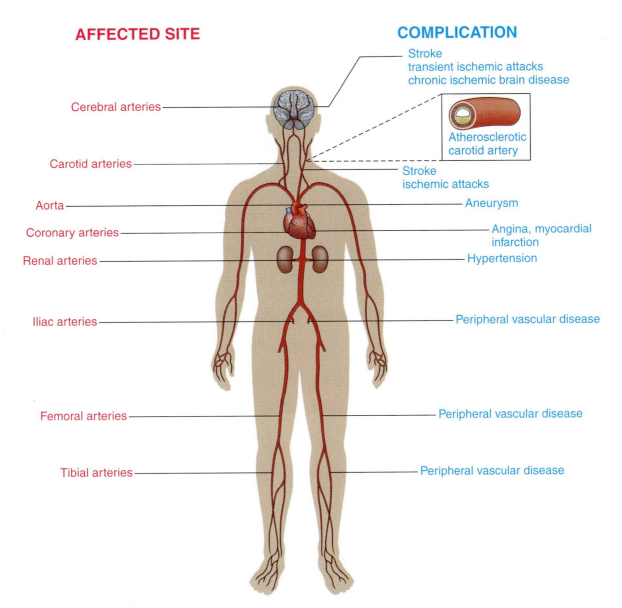

FIGURE 14-10 *Arteries affected by and resulting complications of atherosclerosis*

are stress, smoking, overweight, diets high in fat, and a family history of the disease. Treatment consists of relaxation techniques, reducing fat in the diet, exercise, weight loss, and medication to control blood pressure. In the treatment of hypertension, patients do not understand the disease and its risks. They frequently stop taking their medication because of costs and side effects. Health care workers must realize that better education and commu-

nication will lead to more effective treatment and a higher level of compliance by patients.

Hypotension is low blood pressure; usually, the systolic reading is under 100 millimeters of mercury.

Transient ischemic attacks (TIA's) are temporary interruptions of the blood flow (ischemia) to the brain. The cause is usually a narrowing of the carotid artery due to an accumulation of fat. Patients may experience stroke-like symptoms such as dizziness, weakness, or temporary paralysis which lasts less than twenty-four hours. About 50% of people who have TIA's have a major stroke within the following year.

Cerebral vascular accident (**CVA**) or **stroke** is the sudden interruption of the blood supply to the brain. This results in a loss of oxygen to brain cells causing impairment of the brain tissue and/or death. Stroke is the third leading cause of death in the United States. Based on statistics from the American Heart Association, about 525,000 Americans are affected per year with about 155,000 resulting in death.

Risk factors include smoking, hypertension, heart disease, and family history. About 90% of strokes are caused by blood clots. The clots become lodged in the carotid arteries, choking off the blood supply to the brain. The remaining 10% of strokes called hemorrhagic strokes are caused when blood vessels within the brain rupture.

Symptoms depend on which side of the brain has its blood supply interrupted. Loss of blood supply to the right cerebrum will result in weakness or **hemiplegia** (paralysis) on the left side of the body. Loss of blood supply to the left brain will result in right side paralysis. Other symptoms include sudden severe headache, dizziness, sudden loss of vision in one eye, **aphasia** (loss of speech), **dysphasia** (inability to say what one wishes), coma, and possible death.

For treatment to be effective it should begin as soon as possible and within four hours after the stroke.[1] On arrival at the hospital a CT scan is done to determine if the cause is a blood clot or a ruptured blood vessel. If the cause is a blood clot a drug such as tPA is used to dissolve the clot, restoring the blood supply to the brain.

Physicians are exploring ways to prevent strokes. Patients who have had TIA's are being examined to check the patency of the carotid

MEDICAL HIGHLIGHT: TECHNOLOGY

Diagnostic Tests for Circulatory Problems

Cardiac catherization is the insertion of a catheter usually into the femoral artery or vein. The catheter tip is fed up into the chambers of the heart. Dye is inserted and pictures are taken as the fluid moves through the chambers of the heart. The patient may experience a warm or flushing sensation as the dye moves through the circulatory system; this lasts only a few seconds. This test is useful to determine patency of the coronary blood vessels as well as the efficiency of the structures of the heart. Patients must be asked if they have any allergies, especially to shellfish. The procedure usually only takes two hours.

Angiography is a specialized x-ray taken of a blood vessel. The procedure is similar to the cardiac catheterization. A catheter is inserted usually into the femoral artery or vein and guided into the blood vessels to be visualized. X-ray pictures are taken. This test is done to indicate the status of blood flow, collateral circulation, an aneurysm, or a hemorrhage. Patients must be asked if they have any allergies, especially to shellfish.

Stress tests determine how the physiological stress of vigorous exercise affects the heart. The test is done while a patient is exercising on a bicycle or treadmill under careful supervision. Any abnormalities may be seen on an electrocardiogram. Scientists are now reporting, however, that psychological stress may be a better determination of how the heart muscles react to stress.

[1]Dr. J. Donald Easton of Rhode Island at the American Heart Association meeting, 1997

artery to see if they would benefit from a balloon angioplasty. In 39% of patients who have had TIA, one aspirin per day seems to have prevented a stroke. Other drugs are currently being tested to determine whether they can prevent or reverse the damage by a stroke. To reduce risk factors, encourage patients to stop smoking, get exercise, and control hypertension. Be aware of the signs and symptoms of stroke and get to a hospital immediately if they occur. A stroke occurs suddenly and a patient who wakes up paralyzed and unable to speak will be very frightened. A health care worker must be very supportive to the patient.

● REVIEW QUESTIONS

Select the letter of choice that best completes the statement.

1. The name of the blood vessel that supplies the myocardium is the:
   a. coronary artery
   b. brachial artery
   c. aorta
   d. subclavian artery

2. Special circulation that collects blood from the organs of digestion and takes it to the liver is the:
   a. coronary
   b. fetal
   c. cardiopulmonary
   d. portal

3. In fetal circulation, the opening between the right atrium and the left atrium is the:
   a. umbilical artery
   b. foramen ovale
   c. umbilical vein
   d. ductus asteriosus

4. The blood vessel that carries blood away from the heart to the lungs is called:
   a. pulmonary artery
   b. pulmonary vein
   c. coronary sinus
   d. coronary artery

5. The inner layer of the artery is called:
   a. tunica adventitia
   b. tunica intima
   c. tunica media
   d. externa

6. The blood supply to the brain is carried by which artery?
   a. external carotid
   b. popliteal
   c. internal carotid
   d. coronary

7. The blood supply returns from the legs through which vein?
   a. saphenous
   b. external jugular
   c. superior vena cava
   d. hepatic

8. A build up of fat in the arterial walls can cause the disease of:
   a. gangrene
   b. atherosclerosis
   c. arteriosclerosis
   d. aneurysm

9. An inflammation of the lining of the vein is called:
   a. hemorrhoid
   b. thrombus
   c. embolism
   d. phlebitis

● MATCHING

Match each term in Column I with its correct description in Column II.

Column I	Column II
_____ 1. arteries	a. small arteries that lead to capillaries
_____ 2. capillaries	b. permit blood to flow in only one direction
_____ 3. valves	c. blood vessels that carry blood back to the heart
_____ 4. veins	d. connect arterioles with venules
_____ 5. arterioles	e. large, thick, muscle-walled blood vessels that carry blood away from the heart
_____ 6. aorta	
_____ 7. atria	f. lower chambers of the heart
_____ 8. cardiac	g. loss of elasticity in the artery
_____ 9. coronary	h. referring to the lungs
_____ 10. hypertension	i. largest artery in body
_____ 11. atherosclerosis	j. traveling blood clot
_____ 12. aneurysm	k. upper chambers of heart
_____ 13. arteriosclerosis	l. enlargement of a blood vessel
_____ 14. pericardium	m. circulation through kidneys
_____ 15. portal circulation	n. blood pressure over 140/90
_____ 16. pulmonary	o. arteries that nourish heart
_____ 17. embolism	p. largest vein in body; returns to right atrium
_____ 18. vena cava	q. deposit of fatty substance in the arteries
(superior and	r. pertaining to the heart
inferior)	s. goes to liver from small intestine
_____ 19. ventricles	t. covering of heart
	u. membrane that lines the chest cavity

● APPLYING THEORY TO PRACTICE

1. You are a red blood cell and you are leaving the arch of the aorta. Trace your journey to the right great toe. Name all the blood vessels you will travel through.

2. You are a red blood cell in the left finger. You need oxygen and you must get to the lungs. Trace your journey from the finger to the lungs. Name all the blood vessels and structures you will travel through.

3. You have just heard about a friend's grandmother who has arteriosclerosis of the brain. Your friend asks you to explain the disease and how her grandmother will act.

4. The fetal heart is unique. Why is it different and describe the structures of the fetal heart which change at birth.

5. Take the pulse and blood pressure of a twenty-year-old, a forty-year-old and a seventy-year-old. Compare the results; if they are different, why are they different?

6. A patient arrives in the emergency room, cannot speak, and has weakness on his right side. He appears frightened and confused. How would you reassure and help this patient? The ER doctor diagnoses the patient with having a CVA. Explain what this means, the symptoms, and treatment.

CHAPTER

15

The Lymphatic System and Immunity

OBJECTIVES

- Describe the lymphatic system
- Define the components of the lymphatic system
- Outline the function of the lymph nodes
- Explain what is meant by immunity
- Identify the causative agents of AIDS
- List the symptoms of AIDS
- Describe the modes of AIDS transmission and measures used to prevent its transmission and acquisition
- Describe standard precautions
- Define the key words that relate to this chapter

KEY WORDS

acquired immunity
acquired immuno-
  deficiency syn-
  drome (AIDS)
active acquired
  immunity
adenitis
allergen
anaphylactic shock
anaphylaxis
artificial acquired
  immunity
autoimmune disor-
  der
autoimmunity
axillary node
hepatomegaly
HIV-Human immun-
  odeficiency virus

Hodgkin's disease
hypersensitivity
immunity
immunization
immunoglobulin
immunosuppressed
incubation period
infectious mononu-
  cleosis
interstitial
Kaposi's sarcoma
leukopenia
lymph
lymphadenitis
lymphadenopathy
lymph nodes
lymph vessels
lymphatic
  system

lymphoma
natural acquired
  immunity
natural immunity
opportunistic
  infection
passive acquired
  immunity
right lymphatic
  duct
spleen
splenomegaly
standard precau-
  tions
thoracic duct (left
  lymphatic duct)
tonsils
tonsillitis

The **lymphatic system** can be considered a supplement to the circulatory system. It is composed of lymph, lymph nodes, lymph vessels, the spleen, the thymus gland, lymphoid tissue in the intestinal tract, and the tonsils. Unlike the circulatory system, it has no muscular pump or heart.

FUNCTIONS OF THE LYMPHATIC SYSTEM

1. *Lymph fluid* acts as an intermediary between the blood in the capillaries and the tissue.

2. *Lymph vessels* transport the excess tissue fluid back into the circulatory system.

3. *Lymph nodes* produce lymphocytes and filter out harmful bacteria.

4. *Spleen*
   - produces lymphocytes and monocytes.
   - acts as a reservoir for blood in case of emergency.
   - works as a recycling plant, destroying and removing old red blood cells, preserving the hemoglobin.

5. *Thymus gland* produces T-lymphocytes necessary for the immune system.

LYMPH

Lymph is a straw-colored fluid, similar in composition to blood plasma. Plasma is what diffuses from the capillaries into the tissue spaces. Since lymph bathes the surrounding spaces between tissue cells it is also referred to as intercellular, **interstitial fluid** or tissue fluid. Lymph is composed of water, lymphocytes, some granulocytes, oxygen, digested nutrients, hormones, salts, carbon dioxide, and urea. It does not contain any red blood cells or protein molecules too large to diffuse through the capillaries.

Lymph acts as an intermediary between the blood in the capillaries and the tissues. It carries digested food, oxygen, and hormones to the cells. It also carries metabolic waste products

(carbon dioxide, urea wastes) away from the cells and back into the capillaries for excretion.

Since the lymphatic system has no pump, other factors operate to push lymph through the lymph vessels. The contractions of the skeletal muscles against the lymph vessels cause the lymph to surge forward into larger vessels. The breathing movements of the body also cause lymph to flow. Valves located along the lymph vessels prevent backward lymph flow.

LYMPH VESSELS

The **lymph vessels** accompany and closely parallel the veins. They form an extensive, branch-like system throughout the body which may be considered as an auxiliary to the circulatory system.

Lymph vessels are located in almost all the tissues and organs that have blood vessels. They are not found in the cuticle, nails, and hair. Lymphatic capillaries are not in the cartilage, central nervous system, epidermis, eyeball, the inner ear, or the spleen.

The lymph surrounding tissue cells enters small lymph vessels, Figure 15-1. These, in turn, join to form larger lymph vessels called lymphatics. They continue to unite, forming larger and larger lymphatics, until the lymph flows into one of two large, main lymphatics.

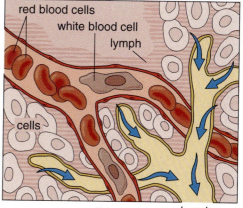

FIGURE 15-1 *Lymph circulation*

They are the thoracic duct and the right lymphatic duct.

The thoracic duct, also called the left lymphatic duct, receives lymph from the left side of the chest, head, neck, abdominal area and lower limbs. Lymph in the thoracic duct is carried to the left subclavian vein, and from there to the superior vena cava and the right atrium. In this manner, lymph carrying digested nutrients and other materials can return to the systemic circulation. Lymph from the right arm, right side of the head and upper trunk enters the right lymphatic duct. From there, it enters the right subclavian vein at the right shoulder, then flows into the superior vena cava, Figure 15-2.

Unlike the circulatory system, which travels in closed circuits through the blood vessels, lymph travels in only one direction: from the body organs to the heart. It does not flow continually through vessels forming a closed circular route.

LYMPH NODES

Lymph nodes are tiny, oval-shaped structures ranging from the size of a pinhead to that of an almond, Figure 15-3. They are located alone or grouped in various places along the lymph vessels throughout the body. Their function is to provide a site for lymphocyte

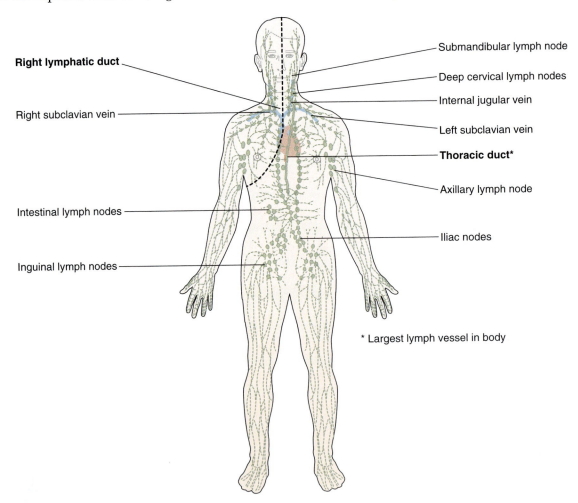

Right lymphatic duct

Right subclavian vein

Intestinal lymph nodes

Inguinal lymph nodes

Submandibular lymph node

Deep cervical lymph nodes

Internal jugular vein

Left subclavian vein

Thoracic duct*

Axillary lymph node

Iliac nodes

* Largest lymph vessel in body

FIGURE 15-2 *Lymph drainage. Most of the lymph enters the circulation system via the thoracic duct, but the right lymphatic duct drains lymph from the right side of the head, right half of the thorax, and the right arm. (From Human Anatomy and Physiology by Joan G. Creager. Copyright 1983 by Wadsworth, Inc. Reprinted by permission of Wadsworth Publishing Company, Belmont, California, 94002.)*

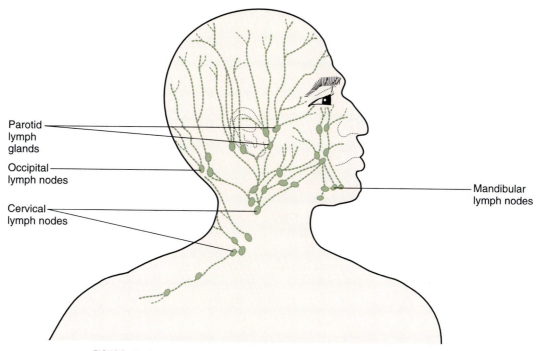

FIGURE 15-3 *Lymph nodes and lymph vessels found in the head*

production and to serve as a filter for screening out harmful substances (such as bacteria or cancer cells) from the lymph. If the harmful substances occur in such large quantities that they cannot be destroyed by the lymphocytes before the lymph node is injured, the node becomes inflamed. This causes a swelling in the lymph glands, a condition known as adenitis.

Knowledge of the location of lymph nodes is important to any health care provider. For example, when giving care to patients with severe infections of the upper leg or thigh, the lymph nodes of the groin (inguinal) and the popliteal area are checked for tenderness and swelling.

Another example of care based on knowledge may be applied to patients with breast cancer. In such cases, lymph nodes under the arms (axillary nodes) and near the breasts may contain entrapped cancer cells. These cancer cells are filtered out of the lymph that comes from the breast area.

Early detection of unusual lumps in the breast is possible through monthly self-examination and routine mammography. Early detection and treatment are *vital*. If discovered too late, the cancer cells may have spread (metastasized) to other areas. It is the lymphatic vessels which spread them.

TONSILS

Tonsils are masses of lymphatic tissues which are capable of producing lymphocytes and filtering bacteria. There are three pairs of tonsils. The most common tonsils are the palatine, which are located on the sides of the soft palate. The tonsils located in the upper part of the throat are more commonly known as adenoids. The third pair, lingual, may be found at the back of the tongue.

During childhood the tonsils frequently become infected, enlarged, and cause difficulty in swallowing, severe sore throat, elevated temperature, and chills. This condition is known as tonsillitis. Surgery is done in only extreme cases since the tonsils have an important role in the line of defense against infection. The tonsils get smaller in size as a person gets older.

SPLEEN

The **spleen** is a sac-like mass of lymphatic tissue. It is located near the upper left area of the abdominal cavity, just beneath the diaphragm. The spleen forms lymphocytes and monocytes. Blood passing through the spleen is filtered, as in any lymph node.

The spleen stores large amounts of red blood cells. During excessive bleeding or vigorous exercise, the spleen contracts, forcing the stored red blood cells into circulation. It also destroys and removes old or fragile red blood cells, and forms erythrocytes in the embryo.

THYMUS GLAND

The **thymus gland** is located in the upper anterior part of the thorax, above the heart. Its function is to produce lymphocytes. These lymphocytes are called T-lymphocytes. The thymus is often classified with the lymphatic organs because it is composed largely of lymphatic tissue. It is also considered an endocrine gland because it secretes a hormone called thymosin which stimulates production of lymphoid cells.

DISORDERS OF THE LYMPH SYSTEM

Lymphadenitis is an enlargement of the lymph nodes. This frequently occurs when an infection is present and the body is attempting to fight the infection. The term "swollen glands" is used frequently for this condition.

Hodgkin's disease is a form of cancer of the lymph nodes. The most common early symptom of this disease is painless swelling of the lymph nodes. Treatment of Hodgkin's disease is chemotherapy and radiation with very good results.

Infectious mononucleosis is a disease caused by the Epstein-Barr virus. It frequently occurs in young adults and children. This dis-

ease is spread by oral contact and is frequently called the "kissing disease" or "mono." The symptoms are enlarged lymph nodes, fever, physical and mental fatigue. There is a marked increase in the number of leukocytes. This illness is treated symptomatically (you treat the symptoms as they appear). Bed rest is essential in the treatment of "mono." In some cases the liver may be affected and hepatitis can result.

IMMUNITY

Sometimes pathogens and foreign materials succeed in penetrating a person's first line of defense, the unbroken skin. The body's ability to resist these invaders and the diseases they cause is called **immunity**. Individuals differ in their ability to resist infection. In addition, an individual's resistance varies at different times.

NATURAL AND ACQUIRED IMMUNITIES

There are two general types of immunity: natural and acquired, Table 15-1. **Natural immunity** is the immunity with which we are born. It is inherited and is permanent. This inborn immunity consists of anatomical barriers, such as the unbroken skin, and cellular secretions, such as mucus and tears. Blood phagocytes and local inflammation are also part of one's natural immunity.

When the body encounters an invader, it tries to kill the invader by creating a specific substance to combat it. The body also tries to make itself permanently resistant to these intruders. **Acquired immunity** is the reaction that occurs as a result of exposure to these invaders. This is the immunity developed during an individual's lifetime. It may be passive or active.

Passive acquired immunity is borrowed immunity. It is acquired artificially by injecting antibodies from the blood of other individuals or animals into a person's body in order to protect him or her from a specific disease. The immunity produced is immediate in its effect.

TABLE 15-1 ● *Types of Immunity*

NATURAL IMMUNITY	ACQUIRED IMMUNITY	
Lasts a lifetime	Reaction as a result of exposure	
Born with it	**ACTIVE:** Lasts a long time.	**PASSIVE:** Borrowed; lasts a short time.
Inherited	*Natural*—Get the disease and recover or mild form of disease with no symptoms and recovery.	*Natural*—baby gets from mother's placenta or mother's milk.
	Artificial—vaccination; immunization.	*Artificial*—Serum from another; immunoglobulin; anti-toxin.

However, it lasts only from three to five weeks. After this period, the antibodies will be inactivated by the individual's own macrophages.

Because it is immediate, passive immunity is used when one has been exposed to a virulent disease, such as measles, tetanus, and infectious hepatitis, and has not acquired active immunity to that disease. The borrowed antibodies will confer temporary protection.

A baby has temporary passive immunity from the mother's antibodies. These antibodies pass through the placenta to enter the baby's blood. In addition, the mother's milk also offers the baby some passive immunity. Thus a newborn infant may be protected against poliomyelitis, measles, and mumps. Measles and mumps immunity may last for nearly a year. Then the child must develop his or her own active immunity.

Active acquired immunity is preferable to passive immunity because it lasts longer. There are two types of active acquired immunity: natural acquired immunity and artificial acquired immunity. Here is how these two types of immunity are acquired:

● **Natural acquired immunity** is the result of having had and recovered from the disease. For example, a child who has had measles and has recovered will not ordinarily get it again because the child's body has manufactured antibodies. This form of immunity is also acquired by having a series of unnoticed or mild infections. For example, a person who has had a mild form of a disease one or more times and has fought it off, sometimes unnoticed, is later immune to the disease.

● **Artificial acquired immunity** comes from being inoculated with a suitable vaccine, antigen, or toxoid. For example, a child vaccinated for measles has been given a very mild form of the disease; the child's body will thus be stimulated to manufacture its own antibodies.

Immunization is the process of increasing an individual's resistance to a particular infection by artificial means. An antigen is a substance that is injected to stimulate production of antibodies. For example, toxins produced by bacteria, dead or weakened bacteria, viruses, and foreign proteins are examples of antigens. Toxin stimulates the body to produce antibodies, while the antitoxin weakens or neutralizes the effect of the toxin.

An **immunoglobulin** is a protein that functions specifically as an antibody. There are five classes of immunoglobulins; immunoglobulin G (IgG), and the others, IgM, IgA, IgD, and IgE.

Autoimmunity

Autoimmunity is when an individual's immune system goes awry. It forms antibodies to its own tissues which destroy these tissues. This is also known as an **autoimmune disorder**.

A well-known example of this disorder is rheumatic fever. A person may get a streptococcal infection as in a "strep" throat, that slightly alters heart tissue. Later streptococcal infections can cause further heart damage. This is because the antibodies formed against the streptococci will also attack the altered heart tissue. This type of heart damage is known as rheumatic heart disease.

Hypersensitivity

Hypersensitivity occurs when the body's immune system fails to protect itself against foreign material. Instead, the antibodies formed irritate certain body cells. A hypersensitive or allergic individual is generally more sensitive to certain allergens than most people.

An **allergen** is an antigen that causes allergic responses. Examples of allergens include grass, ragweed pollen, ingested food, penicillin and other antibiotics, and bee and wasp stings. Such allergens stimulate antibody formation, some of which are known as the IgE antibodies. Antibodies are found in individuals who are allergic, drug sensitive, or hypersensitive. The antibodies bind to certain cells in the body, causing a characteristic allergic reaction.

In asthma, the IgE antibodies bind to the bronchi and bronchioles; in hay fever they bind to the mucous membranes of the respiratory tract and eyes, causing runny nose and itchy eyes. In hives and rashes, they bind to the skin cells.

An even more severe and sometimes fatal allergic reaction is called **anaphylaxis** or **anaphylactic shock**. It is the result of an antigen-antibody reaction that stimulates a massive secretion of histamine. Anaphylaxis can be caused by insect stings and injected drugs like penicillin. A person suffering from anaphylaxis experiences breathing problems, headache, facial swelling, falling blood pressure, stomach cramps, and vomiting. The antidote is an injection of either adrenaline or antihistamine. If proper care is not given right away, death may occur in minutes.

Health care professionals should always ask patients whether they are sensitive to any allergens or drugs. This precaution is necessary to prevent negative and sometimes fatal allergic responses to injected drugs. People with such hypersensitivities should wear a Med-Alert tag about the neck or wrist. This will alert health professionals in the event of an emergency. Such tags have saved the lives of patients rendered unconscious or otherwise unable to communicate.

AIDS/HIV

Discovery of AIDS

Between October 1980 and May 1981, five young, previously healthy homosexual men were treated for a pneumonia caused by a parasite, *Pneumocystis carinii*. Before this, P. carnii pneumonia occurred only in **immunosuppressed** (suppression of the immune system so there is a decreased ability to fight disease and infections) patients, especially those receiving cancer therapy. At the same time, a rare and unusual blood vessel malignancy called **Kaposi's sarcoma** was being diagnosed with increasing frequency in young homosexual males. In 1981, twenty-six cases of Kaposi's sarcoma had been diagnosed in young homosexual males. These cases were an early indication of an epidemic of a previously unknown disease. Later, it was called the **Acquired Immunodeficiency Syndrome** (AIDS). It is said to be the third leading cause of death in young people.

Causative Agent of AIDS

The causative agent of AIDS is called HTLV-III. HTLV-III stands for *h*uman *T*-lymphotrophic *v*irus type *III*. The most common name is **HIV** or **Human immunodeficiency virus**.

HIV Statistics

HIV is no longer a disease of only homosexual males. In its second decade, it is in the mainstream of America. More than one million Americans—one in every 250—are believed to be infected with the HIV virus. The World Health Organization estimates that by the year 2000, thirty-forty million people will be HIV positive and twelve-eighteen million will have AIDS.

Symptoms of AIDS

AIDS is a disease that suppresses the body's natural immune system. A patient with AIDS cannot fight off cancers and most infections. The term AIDS or Acquired Immunodeficiency Syndrome stands for:

- *A-Acquired*—The disease is not inherited or caused by any form of medication
- *I-Immuno*—Refers to the body's natural defenses against cancers, disease, and infections
- *D-Deficiency*—Lacking in cellular immunity
- *S-Syndrome*—The set of diseases or conditions that are present to signal the diagnosis.

There are three possible outcomes that can result from infection with the HIV virus. One is the actual development of AIDS, the second is the development of a condition called AIDS-Related Complex (ARC), and the third condition is known as an asymptomatic infection.

Screening Tests for HIV/AIDS

- *HIV antibody test* detects the presence of antibodies in the blood. From two weeks to three months following infection, antibodies to HIV viruses can be detected in the blood. A positive result may indicate that the person has fought off the infection and is now immune to AIDS, the person is carrying the infection but is not sick, or the person may be developing or already have AIDS.
- *Enzyme linked immunosorbent* (*ELISA*) test is an AIDS antibody indicator. It can detect antibodies for the AIDS virus but not the virus itself.
- *Western Blot* is a follow-up test to confirm the ELISA test.

In June of 1996 the FDA approved two new tests for HIV/AIDS:

- *Orasure* is the first oral test for HIV antibodies. A treated cotton pad is used to scrape a tissue sample between the gums and teeth. The sample is then checked for HIV antibodies. Physicians feel that more people will have this test done since it does not require a blood sample.
- *Amplior test* is for people who have already tested HIV positive. Doctors can gauge AIDS progression or the effectiveness of treatment by measuring the levels of the immune cell called CD4 (the CD4 lymphocyte cell is the main target of the AIDS virus).

ACQUIRED IMMUNODEFICIENCY SYNDROME (AIDS)

AIDS is the most severe type of HIV infection. When a patient has AIDS, the immune system is severely suppressed. The person becomes highly susceptible to certain cancers and opportunistic infections. (An opportunistic infection can normally be fought off by a healthy individual with a normal functioning immune system but infects a person with immune dysfunction.) The opportunistic conditions include:

- Cancers, especially Kaposi's sarcoma and at times primary lymphoma (tumors) of the brain.
- Parasitic infections such as *Pneumocystis carinii* pneumonia and *toxoplasmosis*.*

---

* *Toxoplasmosis* is a disease by a sporozoan protozoa called *Toxoplasma gondii*. Orally acquired toxoplasmosis seldom causes illness and may often go undetected, marked only by fatigue and muscle pains. Acute toxoplasmosis is rare. Symptoms range from fever, lymphadenopathy (lymph node enlargement), muscle fatigue, and pain, to cerebral infection. Its symptoms can mimic aseptic meningitis, hepatitis, myocarditis, or pneumonia, depending on the site of the parasite.

- Fungal infections such as candidiasis and *histoplasmosis.**
- Viral infections such as *cytomegalovirus* (*CMV*) disease,* herpes simplex, hepatitis B, and non-A, non-B hepatitis.
- Persons who are HIV positive are at a higher risk for tuberculosis and syphilis.
- Women who are HIV positive are also at a higher risk for cervical cancer.

The symptoms of AIDS are often non-specific. These symptoms are often similar to illnesses like the common cold or the flu. Unfortunately, these symptoms usually do not go away. They include:

- Prolonged fatigue that is not due to physical exertion or other disorders
- Persistent fevers or night sweats
- A persistent, unexplained cough
- A thick, whitish hairlike coating in the throat or on the tongue
- Easy bruising or unexplained bleeding
- Recent appearance of discolored or purplish lesions of the mucous membranes or skin that do not go away and slowly increase in size
- Chronic diarrhea
- Shortness of breath
- Unexplained lymphadenopathy (swollen glands) that has persisted over three months
- Unexplained weight loss of ten or more pounds in less than two months.

Incubation Period. The incubation period (the period between becoming infected and the actual development of the disease symptoms for AIDS is quite long, ranging from one month to twelve years. The exact number of people who are HIV positive and later develop the disease is still an unknown.

At present, there is no cure for AIDS. However, the opportunistic infections can be treated. Several antiretroviral drugs are being used on AIDS patients in the United States and Europe. Other doctors and health care professionals are treating patients with only minimal symptoms early in the onset of their disease to see if more serious symptoms can be prevented. There is no known vaccine at present. The most common treatment is with AZT or similar drugs which help to prevent the HIV virus from duplicating itself. They act by slowing down the destruction of T-lymphocytes; therefore the body is able to have a better immune response. In 1996, clinical trials demonstrated that protease inhibitors used with AZT reduce the virus to a level that the immune system can handle.

AIDS-Related Complex (ARC)

An individual can contract the HIV virus and develop other conditions, but not AIDS itself. These conditions are called AIDS-Related Complex (ARC). Symptoms range from chronic diarrhea, to chronic lymphadenopathy, to unexplained weight loss. Some individuals with ARC develop a life-threatening opportunistic infection; when this occurs, the person is then said to have AIDS.

Asymptomatic Infection

Some people who have been infected with the HIV virus do not develop any symptoms. These are known as asymptomatic infections and occur with all viruses, and AIDS is no exception. Only long-term follow-up studies of in-

---

* *Histoplasmosis* is an infection caused by the fungus Histoplasma capsulatum. The symptoms range from a mild respiratory infection to more severe ones such as fever, anemia, **hepatomegaly** (liver enlargement), **splenomegaly** (spleen enlargement), **leukopenia** (reduction of the number of white blood cells in the peripheral blood), pulmonary lesions, gastrointestinal ulcerations, and suprarenal necrosis.

*Cytomegalovirus (CMV) disease is a disease that is particularly severe in immunosuppressed persons, especially those with AIDS. Symptoms range from hepatitis and mononucleosis to pneumonia.

MEDICAL HIGHLIGHT: RESEARCH

Developments in AIDS Research

Vaccine for AIDS

Dr. Anthony Fauci of the National Institute of Allergic and Infectious Diseases (NIAID) states that developing a safe and effective vaccine against HIV is critical to efforts to control HIV and AIDS. At the present time, data that has been collected from animal modes demonstrates that vaccine-induced protection against HIV is possible. The goal of the vaccine is to prevent initial infection and/or disease, be safe and well tolerated, induce a durable immune response, provide protection against exposure at mucosal surfaces and to blood, and be easily administered.

Home Test for HIV/AIDS

Johnson and Johnson Company received approval from the FDA in May of 1996 to market the first at-home test for HIV. The test allows people to take blood samples from their fingertips and then send them to a certified lab for testing. The system, called Confide HIV Testing Service, then allows users to receive confidential results and counseling from the center.

fected, asymptomatic people will show whether or not they will later develop AIDS or ARC.

High-Risk Groups for AIDS

The individuals who are the highest risk of contracting AIDS are:

- Homosexual and bisexual men with multiple sexual partners
- Male and female IV (intravenous) drug users who share needles and syringes
- Infants born to persons who are HIV positive
- Persons who may have received blood or blood products before all blood banks were required to test for the HIV virus

This disease is now more prevalent in heterosexuals and there has been an increase in the number of teenagers who are HIV positive.

Transmission of AIDS

The transmission of the HIV virus occurs in three ways (Figure 15-4):

1. Sexual intercourse where semen enters the body (about 75% of the adults in the

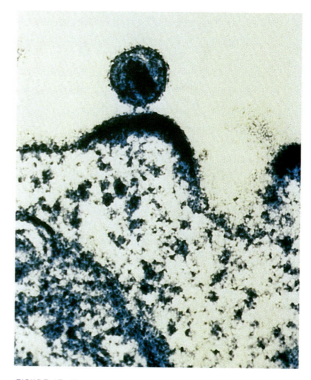

FIGURE 15-4 *HIV that buds out of a T cell migrates through body fluids and infects other cells in the body; the virus is also infectious to others if transmission through body fluids occurs. (Courtesy of National Institute of Allergy and Infectious Diseases.)*

United States who have AIDS contracted it through sexual intercourse)

2. Sharing of hypodermic needles among IV drug users where infected blood is injected into the body (accounts for 17–25% of the AIDS cases in the United States)

3. In utero or at birth from an infected mother to her unborn or newborn infant

Transmission of the HIV virus through transfusion of the blood or blood products has been almost eliminated. This is possible because blood banks now test *all* blood donors to determine whether they have been exposed to the HIV virus. Also, federal guidelines recommend that individuals in the high-risk group do not donate blood or blood products. So far, it seems unlikely that AIDS can be contracted through casual contact. The virus cannot be contracted through air, feces, food, urine, or water. The virus is fragile outside the body and cannot survive. Even close non-sexual contact such as coughing, sneezing, embracing, shaking hands, and sharing eating utensils cannot spread the virus.

Measures to Prevent Transmission and Acquisition

The most important methods in the prevention of AIDS are education and training. It is important to understand that it is not who you are but rather what you do that puts you at risk of contracting the disease. Persons in the risk groups having AIDS must take precautions to reduce the chances of giving the virus to others. At the same time, those in the risk groups must take measures to reduce their chances of contracting AIDS. These measures should be followed by the above mentioned persons:

- Limit the number of sexual contacts because each new sexual partner increases the chance of infection.

- Use latex condoms during sexual intercourse.

- Do not donate blood, blood products, sperm, or any other parts of the body if you are in the high-risk group.

- Abstain from sexual acts where blood or semen are exchanged, as in anal, oral, and vaginal intercourse.

- Do not share hypodermic needles or syringes.

- Make sure that soiled articles, materials, and surfaces are thoroughly cleaned with soap and hot water after incidents involving bleeding.

- Cover an open cut, sore, or wound with a bandage.

- Discuss with your doctor the possible delay of a pregnancy until more is known about the risk of transmitting HIV to the baby.

To prevent the health care worker from contracting AIDS and other diseases, the Center for Disease Control has published guidelines called **Standard Precautions**.

STANDARD PRECAUTIONS

Standard precautions are guidelines to be used during routine patient care and cleaning duties. They must be used when you expect to have contact with blood, any body fluid except sweat, mucous membranes, and non-intact skin.

Handwashing

Handwashing is the single most effective way to prevent infection.

1. Wash hands after touching blood, body fluids, secretions, excretions, and contaminated items, *whether or not gloves are worn.*

2. Wash hands immediately after removing gloves, between patient contacts, and when otherwise indicated in order to avoid transfer of microorganisms to other patients or the surrounding environment.

3. Use a plain (non-antimicrobial) soap for handwashing.

4. Wash hands for a minimum of ten seconds.

Gloves

Wear gloves (clean, non-sterile gloves are adequate) when touching blood, body fluids, secretions, excretions and contaminated items. Put on clean gloves just before touching mucous membranes and non-intact skin. Remove gloves after use and wash hands.

Mask, Eye Protection, and Face Shield

Wear a mask and eye protection or a face shield to protect mucous membranes of the eyes, nose, and mouth during procedures and patient care activities that are likely to generate splashes or sprays of blood, body fluids, secretions, or excretions.

Gown

Wear a clean, non-sterile gown to protect skin and prevent soiling of clothing during procedures and patient care activities that are likely to generate splashes or sprays of blood, body fluids, secretions, or excretions, or cause soiling of clothing. Remove a soiled gown promptly and wash hands to avoid transfer of microorganisms to other patients or the surrounding environment.

Patient Care Equipment

Handle used patient care equipment soiled with blood, body fluids, secretions, or excretions in a manner that prevents skin and mucous membrane exposures, contamination of clothing, and transfer of microorganisms to other patients and environments. Be certain that reusable equipment is properly cleaned and reprocessed before it is used on another patient. Single use items must be discarded properly.

Linens

Handle, transport, and process used linen soiled with blood, body fluids, secretions, or excretions in a manner that prevents skin and mucous membrane exposures and contamination of clothing, and avoids transfer of microorganisms to other patients and environments.

Occupational Health and Bloodbourne Pathogens

1. Take care to prevent injuries from needles, scalpels, and other sharp instruments or devices when handling these sharp instruments after procedures, when cleaning used instruments, and when disposing of used needles. *CAUTION:* never recap used needles or use any technique that involves directing the point of the needle toward any part of the body. Place used disposable syringes, needles, scalpels, and other sharp items in appropriate puncture-resistant containers located as close as practical to the area in which the items were used.

2. Use mouthpieces, resuscitation bags, or other ventilation devices as an alternative to mouth-to-mouth resuscitation methods in areas where there is need for resuscitation.

Patient Placement

Place a patient who contaminates the environment or who does not assist in maintaining appropriate hygiene or environmental precautions in a private room or other relatively isolated area. See Table 15-2.

TABLE 15-2 ● *Examples of Personal Protective Equipment in Common Nursing Tasks*

TASK	GLOVES	GOWN	GOGGLES/ FACE SHIELD	SURGICAL MASK
Controlling bleeding with squirting blood	Yes	Yes	Yes	Yes
Wiping a wheelchair or shower chair with disinfectant solution	Yes	No	No	No
Emptying a catheter bag	Yes	No	Yes, if facility policy	Yes, if facility policy
Serving a meal tray	No	No	No	No
Giving a back rub to a patient who has intact skin	No	No	No	No
Giving oral care	Yes	No	No	No
Helping the dentist with a procedure	Yes	Yes, if facility policy	Yes	Yes
Cleaning a resident and changing the bed after an episode of diarrhea	Yes	Yes, if facility policy	No	No
Taking an oral temperature	Yes, if facility policy	No	No	No
Taking a rectal temperature	Yes	No	No	No
Taking a blood pressure	No	No	No	No
Cleaning soiled care utensils, such as bedpans	Yes	Yes, if splashing is likely	Yes, if splashing is likely	Yes, if splashing is likely
Shaving a patient with a disposable razor	Yes*	No	No	No
Giving eye care	Yes	No	No	No
Giving special mouth care to an unconscious patient	Yes	No, unless coughing is likely	No, unless coughing is likely	No, unless coughing is likely
Washing a patient's genital area	Yes	No	No	No
Washing the patient's arms and legs when the skin is intact	No	No	No	No

*Because of the high risk of this procedure for contact with blood.

CAREER PROFILES

HOME HEALTH AIDES

Home health aides help elderly, disabled, and ill persons live in their homes instead of in a health care facility.

Home health aides provide housekeeping services, personal care, and emotional support for their clients. Aides may plan meals, shop for food, and cook. Home health aides take vital signs, help get clients in and out of bed, and assist with medication routines. Occasionally, they change non-sterile dressings, use special equipment such as hydraulic lifts and give massages.

Home health aides also provide psychological support. They assist with toilet training for severely mentally handicapped children or just listen to clients talk about their problems. In home care agencies, aides are supervised by a registered nurse, a physical therapist, or a social worker who assigns them their specific duties.

The federal government has enacted guidelines for home health aides who receive reimbursement from Medicare. Federal law requires home health aides to pass a competency test covering twelve areas. Federal law suggests at least seventy-five hours of classroom and practical training supervised by a registered nurse. Home health aides who do not receive reimbursement under Medicare provisions may receive on-the-job training.

Job outlook is good and is expected to be one of the fastest growing occupations in the years ahead.

Health Care Worker and the AIDS Patient

Patients with the AIDS virus may have been treated as "outcasts" by the general public. It is most important that the health care worker be supportive of patients with the AIDS virus or patients who have been diagnosed as HIV positive. Wearing gloves for all patient care is not necessary. In fact, the use of gloves for every normal patient contact is not recommended. Wearing gloves for all care sends a negative message to the patient. It implies that the patient is unclean. Patients need the human touch. Have available for patients any information on support services they may need. A toll free hotline is 1-800-342-AIDS.

● REVIEW QUESTIONS

Select the letter of the choice that best completes the statement.

1. Lymph fluid may also be called:
   a. plasma
   b. blood
   c. interstitial
   d. serum

2. The function of the lymph nodes is to produce:
   a. platelets
   b. lymphocytes
   c. basophils
   d. erythrocytes

3. The name of the vessel through which lymph finally rejoins general circulation is called:
   a. thoracic duct
   b. left lymphatic duct
   c. superior vena cava
   d. right lymphatic duct

4. The organ composed of lymphatic tissue which filters blood and produces white blood cells is called the:
   a. spleen
   b. liver
   c. kidney
   d. stomach

5. The ability of the body to resist disease is known as:
   a. sensitivity
   b. resistance
   c. immunity
   d. non-infection

● MATCHING

Match each term in Column I with its correct description in Column II.

Column I	Column II
_____ 1. natural immunity	a. immunization
_____ 2. acquired active immunity	b. immune globulin
_____ 3. acquired passive immunity	c. inherited
_____ 4. acquired active artificial	d. obtained through mother's milk
_____ 5. acquired passive artificial	e. have the disease and recover

● COMPLETION

Complete the following sentences:

1. A person who is highly sensitive to an allergen is said to be _____.

2. An antigen that causes an allergic response is an _____.

3. A fatal allergic response is _____.

4. A cancer of the lymph nodes is called _____.

5. A mass of lymph tissue in the throat is called _____.

● APPLYING THEORY TO PRACTICE

1. A family member is entering school and must have his immunizations complete. Explain to the parent what this means.

2. Your friend says, "I think I have the kissing disease. What is it?" Explain the disease to your friend and how the disease is transmitted and treated.

3. Your class is putting on an educational forum on AIDS for a local community group. Outline the topic; include description of the disease, causes, high-risk groups, treatment of, confidentiality, standard precautions, and how the disease impacts the patient, family, and society.

4. You go to the doctor because you have swollen glands and a temperature of 101°F. The doctor states that the body is fighting an infection which is causing your swollen glands. What does it mean?

5. A woman is complaining of swelling in her left arm after a mastectomy on her left breast. She also had lymph nodes removed for testing. Explain to the patient why the swelling has occurred.

CHAPTER

16

Respiratory System

OBJECTIVES

- Describe the functions of the respiratory system
- Describe the structures and functions of the organs of respiration
- Explain the breathing and respiratory process
- Discuss how breathing is controlled by neural and chemical factors
- Discuss respiratory disorders
- Define the key words that relate to this chapter

KEY WORDS

alveolar sacs (alveoli)
apnea
asthma
atelectasis
bronchiectasis
bronchitis
bronchiole
bronchoscopy
bronchus
cancer of the larynx
cancer of the lungs
cellular respiration (oxidation)
chemoreceptor
chronic obstructive pulmonary disease (COPD)
cilia
conchae
coughing
diphtheria
dyspnea
emphysema
epiglottis
eupnea
expiration

expiratory reserve volume (ERV)
external respiration
functional residual capacity
glottis
Hering-Brewer reflex
hiccough
hyperpnea
hyperventilation
influenza
inspiration
inspiratory reserve volume (IRV)
internal respiration
laryngitis
larynx
mediastinum
nares
nasal polyps
olfactory nerve
orthopnea
pertussis (whooping cough)
pharyngitis
pharynx

pleural fluid
pleurisy
pneumonia
pneumothorax
pulmonary embolism
rales
residual volume
rhinitis
silicosis
sinus
sinusitis
sneezing
spirometer
sudden infant death syndrome (SIDS)
tachypnea
thoracentesis
tidal volume
total lung capacity
trachea
tuberculosis
vital lung capacity
wheezing
yawning

INTRODUCTION TO THE RESPIRATORY SYSTEM

The countless millions of cells which make up the human body require a constant supply of energy. This energy is required for cells to perform their many chemical activities in maintaining the body's homeostasis. For this to occur, energy-rich nutrient (fuel) molecules must be transported to the cells. Oxygen facilitates the release of energy stored in nutrient molecules. It must be in constant supply to the body. Without oxygen, a human being can live no more than a few minutes at best.

FUNCTIONS OF THE RESPIRATORY SYSTEM

1. Provides the structures for the exchange of oxygen and carbon dioxide in the body through respiration, which is subdivided into external respiration, internal respiration, and cellular respiration. See Figure 16-1.

2. Responsible for the production of sound, the larynx contains the vocal cords. When air is expelled from the lungs it passes over the vocal cords and produces sound.

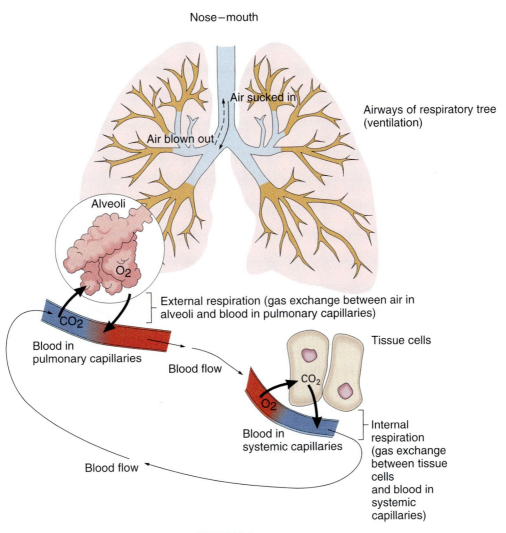

FIGURE 16-1 *Respiration*

Respiration

External respiration is also known as breathing, or ventilation. This is the exchange of oxygen and carbon dioxide between the lungs, body, and the outside environment. The breathing process consists of inspiration (inhalation) and expiration (exhalation). On inspiration, air enters the body and is warmed, moistened, and filtered as it passes to the air sacs of the lungs (alveoli). The concentration of oxygen in the alveoli is greater than in the bloodstream. Oxygen diffuses from the area of greater concentration (the alveoli) to an area of lesser concentration (the bloodstream), then into the red blood cells. At the same time, the concentration of carbon dioxide in the blood is greater than in the alveoli, so it diffuses from the blood to the alveoli. Expiration expels the carbon dioxide from the alveoli of the lungs. Some water vapor is also given off in the process.

Internal respiration includes the exchange of carbon dioxide and oxygen between the cells and the lymph surrounding them, plus the oxidative process of energy in the cells. After inspiration, the alveoli are rich with oxygen and transfer the oxygen into the blood. The resulting greater concentration of oxygen in the blood diffuses the oxygen into the tissue cells. At the same time, the cells build up a higher carbon dioxide concentration. The concentration increases to a point which exceeds the level in the blood. This causes the carbon dioxide to diffuse out of the cells and into the blood where it is then carried away to be eliminated.

Deoxygenated blood, produced during internal respiration, carries carbon dioxide in the form of bicarbonate ions (HCO_3^-). These ions are transported by both blood plasma and red blood cells. Exhalation expels carbon dioxide from the red blood cells and the plasma; it is released from the body in the following manner:

$$H_2CO_3 \longrightarrow H_2O + CO_2$$

(Bicarbonate ions decompose to form water and carbon dioxide)

Cellular respiration, or **oxidation**, involves the use of oxygen to release energy stored in nutrient molecules like glucose. This chemical reaction occurs within the cells. Just as wood, when burned (oxidized), gives off energy in the form of heat and light, so does food give off energy when it is burned, or oxidized in the cells. Much of this energy is released in the form of heat to maintain body temperature. Some of it, however, is used directly by the cells for such work as contraction of muscle cells. It is also used to carry off other vital processes.

Food, when oxidized, gives off waste products including carbon dioxide and water vapor. These waste products are carried away through the process of internal respiration.

RESPIRATORY ORGANS AND STRUCTURES

Figure 16-2 illustrates how air moves into the lungs through several passageways. The following structures are included: nasal cavity, pharynx, larynx, trachea, bronchi, bronchioles, alveoli, lungs, pleura, and mediastinum.

THE NASAL CAVITY

In humans, air enters the respiratory system through two oval openings in the nose. They are called the nostrils, or **anterior nares**. From here, air enters the nasal cavity, which is divided into a right and left chamber, or smaller cavity, by a partition known as the **nasal septum**. Both cavities are lined with mucous membranes.

Protruding into the nasal cavity are three **turbinate**, or nasal conchae bones. These three scroll-like bones (superior, middle, and inferior concha) divide the large nasal cavity into three narrow passageways. The turbinates increase the surface area of the nasal cavity causing turbulence in the flowing air. This causes the air to move in various directions before exiting the nasal cavity. As it moves through the nasal cavity, air is being filtered of dust and dirt particles by the mucous membranes lining the conchal

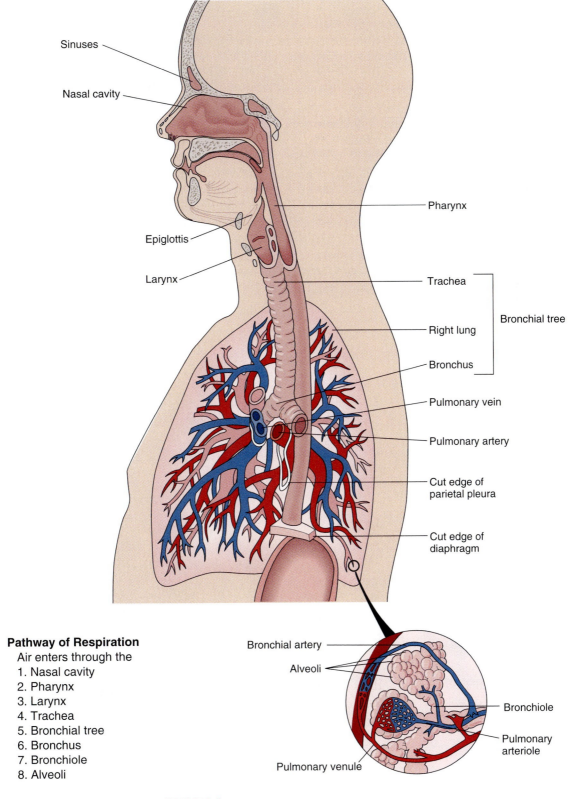

Pathway of Respiration
Air enters through the
1. Nasal cavity
2. Pharynx
3. Larynx
4. Trachea
5. Bronchial tree
6. Bronchus
7. Bronchiole
8. Alveoli

FIGURE 16-2 *Respiratory organs and structures*

and nasal cavity. The air is also moistened by the mucus and warmed by blood vessels which supply the nasal cavity. At the front of the nares are small hairs or **cilia** which entrap and prevent the entry of larger dirt particles. By the time the air reaches the lungs, it has been warmed, moistened, and filtered. Nerve endings providing the sense of smell (**olfactory nerves**) are located in the mucous membrane, in the upper part of the nasal cavity.

The **sinuses**, named frontal, maxillary, sphenoid, and ethmoid, are cavities of the skull in and around the nasal region, Figure 16-3. Short ducts connect the sinuses with the nasal cavity. Mucous membrane lines the sinuses and helps to warm and moisten air passing through them. The sinuses also give resonance to the voice. The unpleasant voice sound of a nasal cold results from the blockage of sinuses.

THE PHARYNX

After air leaves the nasal cavity it enters the **pharynx**, commonly known as the throat. The pharynx serves as a common passageway for air and food. It is about 5″ long and can be subdivided into three sections. The uppermost section, just after the nasal cavity, is the nasopharynx. The left and right eustachian tubes open directly into the nasopharynx, connecting each middle ear with the nasopharynx. Because of this connection, nasopharyngeal inflammation can lead to middle ear infections. The propharynx lies behind the mouth. The lowest portion is known as the laryngopharynx. Air travels down the pharynx on its way to the lungs; food travels this route on its way to the stomach.

When food is swallowed, a cartilage "lid" called the epiglottis is pushed by the base of the

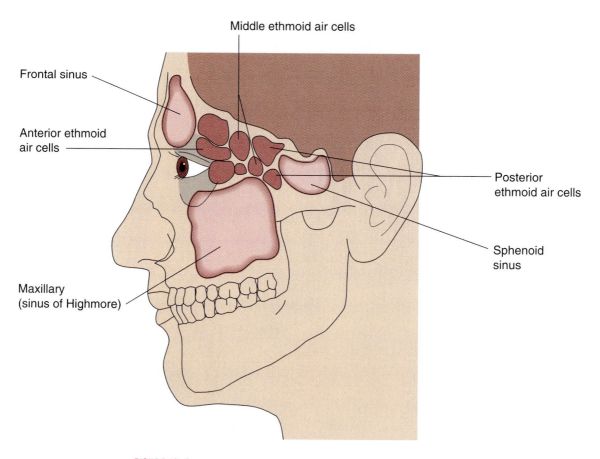

FIGURE 16-3 *Paranasal sinuses, side cross-sectional view*

Labels: Middle ethmoid air cells; Frontal sinus; Anterior ethmoid air cells; Maxillary (sinus of Highmore); Posterior ethmoid air cells; Sphenoid sinus

tongue to cover the opening into the larynx. At the same time, the larynx moves up to help close the opening. With the opening to the larynx covered by the epiglottis, food is directed down the esophagus into the stomach. See Figure 16-4.

THE LARYNX

The larynx, or voice box, is a triangular chamber found below the pharynx. The laryngeal walls are composed of nine fibrocartilaginous plates. The largest of these fibrocartilaginous plates is commonly called the "Adams Apple." During puberty, the vocal cords become larger in the male. Therefore, the Adams Apple is more prominent.

The larynx is lined with a mucous membrane, continuous from the pharyngeal lining above to the tracheal lining below. Within the larynx are the characteristic vocal cords. There is a space between the vocal cords known as the glottis. When air is expelled from the lungs, it passes the vocal cords. This sets off a vibration, creating sound. The action of the lips and tongue on this sound produces speech.

THE TRACHEA

The trachea, or windpipe, is a tube-like passageway some 11.2 centimeters (about 4.5") in length. It extends from the larynx, passes in front of the esophagus, and continues to form the two bronchi (one for each lung). The walls of the trachea are composed of alternate bands of membranes, and fifteen to twenty C-shaped rings of hyaline cartilage. These C-shaped rings are virtually noncollapsible, keeping the trachea open for the passage of oxygen into the lungs. However, the trachea can be obstructed by large pieces of

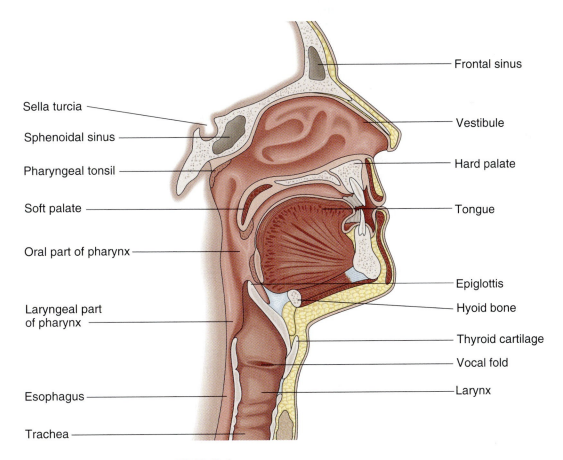

Sella turcia

Sphenoidal sinus

Pharyngeal tonsil

Soft palate

Oral part of pharynx

Laryngeal part of pharynx

Esophagus

Trachea

Frontal sinus

Vestibule

Hard palate

Tongue

Epiglottis

Hyoid bone

Thyroid cartilage

Vocal fold

Larynx

FIGURE 16-4 *Sagittal section of the face and neck*

food, tumorous growths, or the swelling of inflamed lymph nodes in the neck.

The walls of the trachea are lined with both mucous membrane and ciliated epithelium. The function of the mucous is to entrap inhaled dust particles; the cilia then sweep such dust-laden mucous upward to the pharynx. Coughing and expectoration dislodges and eliminates the dust-laden mucous from the pharynx, see Figure 16-4.

THE BRONCHI AND THE BRONCHIOLES

The lower end of the trachea divides in two into the right bronchus and the left bronchus. There is a slight difference between the two bronchi, the right bronchus being somewhat shorter, wider and more vertical in position.

As the bronchi enter the lung, they subdivide into bronchial tubes and smaller bronchioles. The divisions are Y-shaped in form. The two bronchi are similar in structure to the trachea, because their walls are lined with ciliated epithelium and ringed with hyaline cartilage. However, the bronchial tubes and smaller bronchi are ringed with cartilaginous plates instead of incomplete C-shaped rings. The bronchioles lose their cartilaginous plates and fibrous tissue. Their thinner walls are made from smooth muscle and elastic tissue lined with ciliated epithelium. At the end of each bronchiole, there is an alveolar duct which ends in a sac-like cluster called **alveolar sacs** (**alveoli**).

THE ALVEOLI

The alveolar sacs consist of many alveoli and are composed of a single layer of epithelial tissue. There are about 500 million alveoli in the adult lung, about three times the amount necessary to sustain life. Each alveolus forming a part of the alveolar sac possesses a globular shape. Their inner surfaces are covered with a lipid material known as **surfactant**. The surfactant helps to stabilize the alveoli, preventing their collapse. Each alveolus is encased by a network of blood capillaries.

It is through the moist walls of both the alveoli and the capillaries that rapid exchange of carbon dioxide and oxygen occurs. In the blood capillaries, carbon dioxide diffuses from the erythrocytes, through the capillary walls, into the alveoli, and is exhaled through the mouth and nose.

The opposite process occurs with oxygen, which diffuses from the alveoli into the capillaries, and from there into the erythrocytes.

THE LUNGS

The lungs are fairly large, cone-shaped organs filling up the two lateral chambers of the thoracic cavity. They are separated from each other by the mediastinum and the heart. The upper part of the lung, underneath the collarbone, is the apex; the broad lower part is the base. Each base is concave, allowing it to fit snugly over the convex part of the diaphragm.

Lung tissue is porous and spongy, due to the alveoli and the tremendous amount of air it contains. If you were to place a specimen of a cow lung into a tankful of water, for example, it would float quite easily.

The right lung is larger and broader than the left because the heart inclines to the left side. The right lung is also shorter due to the diaphragm's upward displacement on the right in order to accommodate the liver. The right lung is divided by fissures (clefts) into three lobes: superior, middle and inferior.

The left lung is smaller, narrower, and longer than its counterpart. It is subdivided into two lobes: superior and inferior.

THE PLEURA

The lungs are covered with a thin, moist, slippery membrane made up of tough endothelial cells, or **pleura**. There are two pleural membranes. The one lining the lungs and dipping between the lobes is the pulmonary, or visceral pleura. Lining the thoracic cavity and the upper surface of the diaphragm is the parietal pleura. Consequently, each lung is enclosed in a double-walled sac. **Pleurisy** is an inflammation of this lining.

The space between the two pleural membranes is the pleural cavity, filled with serous fluid called **pleural fluid**. This fluid is necessary to prevent friction as the two pleural membranes rub against each other during each breath.

The pleural cavity may, on occasion, fill up with an enormous quantity of serous fluid. This occurs when there is an inflammation of the pleura. The increased pleural fluid compresses and sometimes even causes parts of the lung to collapse. This obviously makes breathing extremely difficult. To alleviate the pressure, a **thoracentesis** may be performed. This procedure entails the insertion of a hollow, tube-like instrument through the thoracic cavity and into the pleural cavity, so as to drain the excess fluid.

Another disorder which can affect the pleural cavity is **pneumothorax**. This condition occurs if there is a buildup of air within the pleural cavity on one side of the chest. The excess air increases pressure on the lung, causing it to collapse. Breathing is not possible with a collapsed lung, but the unaffected lung can still continue the breathing process.

THE MEDIASTINUM

The **mediastinum**, also called the interpleural space, is situated between the lungs along the median plane of the thorax. It extends from the sternum to the vertebrae. The mediastinum contains the thoracic viscera: the thymus gland, heart, aorta and its branches, pulmonary arteries and veins, superior and inferior vena cava, esophagus, trachea, thoracic duct, lymph nodes and vessels.

MECHANICS OF BREATHING

Pulmonary ventilation (breathing) of the lungs is due to changes in pressure which occur within the chest cavity. The normal pressure within the pleural space is always negative, less than atmospheric pressure. The negative pressure helps to keep the lungs expanded. The variation in pressure is brought about by cellular respiration and mechanical breathing movements.

THE BREATHING PROCESS

Pulmonary ventilation allows the exchange of oxygen between the alveoli and erythrocyte, and eventually between the erythrocyte and cells.

Inhalation/Inspiration

There are two groups of intercostal muscles: external intercostals and internal intercostals. Their muscle fibers cross each other at an angle of 90°. During inhalation, or **inspiration**, the external intercostals lift the ribs upward and outward, Figure 16-5. This increases the volume of the thoracic cavity. Simultaneously, the sternum rises along with the ribs and the dome-shaped diaphragm contracts and becomes flattened, moving downward. As the diaphragm moves downward, pressure is exerted on the abdominal viscera. This causes the anterior muscles to protrude slightly, increasing the space within the chest cavity in a vertical direction. As a result, there is a decrease in pressure. Since atmospheric pressure is now greater, air rushes in all the way down to the alveoli, resulting in inhalation.

Exhalation/Expiration

In exhalation, or **expiration**, just the opposite takes place. Expiration is a passive process; all the contracted intercostal muscles and diaphragm relax. The ribs move down, the diaphragm moves up. In addition, the surface tension of the fluid lining the alveoli reduces the elasticity of the lung tissue and causes the alveoli to collapse. This action, coupled with the relaxation of contracted, respiratory muscles, relaxes the lungs; the space within the thoracic cavity decreases, thus increasing the

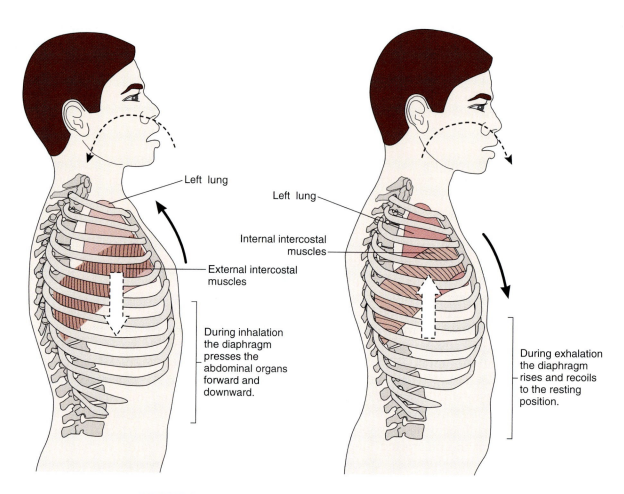

FIGURE 16-5 *Mechanics of breathing--inhalation and exhalation*

internal pressure. Increased pressure forces air from the lungs, resulting in exhalation.

The lungs are extremely elastic. They are able to change capacity as the size of the thoracic cavity is altered. This ability is known as compliance. When lung tissue becomes diseased and fibrotic, the lung's compliance decreases and ventilation decreases.

Respiratory Movements and Frequency of Respiration

The rhythmic movements of the rib cage where air is drawn in and expelled from the lungs makes up the respiratory movements. Inspiration and expiration combined is count-ed as one respiratory movement. Thus, the normal rate in quiet breathing for an adult is about fourteen to twenty breaths per minute. This rate is changeable. The respiratory rate can be increased by muscular activity, increased body temperatures, and in certain pathological disorders like hyperthyroidism. It changes with sex, females having the higher rate at sixteen to twenty breaths per minute. *Age* will also change the respiratory rate. For example, at birth the rate is forty to sixty breaths per minute; at five years, twenty-four to twenty-six breaths. The *body's position* also affects the respiration rate. When the body is asleep or prone, the rate is twelve to fourteen breaths per minute; in a sitting position, it is eighteen, and in a standing position, it is twenty to twenty-two breaths per minute. *Emotions* play a role in decreasing or increasing the respiratory rate, probably through the hypothalamus and pons. See Chapter 8 on the Nervous System.

Other situations that can affect the respiratory rate are:

- *Coughing*—a deep breath is taken followed by a forceful exhalation from the mouth to clear the lower respiratory tract.

- *Hiccoughs* (hiccups)—caused by a spasm of the diaphragm and a spasmodic closure of the glottis. It is believed to be the result of an irritation to the diaphragm or the phrenic nerve.

- *Sneezing*—occurs like a cough except air is forced through the nose to clear the upper respiratory tract.

- *Yawning*—a deep, prolonged breath that fills the lungs, believed to be caused by the need to increase oxygen within the blood.

CONTROL OF BREATHING

The rate of breathing is controlled by neural (nervous) and chemical factors. Although both have the same goal—that of respiratory control—they function independently of one another.

Neural Factors

The respiratory center is located in the medulla oblongata in the brain, see Figure 16-6. It is subdivided into two centers: one to regulate inspiration, the other for expiratory control.

The upper part of the medulla contains a grouping of cells that is the seat of the respiratory center. An increase of CO_2 or lack of O_2 in the blood will trigger the respiratory center.

Two neuronal pathways are involved in breathing. One group of motor nerves, called the phrenic nerves, leads to the diaphragm and the intercostal muscles. The other nerve

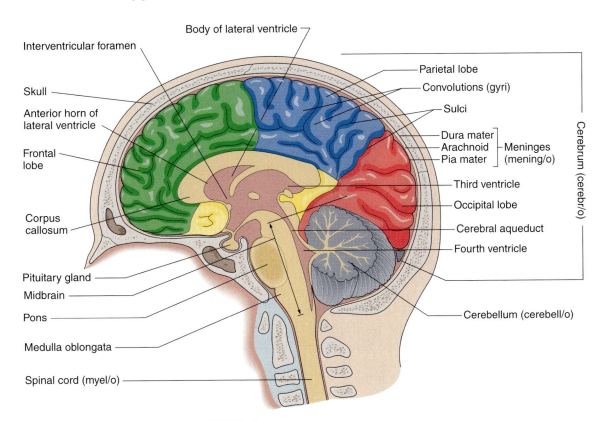

FIGURE 16-6 *Cross section of the brain*

pathway carries sensory impulses from the nose, larynx, lungs, skin, and abdominal organs via the vagus nerve in the medulla.

The rhythm of breathing can be changed by stimuli originating within the body's surface membranes. For example, a sudden drenching with cold water can make us gasp, while irritation to the nose or larynx can make us sneeze or cough.

Although the medulla's respiratory center is primarily responsible for respiratory control, it is not the only part of the brain that controls breathing. A lung reflex, called the **Hering-Brewer reflex**[1], is involved in preventing the overstretching of the lungs. When the lungs are inflated, the nerve endings in the walls are stimulated. A nerve message is sent from the lungs to the medulla by way of the vagus nerve, inhibiting inspiration and stimulating expiration. This mechanism prevents over-inflation of the lungs, keeping them from being ripped apart like an over-inflated balloon. Also it prevents the lungs from taking up too much blood, and so depriving the left side of the heart of its blood supply.

Chemical Factors

Chemical control of respiration is dependent upon the level of carbon dioxide in the blood. When blood circulates through active tissue, it receives carbon dioxide and other metabolic waste products of cellular respiration. As blood circulates through the respiratory center, the respiratory center senses the increased carbon dioxide in the blood and increases the respiratory rate. For example, a person performing vigorous exercise or physical labor breathes more deeply and quickly to cope with the need for more oxygen and the production of extra carbon dioxide.

Other chemical regulators of respiration are the chemoreceptors which are found in carotid arteries and the aorta. These chemoreceptors are sensitive to the amount of the blood oxygen levels. As the arterial blood flows around these carotid and aortic bodies, the chemoreceptors are particularly sensitive to the amount of oxygen present. If oxygen declines to very low levels, impulses are sent from the carotid and aortic bodies to the respiratory center, which will stimulate the rate and depth of respiration. The respiratory center can be affected by drugs such as depressants, barbituates, and morphine.

A&P CHALLENGE

LUNG CAPACITY AND VOLUME

Have you ever held your breath for so long that you thought you would burst? To measure how much air you can hold (your lung capacity), use a device called a **spirometer**. A spirometer measures the volume and flow of air during inspiration and expiration. By comparing the reading with the norm for a person's age, height, weight, and sex, it can be determined if any deficiencies exist. Disease processes like chronic obstructive pulmonary disease (COPD) affect lung capacity, Figure 16-7.

- **Tidal volume** is the amount of air that moves in and out of the lungs with each breath. The normal amount is about 500ml.

- **Inspiratory reserve volume** (IRV) is the amount of air you can force a person to take in over and above the tidal volume. The normal amount is 2100-3000ml.

- **Expiratory reserve volume** (ERV) is the amount of air you can force a person to exhale over and above the tidal volume. The normal amount is 1000ml.

- **Vital lung capacity** is the total amount of air involved with tidal volume, inspiratory reserve volume, and expiratory reserve volume. The normal vital capacity is 4500ml.

- **Residual volume** is the amount of air that cannot be voluntarily expelled in the lungs. It allows for the continuous exchange of

---

[1]Karl Hering (1834-1918), German physiologist and Josef Brewer (1842-1925), Austrian psychiatrist.

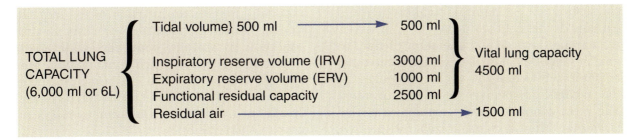

FIGURE 16-7 *Lung capacity and volume*

gases between breaths. The normal residual volume is 1500ml.

- **Functional residual capacity** is the sum of the expiratory reserve volume plus the residual volume. The normal amount is 2500ml.

- **Total lung capacity** includes tidal volume, inspiratory reserve, expiratory reserve, and residual air. The normal amount is 6000ml.

TYPES OF RESPIRATION

The health care professional should be aware of the various changes to the respiratory rate and sounds of human respiration. These changes can alert a health professional to an abnormal respiratory condition in a patient they are caring for or treating. The following conditions describe various kinds and conditions of respiration.

Apnea is the temporary stoppage of breathing movements.

Dyspnea is difficult, labored or painful breathing, usually accompanied by discomfort and breathlessness.

Eupnea is normal or easy breathing with the usual quiet inhalations and exhalations.

Hyperpnea is an increase in the depth and rate of breathing accompanied by abnormal exaggeration of respiratory movements.

Orthopnea is difficult or labored breathing when the body is in a horizontal position. It is usually corrected upon taking a sitting or standing position.

Tachypnea is an abnormally rapid and shallow rate of breathing.

Hyperventilation is a condition that can be caused by disease or stress. Rapid breathing occurs which causes the body to lose carbon dioxide too quickly. The blood level of carbon dioxide is lowered which leads to alkalosis. Symptoms are dizziness and possible fainting. To correct this condition, have the person breathe into a paper bag. The exhaled air contains more carbon dioxide; the air breathed in will have higher levels of carbon dioxide, so this activity will restore the normal blood levels of carbon dioxide.

DISORDERS OF THE RESPIRATORY SYSTEM

Infectious Causes

The respiratory system is subject to various infections and inflammations caused by bacteria, viruses, and irritants.

The greatest loss in production hours each year is caused by the *common cold*. This respiratory infection spreads quickly through the classroom, factory, or business office. It is often the basis for more serious respiratory disease. It lowers body resistance, making it subject to infection. The direct cause of a cold is usually a virus. Indirect causes include: chilling, fatigue, lack of proper food, and not enough sleep. A person who has a cold should stay in bed, drink warm liquids and fruit juice, and eat wholesome, nourishing foods.

Pharyngitis is a red, inflamed throat which may be caused by one of several bacteria or viruses. It also occurs as a result of irritants such as too much smoking or speaking. It is characterized by painful swallowing and extreme dryness of the throat.

Laryngitis is an inflammation of the larynx, or voice box. It is often secondary to other respiratory infections. It can be recognized by the incidence of hoarseness or loss of voice. The most common form is chronic catarrhal laryngitis. This is characterized by dryness, hoarseness, sore throat, coughing and dysphagia (difficulty in swallowing).

Sinusitis is an infection of the mucous membrane which lines the sinus cavities. One or several of the cavities may be infected. Pain and nasal discharge are symptoms of this infection which, if severe, may lead to more serious complications. The sinuses affected can be the ethmoid, frontal, sphenoid, and maxillary sinuses.

Bronchitis is an inflammation of the mucous membrane of the trachea and the bronchial tubes which produces excessive mucous. It may be acute or chronic and often follows infections of the upper respiratory tract. Acute bronchitis can be caused by the spreading of an inflammation from the nasopharynx, or by inhalation of irritating vapors. This condition is characterized by a cough, fever, substernal pain and by **rales** (raspy sound).

Chronic bronchitis usually occurs in middle or old age. Cigarette smoking is the most common cause of chronic bronchitis. Acute bronchitis may become chronic after many episodes. Symptoms include a severe and persistent cough and large amounts of discolored sputum. In order to be termed "chronic," the cough must last for three months and have occurred for two consecutive years. Treatment is symptomatic; the patient must stop smoking.

Influenza or "flu" is a viral infection characterized by inflammation of the mucous membrane of the respiratory system. The infection is accompanied by fever, a mucopurulent discharge, muscular pain, and extreme exhaustion. Complications such as bronchopneumonia, neuritis, otitis media (middle ear infection), and pleurisy often follow influenza. Treat the symptoms.

Pneumonia is an infection of the lung. It may be caused by a bacteria or virus. In this condition, the alveoli become filled with a thick fluid called exudate which contains both pus and red blood cells. The symptoms of pneumonia are chest pain, fever, chills and dyspnea. Treatment may require the administration of oxygen and antibiotics.

Tuberculosis is an infectious disease of the lungs, caused by the tubercle bacillus, *Mycobacterium tuberculosis*. The organs usually most affected in TB are the lungs; however, the organism may also affect the kidney, bones, and lymphs. In pulmonary TB, lesions called tubercles form within the lung tissue. Symptoms of TB are cough, low grade fever in the afternoon, weight loss, and night sweats. The diagnostic test for TB is the Mantoux test— a skin test which is read within forty-eight to seventy-two hours by a health care professional. A positive skin test must be followed by a chest x-ray and sputum sample.

The incidence of TB had been declining because of early detection, treatment with drugs, and patient education. The Center for Disease Control, however, now sees an increase in the number of cases. The reasons for the increase include illegal immigration[1], an increase in the number of homeless and poor, and the spread of AIDS. In addition, there is a new strain of the TB bacteria which is resistant to treatment. People with TB must stay on the drug INH for a long time. Many people stop taking the drug which then leads to drug-resistant organisms. There is concern we will once again see tuberculosis as a widespread infectious disease.

Diphtheria is a very infectious disease caused by the *Corynebacterium diphtheria*. As part of the normal immunization process, children receive a vaccine which is effective against diphtheria.

Pertussis (**whooping cough**) is characterized by severe coughing attacks that end in a "whooping" sound and dyspnea. The widespread use of the pertussis vaccine limits the number of cases in the United States to about

---

[1]Illegal immigrants do not go through a screening process for tuberculosis.

4,000 each year; worldwide pertussis attacks fifty million children. In August of 1996, the Food and Drug Administration gave their approval for a new vaccine called Trepedia which contains diphtheria and tetanus toxoids and acellular pertussis vaccine. Safety data shows that acellular pertussis vaccines cause fewer adverse reactions than whole cell vaccines.

Noninfectious Causes

Respiratory ailments which are unrelated to infectious causes sometimes develop in the respiratory system.

Rhinitis is the inflammation of the nasal mucous membrane causing swelling and increased secretions. Various forms include acute rhinitis and allergic rhinitis caused by any allergen (more commonly known as hay fever).

Asthma is a disease in which the airway becomes obstructed due to an inflammatory response to a stimuli. It was previously thought that the obstruction was due primarily to bronchoconstriction. The stimuli may be an allergen or psychological stress. About 5% of the American population have asthma, which is an increase over the past ten years. The symptoms include difficulty in exhaling, dyspnea, **wheezing** (sound produced by a rush of air through a narrowed passageway), and tightness in the chest. Treatment is with anti-inflammatory drugs. An inhaled bronchodilator may be used as supplemental therapy.

Atelectasis is a condition in which the lungs fail to expand normally due to bronchial occlusion.

Bronchiectasis is the dilation of a bronchus caused by an inflammation, accompanied by heavy pus secretion.

Silicosis is caused by breathing dust containing silicon dioxide over a long period of time. The lungs become fibrosed which results in a reduced capacity for expansion. Silicosis is also called *chalicosis, lithosis, miner's asthma,* or *miner's disease.*

Nasal polyps are growths which sometimes occur in the sinus cavity and cause an obstruction of the air pathway. The polyps may

MEDICAL HIGHLIGHT: TREATMENTS

Emphysema and Asthma

Emphysema

Surgery for emphysema is not a cure but a type of treatment to improve the quality of life, say the doctors at Rose Medical Center in Denver, Colorado. Over two million people in the United States have emphysema. In emphysema, millions of alveoli enlarge and break down, the lungs become overstretched, and the elasticity is lost. Dr. John Simon's combined technique is to make small incisions around the scapula area using optical devices, surgical lasers, and a special stapling device to treat and/or remove the diseased overinflated portion of the lung. This allows the normal portion of the lung more space in which to function, and a smaller more elastic lung makes the work of breathing easier.

Acupuncture for Asthma

Acupuncture may reduce the severity as well as reduce the amount of medication the asthma patient may have to take, says Dr. Kim Jobst from Oxford University, England. Patients should not stop taking their asthma medication but there is evidence that acupuncture can be effective in reducing the severity of the disease. Doctors cannot explain exactly how acupuncture is effective but suggest it may have a relaxing effect on patients. Acupuncture is no longer considered an investigational medical treatment by the FDA. Acupuncture is approved to be used by qualified practitioners. Each state sets the criteria for "qualified practitioner."

be surgically removed which will correct the condition.

Chronic Obstructive Pulmonary Disease (**CDPD**) is a term which health care professionals use to indicate chronic lung conditions, especially emphysema and chronic bronchitis.

In **emphysema**, the alveoli of the lung become over dilated, lose their elasticity and cannot rebound. The alveoli may eventually rupture. In this process, air becomes trapped, is difficult to exhale, forced exhalation is required, and there is a reduced exchange of carbon dioxide and oxygen. The patient with emphysema experiences dyspnea which becomes more severe as the disease progresses.

The goal of treatment in COPD is to alleviate the symptoms as much as possible. Persons with COPD need to reduce their exposure to respiratory irritants, prevent infections, and restructure their activity to minimize their need for oxygen.

Cancer of the lungs is caused by a small cell (also known as an oat cell) which spreads rapidly to other organs. This type is found mainly in people who are smokers. The other types of lung cancer are *squamous cell* or *adenocarcinoma* which do not spread as rapidly. Symptoms include cough and weight loss. Diagnosis is made by x-ray and white-light **bronchoscopy**. A small, flexible tube is passed through the mouth or nose into the bronchi and into the lung. The area is flooded with a white light in order to find abnormal tissue; then, a piece of tissue is obtained for study. It is important for the heath care worker to know that the throat may be anesthetized for this procedure and that the cough reflex must have returned before the person can have fluid or food. Treatment of the cancer may be surgery, chemotherapy, and/or radiation. See Figure 16-8.

Cancer of the larynx is curable if early detection is made of the disorder. It is found most frequently in men over fifty.

Pulmonary embolism occurs when a blood clot (embolism) breaks off and travels to the lung. This condition may occur after surgery or if a person has been on bed rest. Symptoms include a sudden severe pain in the chest and dyspnea. Diagnosis is confirmed by a lung scan. Treatment includes anti-coagulant

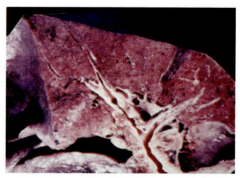
Normal lung

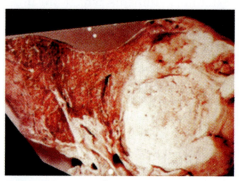
Cancer

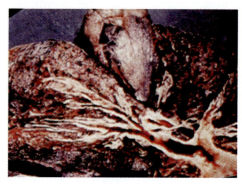
Emphysema

FIGURE 16-8 *Normal and diseased lung tissue (Courtesy of American Cancer Society)*

therapy. To prevent this, early ambulation (or walking) after surgery is important.

Sudden Infant Death Syndrome (**SIDS**) is also known as "crib death," and usually occurs between two weeks and one year of age. The infant stops breathing during sleep. The exact cause of SIDS is unknown; however, evidence suggests that there is a disturbance of the respiratory control center in the brain. If there is any indication that SIDS may occur, the infant is monitored so that an alarm sounds if the infant stops breathing.

Professional health care in many of these respiratory ailments is directed toward maintaining external respiration while making the patient as comfortable as possible. In addition, sufficient rest and proper nourishment are essential.

● REVIEW QUESTIONS

Select the letter of the choice that best completes the statement.

1. The exchange of oxygen and carbon dioxide between the body and the air we breathe in is called:
   a. cellular respiration
   b. external respiration
   c. internal respiration
   d. breathing

2. Oxygen moves from an area of higher concentration through a process called:
   a. active transport
   b. osmosis
   c. diffusion
   d. filtration

3. When air travels through the nose it is filtered and:
   a. warmed and moistened
   b. warmed and exchanged for carbon dioxide
   c. cooled and exchanged for carbon dioxide
   d. cooled and moistened

4. The structure responsible for giving tone to the voice is:
   a. nares
   b. nasal septum
   c. glottis
   d. conchae

5. This structure contains fifteen to twenty cartilage rings and serves as a passageway for air; it is known as:
   a. nasopharynx
   b. trachea
   c. pharynx
   d. larynx

6. The structure at the end of the bronchial tree where the exchange between oxygen and carbon dioxide occurs is the:
   a. alveolar ducts
   b. alveoli
   c. bronchiole
   d. bronchial tree

7. Collapse of the lung is called:
   a. pleurisy
   b. pneumonia
   c. pneumothorax
   d. thoracentesis

8. The rate of breathing is affected by which part of the brain?
   a. cerebrum
   b. medulla
   c. cerebellum
   d. frontal lobe

9. Difficult or labored breathing is known as:
   a. eupnea
   b. dyspnea
   c. orthopnea
   d. hyperpnea

10. Pharyngitis is the inflammation of the:
    a. throat
    b. voice box
    c. windpipe
    d. upper nose

11. An inflammation of the lining of the lung is called:
    a. pneumonia
    b. pleurisy
    c. sinusitis
    d. tuberculosis

12. The vaccine used to protect children against "whooping cough" is:
    a. MMR
    b. Mantoux
    c. Trepedia
    d. Salk

13. Chronic obstructive pulmonary disease means the person has:
    a. asthma
    b. pneumonia
    c. bronchiectasis
    d. emphysema

14. A respiratory disorder with wheezing and dyspnea is known as:
    a. acute bronchitis
    b. atelectasis
    c. asthma
    d. SIDS

15. A respiratory disease that has shown a marked increase in the past few years is:
    a. asthma
    b. cancer of the lung
    c. tuberculosis
    d. COPD

● MATCHING

Match each term in Column I with its function or description in Column II.

Column I	Column II
_____ 1. respiratory control center	a. opposite of inhalation
_____ 2. inspiration and expiration	b. measures of the ability to inspire and expire air
_____ 3. vagus nerve	c. complemental air
_____ 4. exhalation	d. located in the medulla
_____ 5. increased respiratory rate	e. occur from sixteen to twenty-four times a minute
_____ 6. diaphragm	f. result of increase in carbon dioxide content of the blood
_____ 7. intercostal muscles	g. becomes flattened and moves downward during inhalation
_____ 8. tidal air	h. air which cannot be forcibly expelled from the lungs
_____ 9. residual volume	i. less than atmospheric pressure
_____ 10. pressure in pleural space	j. air inhaled and exhaled during rest
	k. muscles in between the ribs which contract during inhalation
	l. inhibits inspiration and stimulates expiration

● APPLYING THEORY TO PRACTICE

1-A. You are a little molecule of oxygen, floating in the air. Suddenly you feel a whoosh, and you are in this dark tube with little hairs tickling you. Is this that thing called the nose? Trace your journey from there to the alveoli of the lung; you will recognize it when you get there. It looks like a bunch of grapes. Name the structures along the way.

1-B. To go even further, after you arrive at the alveoli, squeeze into the capillary around the alveolus and get to the pulmonary vein. You can now begin a new journey to the left knee; trace that journey. Name the structures and vessels you go through.

2. You have a cold, sinusitis, and you talk funny. What is happening? How do you explain it?

3. Take a breath; now breathe deeper, deeper, deeper. Name the process you have just experienced. Let the breath out; force more and more air out until you gasp. Name the process you have experienced.

4. Tuberculosis is a disease that has been with mankind for a long time. Scientists thought that it was a disease that was responding to treatment. However, in the past few years there has been an increase in the number of cases of tuberculosis. Explain the reason for this increase.

5. Breathe on a mirror. Note the moisture which appears from the exhaled air. Discuss the fact that carbon dioxide, heat, and water vapor are given off in exhalation.

6. Jog in place. Note the effect of body activity on the rate of breathing. How does exercise change breathing? Why?

7. Why does a young child breathe more rapidly than an aged person?

C H A P T E R

17

Digestive System

KEY WORDS

absorption
accessory organs
alimentary canal
amylase
amylopsin
anus
appendicitis
bicuspids
bile
bilirubin
bolus
buccal cavity
canines
cardiac sphincter
cecum
cholecystitis
chyme
cirrhosis
colitis (IBS)
colon
colostomy
common bile duct
constipation
crown
cystic duct
deciduous
defecation
deglutition
dentin
diarrhea
digestion
diverticulosis
duodenum
emulsified

enamel
enteritis
esophagus
feces
flatulence
gallbladder
gallstones
gastritis
gastroenteritis
gastroesophageal
  reflux
gingivae
glycogen
greater omentum
heartburn
hemoccult
hemorrhoids
hepatic duct
hepatitis
histamine
ileo cecal-valve
ileum
incisors
intrinsic factor
jaundice
jejunum
lipase
liver
masticate
mesentery
molars
neck of tooth
pancreatitis
pepsin

peptic ulcer
periodontal
  membrane
peristalsis
peritoneum
peritonitis
protease
ptyalin
pulp cavity
pyloric sphincter
pyloric stenosis
pylorospasm
rectum
root
rugae
salivary glands
  parotid
  sublingual
  submandibular
segmented move-
  ment
sigmoid colon
steapsin
stomach
stomatitis
taste buds
trypsin
ulcer
uvula
vermiform appendix
villi
wisdom teeth

All food which is eaten must be changed into a soluble, absorbable form within the body before it can be used by the cells. This means that certain physical and chemical changes must take place to *change the insoluble complex food molecules into simpler soluble ones.* These can then be transported by the blood to the cells and be *absorbed through the cell membranes.* The process of changing complex solid foods into simpler soluble forms which can be absorbed by the body cells is called digestion. It is accomplished by the action of various digestive juices containing enzymes. Enzymes are chemical substances that promote chemical reactions in living things although they themselves are unaffected by the chemical reactions.

Digestion is performed by the digestive system, which includes the alimentary canal and accessory digestive organs. The alimentary canal is also known as the digestive tract or gastrointestinal tract (GI tract). The alimentary canal consists of the mouth (oral cavity), pharynx (throat), esophagus (gullet), stomach, small intestine, large intestine (colon), and the anus, see Figure 17-1. It is a continuous tube some 30 feet (9 meters) in length, from the

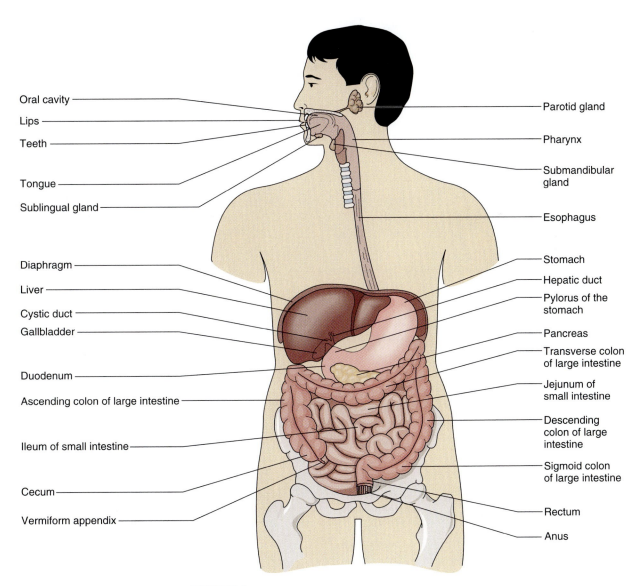

Oral cavity
Lips
Teeth
Tongue
Sublingual gland
Diaphragm
Liver
Cystic duct
Gallbladder
Duodenum
Ascending colon of large intestine
Ileum of small intestine
Cecum
Vermiform appendix

Parotid gland
Pharynx
Submandibular gland
Esophagus
Stomach
Hepatic duct
Pylorus of the stomach
Pancreas
Transverse colon of large intestine
Jejunum of small intestine
Descending colon of large intestine
Sigmoid colon of large intestine
Rectum
Anus

FIGURE 17-1 *Alimentary canal and accessory organs*

mouth to anus. However, during life, the length of the alimentary canal is much shorter (12-15 feet) due to muscle tone.

The accessory organs of digestion are the tongue, teeth, salivary glands, the pancreas, liver, and gallbladder.

The walls of the alimentary canal are composed of four layers: (1) the innermost lining, called the mucosa, is made of epithelial cells, (2) the submucosa, consists of connective tissue with fibers, blood vessels, and nerve endings, (3) the third layer is comprised of circular muscle, (4) the fourth has longitudinal muscle. The mucosa secretes slimy mucous. In some areas, it also produces digestive juices. This slimy mucous lubricates the alimentary canal, aiding in the passage of food. It also insulates the digestive tract from the effects of powerful enzymes while protecting the delicate epithelial cells from abrasive substances within the food.

LINING OF THE DIGESTIVE SYSTEM

The abdominal cavity is lined with a serous membrane called the **peritoneum**. This is a two-layered membrane with the outer side, or *parietal*, lining the abdominal cavity and the inner side, or *visceral*, lining covering the outside of each organ in the abdominal cavity. An inflammation of the lining of this cavity caused by disease-producing organisms is called **peritonitis**.

There are two specialized layers of peritoneum. The peritoneum which attaches to the posterior wall of the abdominal cavity is called the **mesentery**. The small intestines are attached to this layer. In the anterior portion of the abdominal cavity a double fold of peritoneum extends down from the greater curvature of the stomach. This hangs over the abdominal organs like a protective apron. This layer contains large amounts of fat and is called the **greater omentum**. The peritoneal structure between the liver and stomach is called the lesser omentum.

FUNCTIONS OF THE DIGESTIVE SYSTEM

1. To physically break food down into smaller pieces.

2. To chemically change food by digestive juices into the end products of fat, carbohydrates, and protein.

3. To absorb the nutrients into the blood capillaries of the small intestines for use in the body.

4. To eliminate the waste products of digestion.

STRUCTURE OF ORGANS OF DIGESTION

Mouth

Food enters the digestive tract through the mouth (oral or **buccal cavity**). The lips (labia) protect the opening to the mouth. The inside of the mouth is covered with a mucous membrane. Its roof consists of a hard and soft palate. The hard palate is hard because it is formed from the maxillary and palatine bones, which are covered by mucous membrane. Behind the hard palate is the soft palate made from a movable mucous membrane fold. It encloses blood vessels, muscle fibers, nerves, lymphatic tissue and mucous glands. The soft palate is an arch-shaped structure, separating the mouth from the nasopharynx. Hanging from the middle of the soft palate is a cone shaped flap of tissue called the **uvula**. This prevents food from entering the nasal cavity when swallowing, Figure 17-2.

Tongue/Accessory Organ of Digestion

The tongue and its muscles are attached to the floor of the mouth, helping in both chewing and swallowing. The tongue is made from skeletal muscles that lie in many different planes. Because of this, the tongue can be moved in various directions. It is attached to four bones: the hyoid, the mandible, and two

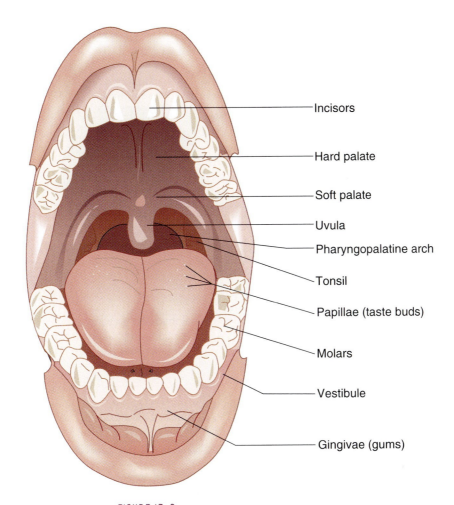

Labels: Incisors, Hard palate, Soft palate, Uvula, Pharyngopalatine arch, Tonsil, Papillae (taste buds), Molars, Vestibule, Gingivae (gums)

FIGURE 17-2 *The mouth and its structures*

temporal bones. On the tongue's epithelial surface are projections called **papillae**, Figure 17-3. There are nerve endings located in many of these papillae forming the sense organs of taste, or **taste buds**. These taste buds respond to bitterness, saltiness, sweetness, and sourness in foods, see Figure 17-3. They are also sensitive to cold, heat, and pressure.

In order for food to be tasted, it must be in solution. The solution passes through the taste bud openings, stimulating the nerve endings in the taste cells.

The sensation of taste is coupled with the sense of smell. When we experience an odor, it stimulates the olfactory nerve endings in the upper part of the nasal cavity. We may confuse the odor of a food with its flavor when it is simultaneously present in the mouth. A bad cold, with nasal congestion, frequently impedes the ability to taste the flavor of foods. This is because increased mucous secretions cover the olfactory nerve endings.

Salivary Glands

Saliva is secreted into the oral cavity by three pairs of salivary glands: the parotid, the submandibular, and the sublingual, Figure 17-4. The **parotid salivary glands** are found on both sides of the face, in front and below the ears. They are the largest salivary glands, the ones that become inflamed during an attack of mumps.

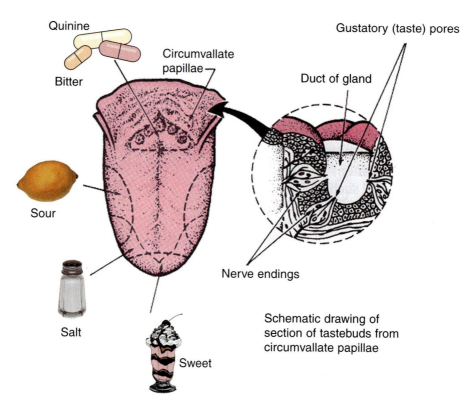

FIGURE 17-3 *There are about 9000 taste buds on the tongue, contained in knob-like elevations called papillae. The taste buds are sensitive to four basic tastes: sweet, sour, salty, and bitter.*

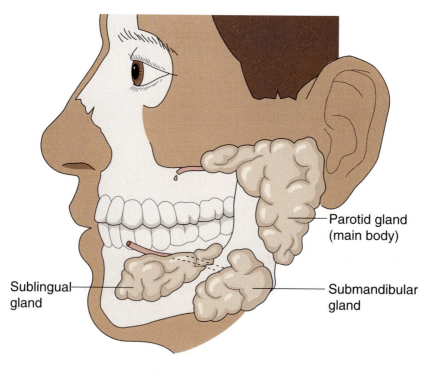

FIGURE 17-4 *Salivary glands*

Chewing, at such times, is painful, because the motion squeezes these tender, inflamed glands. A parotid duct carries its secretion (almost entirely salivary amylase) into the mouth. It opens upon the inner surface of the cheeks, opposite the second molar of the upper jaw.

Below the parotid salivary gland and near the angle of the lower jaw is a **submandibular gland**. This gland is about the size of a walnut and its secretions contain both mucin and ptyalin. The secretions enter the buccal cavity via the submandibular duct at the anterior base of the tongue.

The final pair of salivary glands are the **sublingual glands**, the smallest of the three. They are found under the sides of the tongue. Their secretion consists mainly of mucous and contains no ptyalin.

TEETH/ACCESSORY ORGAN OF DIGESTION

The **gingivae**, or gums, support and protect the teeth. They are made up of fleshy tissue covered with mucous membrane. This membrane surrounds the narrow portions of the teeth (also called cervix or neck), and covers the structures in the upper and lower jaws.

Food ingested by the mouth must be thoroughly chewed, or **masticated**, by the teeth. Teeth help break food down into very small morsels, increasing the food's surface area. This activity enables the digestive enzymes to digest the food more efficiently and quickly than if it were swallowed without being chewed. During normal growth and development, the human mouth develops two sets of teeth: (1) the deciduous or milk teeth, which are later replaced by (2) the permanent teeth.

Deciduous teeth start to erupt at about six months and continue until around two years of age. In total, twenty deciduous teeth are cut during the first two years—ten in the upper and ten in the lower jaw. They are: four incisors, two canines, and four molars. This relationship is expressed in the dentition formula as shown in Figure 17-5. The **incisors** have sharp edges for biting, the **canines** are pointed for tearing, and the **molars** have ridges, designed for crushing and grinding. There are no premolars among the deciduous teeth. Deciduous teeth may last up to the age of twelve.

Permanent teeth begin developing at this point, pushing out their deciduous predecessors. The first molars lead the way between the fifth and seventh years. The last to emerge are the third molars, or "**wisdom teeth**," which may appear anywhere from seventeen to twenty-five years of age. In total, the adult mouth develops thirty-two teeth, sixteen in each jaw, Figure 17-5.

A. The dentition formula for deciduous teeth is:

	Molars	Canine	Incisors	Canine	Molars
Upper Jaw	2	1	4	1	2
Lower Jaw	2	1	4	1	2

B. The dentition formula for permanent teeth is:

	Molars	Premolars	Canine	Incisors	Canine	Premolars	Molars
Upper jaw	3	2	1	4	1	2	3
Lower jaw	3	2	1	4	1	2	3

FIGURE 17-5 *Dentition formulas for deciduous and permanent teeth*

Based on the dentition formula, the adult mouth has eight premolars, or **bicuspids**: four in the upper and four in the lower jaw. Bicuspids are broad, with two ridges on each crown, and have only two roots. Their design is ideal for grinding food. Figure 17-6 shows the arrangement of the deciduous and permanent teeth, and the years during which they normally erupt.

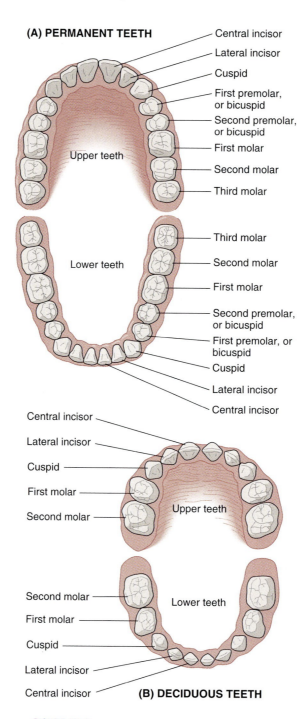

(A) PERMANENT TEETH

Central incisor
Lateral incisor
Cuspid
First premolar, or bicuspid
Second premolar, or bicuspid
First molar
Second molar
Third molar

Upper teeth

Third molar
Second molar
First molar
Second premolar, or bicuspid
First premolar, or bicuspid
Cuspid
Lateral incisor
Central incisor

Lower teeth

Central incisor
Lateral incisor
Cuspid
First molar
Second molar

Upper teeth

Second molar
First molar
Cuspid
Lateral incisor
Central incisor

Lower teeth

(B) DECIDUOUS TEETH

FIGURE 17-6 *Teeth and their eruption times*

CAREER PROFILES

DENTAL HYGIENISTS

Dental hygienists clean teeth and provide other preventive dental care as well as teach patients how to practice good oral hygiene. Hygienists examine teeth, remove plaque, take and develop x-rays, remove sutures, and smooth and polish restorations.

Dental hygienists must be licensed by the state in which they practice. To qualify for licensure, a candidate must graduate from an accredited dental hygiene school and pass both a written test and a clinical examination. Some programs lead to a bachelor's degree but most grant an associate's degree. Dental hygienists should have manual dexterity because they use dental instruments with little room for error within the patient's mouth.

Employment is expected to grow faster than the average for all occupations in response to increasing demand for dental care and the greater substitution of hygienists for services previously performed by a dentist.

DENTAL ASSISTANTS

Dental assistants perform a variety of patient care and laboratory duties. They work at the chairside to assist while the dentist examines and treats patients. Assistants keep patient's mouths dry and clear by using suction or other devices.

Those with laboratory duties make casts of teeth and mouth from impressions taken by the dentist. Dental assistants with office duties schedule and confirm appointments, receive patients, keep treatment records, send bills, receive payments, and order supplies and materials.

Programs in dental assisting take one year or less and are offered at community colleges, vocational schools, and technical institutes. Assistants must be a dentist's "third hand"; therefore, dentists look for people who are reliable, can work with others, and have manual dexterity.

Employment is good. Population growth and greater retention of natural teeth by middle-aged and older people will fuel the demand for dental services.

DENTAL LABORATORY TECHNICIANS

Dental laboratory technicians fill prescriptions from dentists for crowns, bridges, dentures, and other dental prosthetics.

Training in dental laboratory technology is available through community colleges, vocational schools, and technical institutes. Programs vary in length. A high degree of manual dexterity, good vision, and the ability to recognize very fine color shadings and variations in shape are necessary.

A&P CHALLENGE

Structure of a Tooth

Each tooth may be divided into three major parts: the crown, the neck, and the root (see Figure 17-7). The **crown** portion is the part of the tooth which is visible; the **neck** is where the tooth enters the gumline; the **root** is embedded in the alveolar processes of the jaw. Helping to anchor the tooth in place is the **periodontal membrane**.

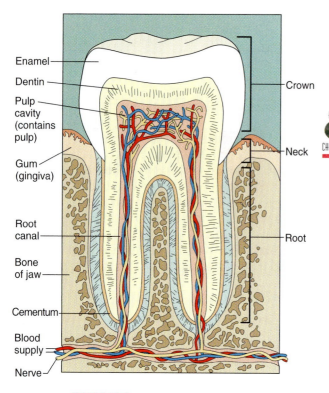

Enamel

Dentin

Pulp cavity (contains pulp)

Gum (gingiva)

Root canal

Bone of jaw

Cementum

Blood supply

Nerve

Crown

Neck

Root

FIGURE 17-7 *Structure of the tooth*

Inside the tooth is the **pulp cavity** which contains the nerves and blood supply. The pulp cavity is surrounded by calcified tissue called **dentin**. In the crown portion the dentin is covered by **enamel**. Enamel is the hardest substance in the body. If the enamel wears down on the surface of the tooth, bacteria may enter and caries or cavities will develop.

ESOPHAGUS

When food is swallowed it enters the upper portion of the esophagus. The **esophagus** is a muscular tube about 25 centimeters (10″) long. It begins at the lower end of the pharynx, behind the trachea. It continues downward through the mediastinum, in front of the vertebral column, and passes through the diaphragm. From there the esophagus enters the upper part, or cardiac portion, of the stomach. This point can be located at the end of the sternum, near the level of the xiphoid process.

The esophageal walls have four layers: the mucosa, submucosa, muscular, and external serous layer. The muscles in the upper third are voluntary and the lower portion is smooth muscle, or involuntary.

STOMACH

The **stomach** is found in the upper part of the abdominal cavity, just to the left of and below the diaphragm. The shape and position are determined by several factors. These include the amount of food contained within the stomach, the stage of digestion, the position of a person's body, and the pressure exerted upon the stomach from the intestines below.

The stomach is divided into three portions: the upper part or fundus, the middle section called the body or greater curvature; and the lower portion called the pylorus. At the opening into the stomach is found a circular layer of muscle, the **cardiac sphincter**, or lower esophageal sphincter, which controls passage of food into the stomach. It is called the cardiac sphincter because of its proximity to the heart. Toward the other end of the stomach lies the **pyloric sphincter** valve which regulates entrance of food into the **duodenum** (the first part of the small intestine). Sometimes the pyloric sphincter valve fails to relax in infants. In such cases, food remaining in the stomach does not get completely digested and eventually is vomited. This condition is called **pylorospasm**. Another abnormal condition is **pyloric stenosis**, a narrowing of the pyloric sphincter which occurs most often in infants.

The stomach wall consists of four layers: mucous, submucous, muscular and serous layers.

1. The mucous coat is the innermost layer. It is a thick layer made up of small gastric glands embedded in connective tissue. When the stomach is not distended with food, the gastric mucosa is thrown into folds called **rugae**, Figure 17-8(a).

2. The submucosa coat is made of loose areolar connective tissue.

3. The muscular coat consists of three layers of smooth muscle: the outer, longitu-

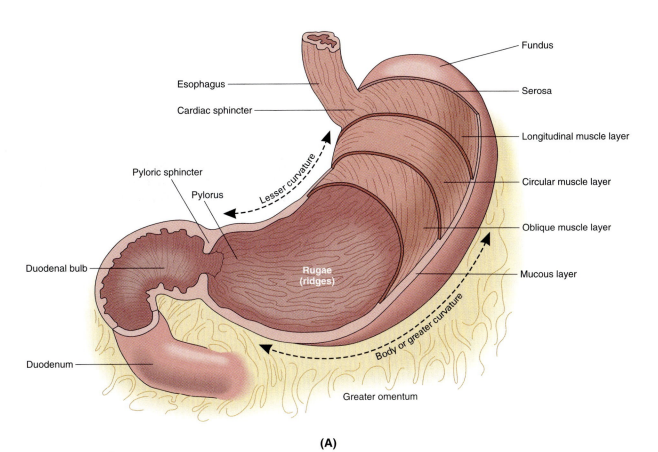

(A)

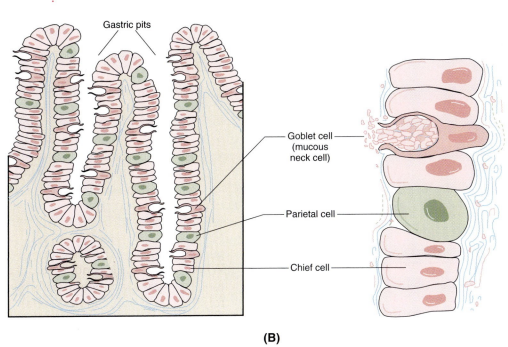

(B)

FIGURE 17-8 *(a) Parts of the stomach, (b) Three types of gastric gland cells make up the gastric glands that line the stomach.*

dinal layer; a middle, circular layer; and an inner, oblique layer, Figure 17-8(a). These muscles help the stomach perform peristalsis which pushes food into the small intestine.

4. The serosa is the thick outer layer covering the stomach. It is continuous with the peritoneum. The serosa and peritoneum meet at certain points, surrounding the organs around the stomach and holding them in a kind of sling.

Gastric Glands

The gastric mucosa contains millions of gastric glands which secrete gastric juice necessary for digestion, Figure 17-8(b).

- Enteroendocrine glands secrete gastrin which in turn stimulates cells to produce hydrochloric acid (HCL) and pepsinogen.

- Parietal cells produce HCL acid which converts pepsinogen into pepsin and destroys bacteria and microorganisms that enter the stomach. It is the body's natural sterilizer.

- Parietal cells also produce the *intrinsic factor*, an element necessary for the absorption of Vitamin B_{12}; without it, a condition known as pernicious anemia exists.

- Chief type cells produce pepsinogen which converts to pepsin. The enzyme pepsin breaks down protein into smaller pieces called protease and peptone.

- Mucous cells secrete alkaline mucous which helps neutralize the effects of HCL acid and the other digestive juices.

- Rennin is found in infants and children, but not adults. It prepares milk proteins for digestion by other enzymes.

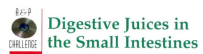

SMALL INTESTINE

The small intestine has the same four layers as the stomach: the mucosa, submucosa, muscle layer, and serosa, Figure 17-9(a).

The final preparation of food to be absorbed occurs in the small intestine. This coiled portion of the alimentary canal can be as long as 20 feet. The small intestine is divided into three sections: the **duodenum**, the **jejunum**, and the **ileum**. The small intestine is held in place by the mesentery. The small intestine lining secretes digestive juices and is covered with villi which absorb the end products of digestion, Figures 17-9(b) and (c).

The first segment of the small intestine is the duodenum. This 12″ structure curves around the head of the pancreas. A few inches into the duodenum is the ampulla of Vater, which is the site where the pancreatic duct and the common bile duct of the liver enter. The pancreatic duct empties the digestive juices of the pancreas and the common bile duct empties bile from the liver.

The next section of the small intestine is the jejunum, which is about eight feet long, and the ileum, which is about ten to twelve feet long.

Digestive Juices in the Small Intestines

- Enzymes, secretin, and cholecystokinin stimulate the digestive juices of the pancreas, liver, and gallbladder.

- Pancreatic juices, namely **protease** or **trypsin** which breaks down protein to amino acids, **amylase** or **amylopsin** which breaks down starches to glucose, and **lipase** or **steapsin** which breaks down fats to fatty acids and glycerol. The pancreatic juices also contain sodium bicarbonate which neutralizes the food content of the stomach which is high in acid.

- **Bile** is necessary to break down or emulsify fat into smaller fat globules to be digested by lipase and steapsin.

- Intestinal juices secreted by the cells of the small intestine including maltase, lactase, and sucrase, change starch into glucose; peptidase changes protease and peptone into amino acids; and steapsin changes fat into fatty acids and glycerol.

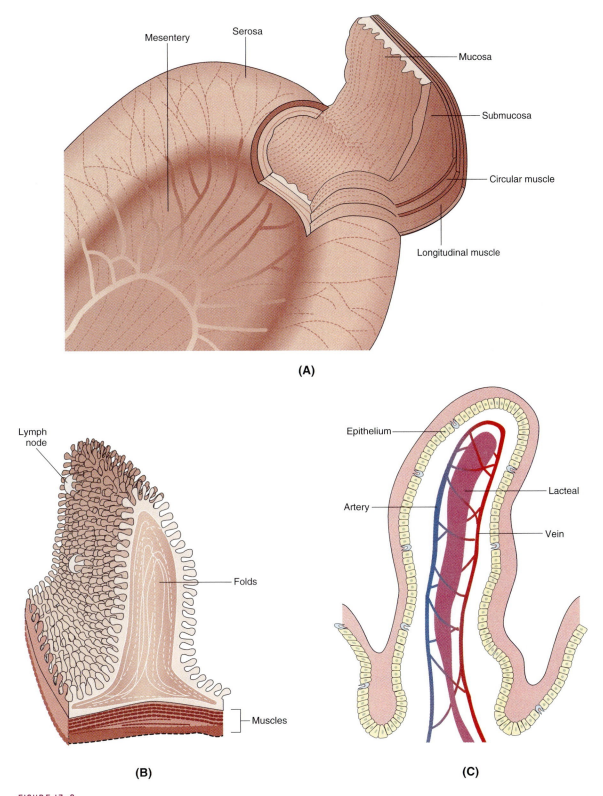

(A)

(B)

(C)

FIGURE 17-9 *(a) Portion of the jejunum showing the inner structure of the small intestine, (b) Diagram of the wall of a portion of the small intestine showing the villi arrangement, and (c) Magnification of a single villus*

CARBOHYDRATES

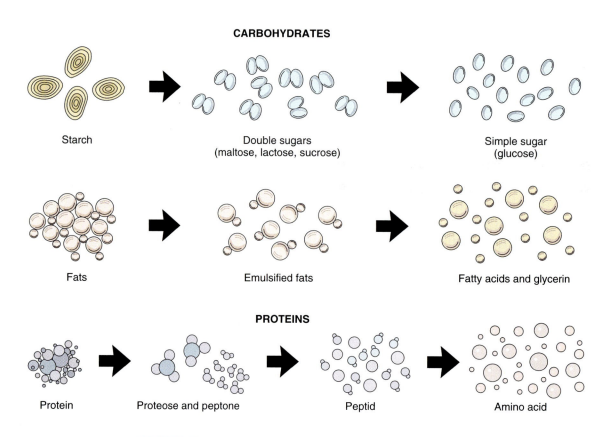

FIGURE 17-10 *Phases in the digestion of starch, fat, and protein*

The combined action of pancreatic juice, bile, and intestinal juice completes the process of changing carbohydrates first into starch then into glucose, protein into amino acids, and fats into fatty acids and glycerol, Figure 17-10. The end products of digestion are now ready for absorption. See Table 17-1.

Absorption in the Small Intestine

Absorption is possible because the lining of the small intestine is not smooth. It is covered with millions of tiny projections called **villi**. Each microscopic villus contains a network of blood and lymph capillaries, Figure 17-9(b). The digested portion of the food passes through the villi into the bloodstream and on to the body cells. The undigestible portion passes on to the large intestine.

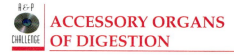

ACCESSORY ORGANS OF DIGESTION

Pancreas

The pancreas is a feather-shaped organ located behind the stomach, see Figure 17-11, page 286. It functions both as an exocrine gland, meaning it has a duct which carries away its secretion, and as an endocrine gland, meaning it is ductless and the secretions are emptied directly into the bloodstream. The digestive juices are carried by the pancreatic duct into the duodenum.

Liver

The liver is the largest organ in the body. It is located below the diaphragm, in the upper

TABLE 17-1 • *Summary of Digestive Enzymes Involved in Human Digestion*

ORGAN	JUICE	GLAND	ENZYME(S)	ACTION	ADDITIONAL FACTS
Mouth	Saliva	Salivary	Amylase found in ptyalin	Starch → Maltose	Physical as well as chemical hydrolysis Mucus flow starts here and continues throughout digestive tract
Esophagus	Mucus	Mucous	None	Lubrication of food	Peristalsis begins here
Stomach	Gastric juice along with HCl acid	Gastric	Protease, pepsin	Proteins → peptones and proteoses	Gastrin activates the gastric glands HCl supplies an acidic medium and kills bacteria Temporary food storage
Small Intestine	Intestinal	Intestinal	Peptiadases	Peptones and proteoses into amino acids	Absorption of end products occurs in small intestine
			Maltase	Maltose → glucose	Villi facilitates absorption
			Lactase	Lactose → glucose and galactose	
			Sucrase	Sucrose → glucose and fructose	
			Lipase	Fats → fatty acids and glycerol	
	Bile	Liver	None	Emulsifies fat	Neutralizes stomach acid
	Pancreatic	Pancreas	Protease (trypsin)	Proteins → peptones and amino acids	Secretin stimulates the flow of pancreatic juice
			Amylase (amylopsin)	Starch → maltose	
			Lipase (steapsin)	Fats → fatty acids and glycerol	
			Nucleases	Nucleic acids (DNA/RNA) nucleotides	

right quadrant of the abdomen, see Figure 17-11. The *portal vein* carries the products of digestion from the small intestine to the liver. Some of the liver's many functions include:

• Manufacture bile, a yellow to green fluid, which is necessary for the digestion of fat. About 800 to 1000cc of bile is produced daily. Bile contains bile salts, bile pigments

(mainly **bilirubin**, which comes from the breakdown of the hemoglobin molecule), cholesterol, phospholipids, and some electrolytes. The **hepatic duct** from the liver joins with the **cystic duct** of the gallbladder to form the **common bile duct**, which carries the bile to the duodenum. If this duct is blocked, bile may then enter the blood

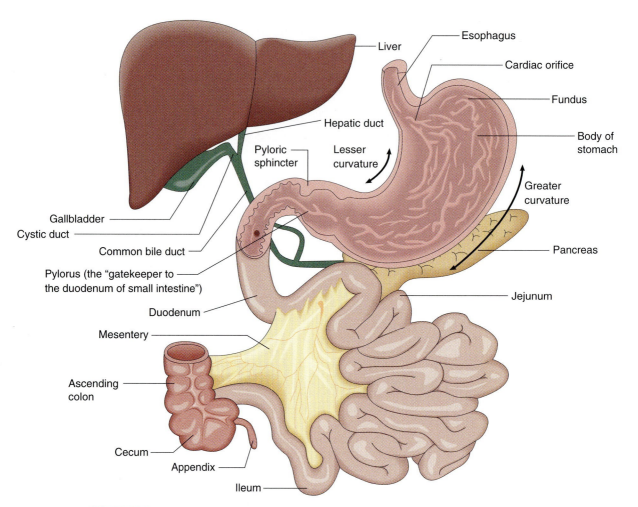

FIGURE 17-11 *Stomach, liver, gallbladder, pancreas, small intestine, and large intestine*

stream causing **jaundice**, which gives the skin and sclera of the eyes a yellow color.

- Produce and store glucose in the form of **glycogen**.

- Detoxify alcohol, drugs, and other harmful substances.

- Manufacture blood proteins such as fibrinogen and prothrombin which are necessary for blood clotting, albumin which is needed for fluid balance in the cells, and globulin which is necessary for immunity.

- Prepare urea, the chief waste product of protein metabolism from the breakdown of amino acids.

- Store Vitamins A, D, and B complex.

Gallbladder

The gallbladder is a small green organ in the inferior surface of the liver, see Figure 17-11. It stores and concentrates bile when it is not needed by the body. When food high in fat enters the duodenum, bile is released by the gallbladder through the cystic duct.

LARGE INTESTINE

The ileum empties its intestinal chyme (semi-liquid food) into the side wall of the large intestine through an opening called the **ileo-cecal valve**. This valve permits passage of the chyme to the large intestine and prevents the backflow of chyme into the ileum. The large

MEDICAL HIGHLIGHT: TECHNOLOGY AND TREATMENT

Laparoscopic Cholecystectomy

Gallbladder surgery, or cholecystectomy, is the most common method for treating gallstones. Each year more than 500,000 Americans have gallbladder surgery. *Laparoscopic cholecystectomy* is a new alternative procedure for gallbladder removal. About 80% of cholecystectomies are performed using this technique.

In this procedure several small incisions are made into the abdomen to allow the insertion of surgical instruments and a small video camera. The camera sends a magnified image from inside the body to a video monitor giving the surgeon a close-up view of the organs and tissues. The surgeon watches the monitor and performs the operation by manipulating the surgical instruments through separate small incisions. The gallbladder is identified and carefully separated from the liver and other structures. Finally, the cystic duct is cut and the gallbladder is removed through one of the small incisions. This type of surgery requires meticulous skill.

Laparoscopic cholecystectomy does not require the stomach muscles to be cut, resulting in less pain, quicker healing, improved cosmetic results, and fewer complications such as infection. Recovery is usually only a night in a hospital and several days recuperation at home. The standard cholecystectomy is a major abdominal surgery requiring a week's stay in the hospital and several weeks at home for recuperation.

A panel convened by the National Institute of Health in September 1992 recommended that laparoscopic cholecystectomy should be performed only by experienced surgeons.

---

intestine is about five feet long and it is approximately 2" in diameter. The **colon**, as it is also called, frames the abdomen, see Figure 17-12.

Cecum and Appendix

Located slightly below the ileo-cecal valve, in the lower right portion of the abdomen, is a blind pouch which we call the **cecum**.

Just below the ileo-cecal valve, to the lower left of the cecum, is the **vermiform appendix**. The appendix is a finger-like projection protruding into the abdominal cavity, see Figure 17-12. It has no digestive function. Because the appendix is a blind sac, it fills up easily, but drains quite slowly; substances can remain within the appendix for prolonged periods. Irritation of the lining of the appendix can make it a suitable area for bacterial growth.

This often leads to the painful inflammatory condition known as **appendicitis**.

Ascending, Transverse and Descending Colon

The colon continues upward, along the right side of the abdominal cavity, to the underside of the liver (hepatic flexure), forming the **ascending colon**. Then it veers to the left of the abdominal cavity, across the abdominal cavity, to a point below the spleen (splenic flexure) forming the **transverse colon**. The **descending colon** travels down from the splenic flexure on the left side of the abdominal cavity. As the descending colon reaches the left iliac region, it enters the pelvis in an S-shaped bend. This section is known as the **sigmoid colon**, which extends some seven or eight inches

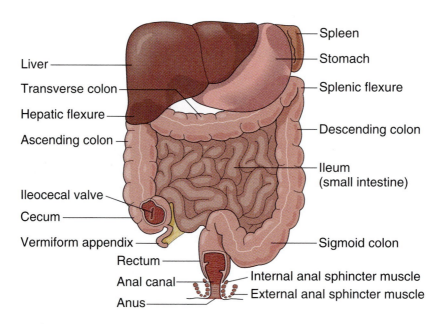

Liver
Transverse colon
Hepatic flexure
Ascending colon
Ileocecal valve
Cecum
Vermiform appendix
Rectum
Anal canal
Anus

Spleen
Stomach
Splenic flexure
Descending colon
Ileum
(small intestine)
Sigmoid colon
Internal anal sphincter muscle
External anal sphincter muscle

FIGURE 17-12 *Accessory organs of digestion: pancreas, liver, and gallbladder*

as the **rectum**. The rectum opens exteriorly into the anus, see Figure 17-12.

Anal Canal

The anal canal is the last portion of the large intestine: its external opening is the **anus**. The anus is guarded by two anal sphincter muscles. One is an internal sphincter of smooth, involuntary muscle, the other an external sphincter of striated, voluntary muscle. Both of these remain contracted to close the anal opening until defecation takes place. The mucous membrane lining the anal canal is folded into vertical folds called rectal columns. Within each rectal column is an artery and a vein. The condition leading to inflammation or enlargement of the rectal column veins is known as **hemorrhoids**.

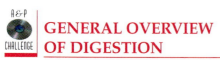

GENERAL OVERVIEW OF DIGESTION

Food enters the gastrointestinal tract via the mouth. In the oral cavity, the food is mechanically digested by the cutting, ripping, and grind-ing action of the teeth. Chemical digestion of carbohydrates is initiated by the secretion of saliva containing a digestive enzyme. Then, the action of the saliva and rolling motion of the tongue turn the food into a soft, pliable ball called a **bolus**. The bolus slides down to the throat (pharynx) to be swallowed. Next it travels through the esophagus into the stomach. Food is pushed along the esophagus by rhythmic, muscular contractions called **peristalsis**. From the stomach, peristaltic contractions continue to push the food into the small intestine. The nervous system stimulates gland activity and peristalsis.

Each part of the alimentary canal contributes to the overall digestive process. Protein digestion, for instance, is initiated by the stomach. Then the small intestine starts and finishes fat digestion, as well as completes the digestion of carbohydrates and proteins. Numerous digestive glands are located in the stomach and small intestine, which secrete digestive juices containing powerful enzymes to chemically digest the food. Due to digestion, insoluble food becomes a soluble fluid substance. This substance is then transported across the small intestinal wall into the bloodstream.

Circulated and absorbed through the blood capillaries into the interstitial fluid and finally into the body cells, the soluble food molecules are utilized for energy, repair, and production of new cells. The remaining undigested substances (**feces**) pass into the large intestine and leave the alimentary canal via the anus. See Figure 17-13.

ACTION IN THE MOUTH

Food enters the mouth and is broken down into smaller pieces by the cutting, ripping, and grinding action of the teeth. The salivary glands fill the mouth with a watery substance called saliva which softens and lubricates the food making it easy to swallow.

Saliva contains **salivary amylase**, also known as **ptyalin**, which converts the starches in carbohydrates into simple sugars. For example, if you place a cracker in your mouth for a few minutes it will have no taste because it is getting broken down into glucose. Saliva is affected by the nervous system; just thinking of food will cause your mouth to water or the opposite effect can occur—a dry mouth when you are nervous or frightened.

ACTION IN THE PHARYNX

Food leaves the mouth and travels to the pharynx, or throat. This structure serves as the common passageway for food and air. See Chapter 12 for a complete description of the pharynx.

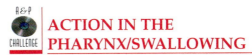

ACTION IN THE PHARYNX/SWALLOWING

Swallowing, or **deglutition**, is a complex process involving the constrictor muscles of the pharynx. It begins as a voluntary process, changing to an involuntary process as the food enters the esophagus. When we swallow, the

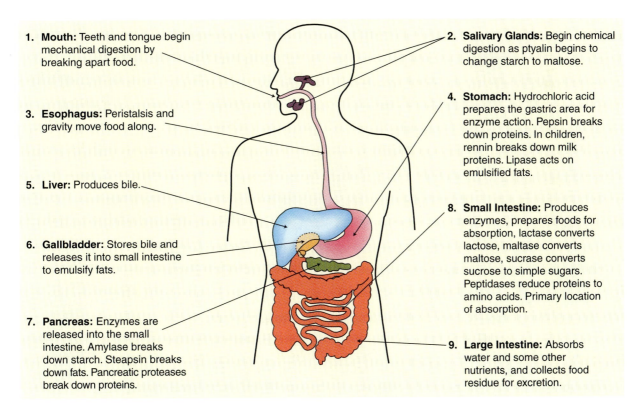

1. **Mouth:** Teeth and tongue begin mechanical digestion by breaking apart food.

2. **Salivary Glands:** Begin chemical digestion as ptyalin begins to change starch to maltose.

3. **Esophagus:** Peristalsis and gravity move food along.

4. **Stomach:** Hydrochloric acid prepares the gastric area for enzyme action. Pepsin breaks down proteins. In children, rennin breaks down milk proteins. Lipase acts on emulsified fats.

5. **Liver:** Produces bile.

6. **Gallbladder:** Stores bile and releases it into small intestine to emulsify fats.

7. **Pancreas:** Enzymes are released into the small intestine. Amylase breaks down starch. Steapsin breaks down fats. Pancreatic proteases break down proteins.

8. **Small Intestine:** Produces enzymes, prepares foods for absorption, lactase converts lactose, maltase converts maltose, sucrase converts sucrose to simple sugars. Peptidases reduce proteins to amino acids. Primary location of absorption.

9. **Large Intestine:** Absorbs water and some other nutrients, and collects food residue for excretion.

FIGURE 17-13 *Overview of digestion*

tip of the tongue arches slightly and moves backward and upward. This action forces the food against the hard palate; simultaneously, the soft palate and the uvula shut off the opening to the nasopharynx. Food is thus prevented from entering the nasopharynx.

In swallowing, the constrictor muscles of the pharynx contract, pushing food into the upper part of the esophagus. At the same time, other pharyngeal muscles raise the larynx causing the epiglottis to cover the trachea (windpipe) to prevent food from entering it. If we talk while eating the epiglottis may not close and food enters the trachea.

The act of swallowing is voluntary. But, as a bolus of food passes over the posterior part of the tongue and stimulates receptors in the walls of the pharynx, swallowing becomes an involuntary reflex action. With the contraction of the pharyngeal muscles, followed by the contraction of the muscles lining the esophagus, food passes down into the stomach. (When you swallow, place your fingers near the trachea; you can feel the structure move upward.)

ACTION IN THE ESOPHAGUS

Food is pushed through the esophagus by the wavelike contractions of the alimentary canal, also called peristalsis. This action explains why you can swallow even standing on your head; once food enters the esophagus it goes to the stomach and it is not affected by gravity.

ACTION IN THE STOMACH

When the food reaches the stomach the *cardiac sphincter* relaxes and allows food to enter. About two to three quarts of digestive juices are produced daily which may explain the gurgling noises you hear at times. When food enters, the gastric juices are released and begin to work on proteins. Salivary amylase continues its work in the stomach.

The action of the gastric juices is helped by the churning of the stomach walls. The semi-liquid food is called chyme. The chyme leaves the stomach through the *pyloric sphincter* which acts as a gate keeper. This action allows a small squirt of chyme into the duodenum from time to time. Food takes about two to four hours to leave the stomach. Food moves through the stomach by peristalsis; vomiting is an action which occurs because of reverse peristalsis. The only known substances to be absorbed in the stomach are alcohol and some medications.

ACTION IN THE SMALL INTESTINE

This the main area of the digestive system. It is in this location that the process of digestion is completed and absorption occurs. Bile emulsifies fat to prepare it for digestion by pancreatic and intestinal juices. Pancreatic juices neutralize the acid chyme and completes the digestion of carbohydrates, fats, and proteins. (Refer to Figure 17-10.) The end products of digestion are:

- Carbohydrates are converted to simple sugars such as *glucose.*

- Proteins are broken down into *amino acids.*

- Fats are changed into *fatty acids* and *glycerol.*

The glucose, amino acids, fatty acids, and glycerol are then absorbed through the villi of the small intestine into the blood and lymph capillaries. The portal vein transports the blood from the small intestine and takes it to the liver where it is distributed to the organs of the body.

The passage of food through the small intestine occurs because of peristalsis and **segmented movement**. Segmented movement is when single segments of the intestine alternate between contraction and relaxation. Because inactive segments exist between active ones, the food is moved forward and backward—it is mixed as well as propelled. It takes about six to eight hours for food to go through the small intestine; undigested foods then reach the ileocecal valve and enter the large intestine.

ACTION IN THE LARGE INTESTINE

The large intestine is concerned with water absorption, bacterial action, fecal formation, gas formation, and defecation. The purpose of these functions is to regulate the body's water balance while storing and excreting waste products of digestion.

Absorption

The large intestine aids in the regulation of the body's water balance by absorbing large quantities of water back into the bloodstream. The water is drawn from the undigested food and indigestible material (like cellulose) that pass through the colon. The large intestine absorbs Vitamins B complex and K.

Bacterial Action

A few hours following the birth of an infant, the lining of the colon starts to accumulate bacteria. These bacteria persist throughout the person's lifetime. The bacteria multiply rapidly, to form the bacterial population or flora, of the colon. The intestinal bacteria are harmless (nonpathogenic) to their host. They act upon undigested food remains, turning them into acids, amines, gases, and other waste products. These decomposed products are excreted through the colon. Another benefit of the bacterial action is the synthesis (formation) of moderate amounts of B-complex vitamins and Vitamin K (needed for blood clotting).

Gas Formation

Most people produce 1-3 pints of gas per day and pass it through the rectum (**flatulence**) about fourteen times a day. Gas is produced by swallowed air and the normal breakdown of food. The unpleasant odor of flatulence comes from bacteria in the large intestine which produces gas containing sulfur or methane. Swallowed air usually remains in the stomach and is relieved by burping and belching.

Research has not shown why some foods produce gas in one person and not another or why some people produce methane gas. Some foods which produce gas are beans, vegetables such as broccoli and cabbage, fruit, whole grains, milk and milk products, and foods containing the artificial sweetener sorbitol.

Lactose is the natural sugar found in milk and milk products. Some people have low levels of the enzyme lactase which is necessary to digest lactose. As people age, their level of lactase decreases, which may explain why older people experience discomfort after using milk products.

Diet modification may reduce the amount of gas produced; however, it is important to remember that some of the foods which produce gas are also essential nutrients.

Fecal Formation

Initially, the undigested or indigestible material in the colon contains a lot of water and is in a liquid state. Due to water absorption and bacterial action, it is subsequently converted into a semisolid form, called feces.

Feces consist of bacteria, waste products from the blood, acids, amines, inorganic salts, gases, mucous, and cellulose. Amines are waste products of amino acids. The gases are ammonia, carbon dioxide, hydrogen, hydrogen sulfide, and methane. The characteristically foul odor of feces derives from these substances.

Cellulose is the fibrous part of plants that humans are unable to digest. It contributes to the bulk of the feces. This bulk stimulates the muscular activity of the colon, resulting in defecation. Regular defecation (regularity) can be promoted by exercising daily and eating foods containing bulk, like whole-grain cereals, fruits, and vegetables. These foods supply the necessary roughage to initiate bowel movements.

Defecation

Once approximately every twelve hours the fecal material moves into the lower bowel (lower colon and rectum) by means of a series of long contractions called mass peristalsis. However, frequency of bowel movements in healthy people varies from three movements a day to three a week. When the rectum becomes distended with the accumulation of feces, a defecation reflex is triggered. Nerve endings in the rectum are stimulated, and a nerve impulse is transmitted to the spinal cord. From the spinal cord, nerve impulses are sent to the colon, rectum, and internal anal sphincter. This causes the colon and rectal muscles to contract and the internal sphincter to relax, resulting in emptying of the bowels.

For defecation to occur, the external anal sphincter must also be relaxed. The external anal sphincter surrounds and guards the outer opening of the anus and is under conscious control. Due to this control, defecation can be prevented when inconvenient, despite the defecation reflex. However, if this urge is continually ignored, it lessens or disappears totally, resulting in constipation. Temporary relief from constipation may be obtained with the use of *laxatives* and *cathartics*. (A laxative is a substance that induces gentle bowel movement; a cathartic stimulates more vigorous movement, which may eventually reduce the bowel's muscle tone.)

COMMON DISORDERS OF THE DIGESTIVE SYSTEM

In times of stress it is not unusual to have "butterflies" in the stomach, nausea, or another type of distress associated with the digestive system. Diseases of the digestive system are responsible for the hospitalization of more people in the United States than any other group of diseases. In recent years, researchers have begun to shed some light on the puzzling aspects of digestive diseases. Diseases once thought to be caused by emotional problems may in fact be caused by viruses interacting with the body's immune system. Some of these diseases are briefly discussed in this unit.

Stomatitis

Stomatitis is an inflammation of the soft tissues of the mouth cavity. Pain and salivation may occur also.

Gastroesophageal Reflux Disease (GERD)

Gastroesophageal Reflux Disease (GERD) is a disorder that affects the lower sphincter muscle connecting the esophagus with the stomach. In GERD, the sphincter muscle is weak or relaxes inappropriately allowing the stomach's contents to flow up into the esophagus. This is a common occurrence in people who suffer from hiatal hernia or heartburn.

Hiatal Hernia

Hiatal hernia, or rupture, occurs when the stomach protrudes above the diaphragm through the esophagus opening. Hiatal hernia is not uncommon in people over the age of fifty. Changes in the diet may relieve the heartburn; surgery is not usually required.

Heartburn

Heartburn or acid indigestion results from a backflow of the highly acidic gastric juice into the lower end of the esophagus. This irritates the lining of the esophagus, causing a burning sensation. Heartburn may be experienced on a daily basis by some people and 25% of all pregnant women experience heartburn.

Temporary relief from heartburn can be obtained by:

- avoiding chocolate and peppermints which may cause the sphincter to relax.
- stopping smoking.
- taking non-prescription antacids to provide temporary relief.
- avoid lying down for two to three hours after eating.
- avoiding coffee, citrus fruits and juices, fried and fatty foods, and tomato products.

Pyloric Stenosis

Pyloric stenosis is a narrowing of the pyloric sphincter at the lower end of the stomach. It is often found in infants. Projectile vomiting may result; surgery is often necessary.

Gastritis

Gastritis is an acute or chronic inflammation on the stomach lining.

Gastroenteritis

Gastroenteritis is the inflammation of the mucous membrane lining of the stomach and intestinal tract. A common cause is a virus which causes diarrhea and vomiting for twenty-four to thirty-six hours. If this condition persists, dehydration may occur. Treatment is symptomatic.

Enteritis

Enteritis is the inflammation of the intestine that may be caused by a bacterial, viral, or protozoan infection. Enteritis can also be caused by an allergic reaction to certain foods or food poisoning.

Peptic Ulcer

An **ulcer** is a sore or lesion that forms in the mucosal lining of the stomach or duodenum where acid and pepsin are present. Ulcers found in the stomach are called gastric ulcers; those in the duodenum are called duodenal ulcers. In general, both types are referred to as **peptic ulcers**.

For almost a century, doctors believed that lifestyle factors such as stress and diet caused ulcers. Today, research shows that most ulcers develop as a result of an infection with bacteria called *Helicobacter pylori* (*H. pylori*). Other factors associated with ulcers include lifestyle, acid, and pepsin; however, *H. pylori* is now considered the primary cause.

Lifestyle factors include cigarette smoking, intake of food and beverages containing caffeine, alcohol consumption, and physical stress associated with major injuries or illness. Researchers believe that the stomach's inability to defend itself against the powerful digestive fluids acid and pepsin contribute to ulcer formation. Non-steroidal anti-inflammatory drugs make the stomach vulnerable to the harmful effects of acid and pepsin.

The most common symptom of an ulcer is a burning pain in the abdomen between the sternum and navel. The pain occurs between meals and in the early hours of the morning. It may be relieved by eating or taking an antacid.

Ulcers are diagnosed by x-ray and testing for the *H. pylori* bacteria. Treatment is dependent on the cause. If the cause is *H. pylori*, antibiotics is the treatment. Elimination of the bacteria means that the ulcer will heal and not recur.

Treatment for ulcers from other causes include the use of H_2 blockers. These drugs reduce the amount of acid the stomach produces by blocking **histamine**, a powerful stimulant of acid secretion. Initially, treatment with H_2 blockers lasts about six to eight weeks. However, since this type of ulcer recurs in about 50 to 80% of cases, many people must continue therapy for years.

Additional treatment includes the use of drugs which stop the stomach's acid pumps, mucosal protective medications, and lifestyle changes.

Colitis or Irritable Bowel Syndrome

Colitis or **IBS** is a condition in which the large intestine or bowel may be inflamed. The exact cause of this disorder is not known. Researchers speculate that IBD may be a viral or bacterial agent which effects the immune system. The person may experience episodes of either constipation or diarrhea. The chronic diarrhea may lead to dehydration and ulceration of the bowel. This condition is an extremely frustrating disorder.

Medication can be given to quiet bowel activity and reduce anxiety.

Irritable bowel syndrome may also be referred to as Krohn's disease.

Appendicitis

Appendicitis occurs when the veriform appendix becomes inflamed. If it ruptures, the bacteria from the appendix can spread to the peritoneal cavity causing peritonitis.

Hepatitis

Hepatitis is an inflammation of the liver. Clinical symptoms are fever, nausea, anorexia, and jaundice.

Hepatitis A

Infectious hepatitis, Hepatitis A, is a viral infection of the liver, often spread through contaminated water or food. Standard precautions are followed.

Hepatitis B or Serum Hepatitis

Serum hepatitis, Hepatitis B, is caused by a virus found only in the blood. It is transmitted by a blood transfusion contaminated with the virus or through the use of inadequately sterilized syringes, needles, or surgical equipment. It is prevalent in drug addicts who use dirty hypodermic needles.

The health care worker is at risk for contracting serum hepatitis; *standard precautions* must be taken at all times (see Chapter 11). A vaccine is now available for Hepatitis B, and it is recommended that health care workers be vaccinated.

Over the past two decades other strains of the hepatitis virus have been identified.

- *Hepatitis C* accounts for 20-40% of acute hepatitis. Most patients have a history of IV drug abuse. Standard precautions are followed. Some cases may be treated with the drug interferon-a.

- *Hepatitis D* requires coinfection with Type B.

- *Hepatitis E* is transmitted through intestinal excretions.

Cirrhosis

Cirrhosis is a chronic, progressive inflammatory disease of the liver, characterized by replacement of normal tissue with fibrous connective tissue. Three-fourths of cirrhosis is caused by excessive alcohol consumption. Where viral hepatitis is common, hepatitis causes cirrhosis.

Cholecystitis

Cholecystitis is the inflammation of the gallbladder. This condition may cause blockage of the cystic duct which would inhibit the release of stored bile.

Gallstones/Enteric

Bile is normally stored in the gallbladder and secreted into the small intestine where fat is emulsified.

Sometimes collections of crystallized cholesterol form in the gallbladder. These are combined with bile salts and bile pigments to form **gallstones**, or cholelithiasis. Gallstones can block the bile duct, causing pain and digestive disorders. Pain may occur in the back between the shoulder blades. In such cases, bile cannot flow into the small intestine to help in fat emulsification, digestion, and absorption. Most gallstones are small and may pass with undigested food. However, the larger and obstructive ones must be surgically removed.

Pancreatitis

Pancreatitis is the inflammation of the pancreas. The pancreas can become edematous, hemorrhagic, or necrotic. One-third of pancreatitis cases are due to unknown causes. Some may be associated with chronic alcoholism.

Diverticulosis

Diverticulosis is a condition in which little sacs (diverticula) develop in the wall of the colon. The majority of people over the age of sixty in the United States have this condition. Most people have no symptoms and would not know they had diverticulosis unless there was an x-ray or intestinal examination. About 20%

of people with this condition may develop **diverticulitis**, which is an inflammation in the wall of the colon.

Diarrhea

If the feces are passed along the colon too rapidly, insufficient water is reabsorbed, and the feces become watery. **Diarrhea** is characterized by loose, watery, and frequent bowel movements. It may result from irritation of the colon's lining by dysentery bacteria, poor diet, nervousness, toxic substances, or from irritants in food (as in prunes, which stimulate intestinal peristalsis).

Chronic Constipation

Feces eliminated through the rectum are normally in a semisolid state. When defecation is delayed, however, the colon absorbs excessive water from the feces rendering them dry and hard. When this occurs, defecation (or evacuation) becomes difficult.

For this reason, suppressing the need to defecate at normal times can lead to **constipation**. Constipation can also be caused by emotions such as anxiety, fear, or fright. Headaches and other symptoms that frequently accompany constipation result from the distension of the rectum, as opposed to toxins from the feces.

Treatment usually consists of eating proper foods, especially cereals, fruits and vegetables, drinking plenty of fluids, getting enough exercise, setting regular bowel habits, and avoiding tension as much as possible.

Stomach Cancer

The initial cancer cells that develop in the stomach quickly grow into masses of tissue known as tumors.

Malignant stomach cancer cells can spread to other body parts, forming new growths or metastases. Even if the original tumor is surgically removed, the cancer may recur when malignant cancer cells have spread.

The initial symptoms of stomach cancer are much like those of other digestive disorders: heartburn, loss of appetite, persistent indigestion, slight nausea, a feeling of bloated discomfort after eating, and occasional mild stomach pain. Later symptoms include traces of blood in the feces, pain, weight loss, and vomiting.

Treatment involves surgical removal of the stomach tumor as soon as possible. Depending upon the size and the extent of growth of the tumor, part or all of the stomach may have to be removed.

If the cancer has spread, chemotherapy (treatment with anticancer drugs) is prescribed. These drugs are administered into the bloodstream, circulating through the body to kill cancerous cells in any location of the body.

Radiation therapy plays a limited role in the treatment of stomach cancer. Very strong radiation doses are needed to kill the cancer cells, and they might also seriously damage neighboring healthy cells.

Cancer of the Colon

Colon cancer is believed to arise from a polypoid lesion. Early detection is critical. The following procedures are recommended for early detection: after the age of forty, an annual digital rectal examination is prescribed; after the age of fifty, a stool slide specimen is obtained, looking for hidden blood (**hemoccult**).

A colon resection may be performed in a patient with colon cancer. Sometimes it may be necessary to perform a **colostomy**. In this procedure, an opening is made through the abdomen into the colon, the cancerous tissue is removed, and the healthy tissue is brought out through the opening onto the skin. A pouch is worn to collect the body's wastes. This procedure causes stress and anxiety. The health care worker must be supportive of a patient with this condition.

● REVIEW QUESTIONS

Select the letter of the choice that best completes the statement.

1. The process of changing complex foods into simpler substances to be absorbed is called:
    a. metabolism
    b. cellular respiration
    c. peristalsis
    d. digestion

2. The walls of the digestive tube which contain mucous are called:
    a. sub-mucosa
    b. mucosa
    c. circular muscle
    d. visceral peritoneum

3. The accessory organs of the alimentary canal are the tongue, teeth, salivary glands, pancreas, liver and:
    a. stomach
    b. esophagus
    c. gallbladder
    d. colon

4. The taste buds are found on projections called:
    a. papillae
    b. parotid
    c. palatine
    d. pharynx

5. The involuntary muscle action of the alimentary canal is called:
    a. pushing
    b. peristalsis
    c. stenosis
    d. contraction

6. Semi-liquid food entering the small intestine is called:
    a. pepsin
    b. ptyalin
    c. chyme
    d. bolus

7. The lining of the abdominal cavity is called:
    a. pleural
    b. peritoneal
    c. submucosa
    d. epithelial

8. The pancreatic enzyme that breaks down starches is called:
    a. trypsin
    b. steapsin
    c. secretion
    d. amylopsin

9. The enzyme that stimulates the liver to produce bile is called:
   a. protease
   b. steapsin
   c. secretin
   d. trypsin

10. Food is absorbed in the small intestine in the:
   a. villi
   b. submucosa
   c. peritoneal lining
   d. colon

● MATCHING

Match each of the terms in Column I with its correct description in Column II

Column I	Column II
_____ 1. papillae	a. substances that promote chemical reactions in living things
_____ 2. enzyme	
_____ 3. digestion	b. bleeding gums
_____ 4. the teeth	c. a small soft structure suspended from the soft palate
_____ 5. enamel	d. gums which protect the teeth
_____ 6. gingivae	e. tract consisting of the mouth, stomach, and intestines
_____ 7. accessory organs and and structures of digestion	f. aids in chewing and swallowing
	g. teeth, tongue, salivary glands, pancreas, liver, gallbladder, and appendix
_____ 8. salivary amylase	h. hardest substance in the body
_____ 9. uvula	i. projections on the surface of the tongue containing the taste buds
_____ 10. alimentary canal	
_____ 11. cirrhosis	j. the process of changing complex solid foods into soluble forms to be absorbed by cells
_____ 12. gastroenteritis	
_____ 13. peptic ulcers	k. the enzyme manufactured by the salivary glands
_____ 14. hiatal hernia	l. frequent liquid bowel movements
_____ 15. heartburn	m. chronic liver disease
_____ 16. diarrhea	n. protrusion of the stomach into the esophagus
_____ 17. cholecystitis	o. viral infection of the liver
_____ 18. infectious hepatitis	p. inflammation of the abdominal cavity
_____ 19. pyloric stenosis	q. obstruction of the hepatic duct
_____ 20. peritonitis	r. inflammation of the stomach and intestinal lining
	s. inflammation of the gallbladder
	t. narrowing of sphincter in the stomach
	u. cardiospasm
	v. lesions which may result from acid secretion
	w. common symptoms characterized by a burning sensation

● TRUE OR FALSE

Read each statement carefully and determine if it is true or false. Encircle the letter *T* for true or *F* for false.

T F 1. The large intestine is called the colon.

T F 2. The large intestine is 20 feet long and 2 inches wide.

T F 3. The cecum is located where the small intestine joins the large intestine.

T F 4. The function of the appendix is unknown.

T F 5. The large intestine stores and eliminates the waste products of digestion.

T F 6. Regulation of water balance occurs in the large intestine because its lining absorbs water.

T F 7. Constipation may be overcome by intensive and long periods of work and exercise.

T F 8. Bulk foods such as whole-grain cereals, fruits, and vegetables may help avoid constipation.

T F 9. The rectum is an extension of the descending colon.

T F 10. The transverse colon lies between the ascending and the descending colon.

● LABELING

Label the teeth on the following diagram. (The teeth on the left are the deciduous ones; those on the right are permanent teeth.)

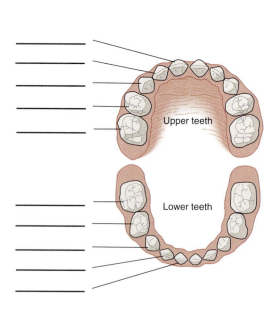

Upper teeth

Lower teeth

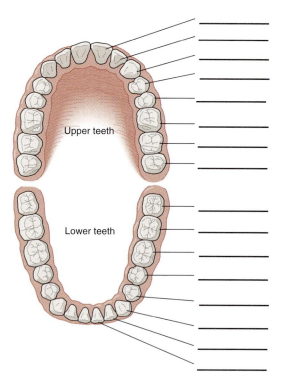

Upper teeth

Lower teeth

● APPLYING THEORY TO PRACTICE

1. You have just eaten a slice of pizza for lunch. In about twelve hours, that slice of pizza will be ready for absorption in the villi of the small intestine. Trace the journey of the pizza, naming all the enzymes involved, where the action takes place, and the end products of carbohydrate, protein, and fat metabolism. Would you consider pizza a good nutritious snack? Explain your answer.

2. Enzymes secreted by the stomach are high in acid content. Explain the reason why the lining of the digestive system does not become ulcerated.

3. Dental checkups make you nervous. Why is it a good health practice to see your dentist at least once a year?

4. A pregnant woman comes into the doctor's office and states, "I have so much heartburn, I know my baby will be born with a full head of hair." Explain to her the reasons for heartburn and why her statement is a myth.

5. In the emergency room a woman, age forty, is complaining of a sharp pain between her shoulder blades on the right side. What is this symptomatic of and what type of treatment is necessary for this condition?

6. You must explain to a patient's family members what the necessary precautions are when caring for patients with hepatitis B. The family wants you to explain what a liver infection is and how it affects a person.

7. Your friend states, "All this stress is going to give me an ulcer." Explain to your friend why this is no longer an accurate statement.

CHAPTER

18

Nutrition

The pace of an active daily life can at times be hectic and stress-filled. This can occasionally cause one to eat "on the run," to "grab a bite" at a fast-food restaurant, or to forget to eat nutritiously.

The food one eats and drinks may or may not be nutritious. For food to be nutritious, it must contain the materials needed by the individual cells for proper cell functioning. These materials or **nutrients** are:

- water
- carbohydrates
- lipids
- proteins
- minerals
- vitamins
- fiber

WATER

Water is an essential component of all body tissues. It has several important functions in the human body:

- Acts as a solvent for all biochemical reactions.
- Serves as a transport medium for substances.
- Functions as a lubricant for joint movement and the digestive tract.
- Controls body temperature by evaporation from the pores of the skin.
- Serves as a cushion for body organs, such as the lungs and brain.

Water makes up between 55 and 65% of our total body weight. The body is continually losing water through evaporation, excretion, and respiration. This water loss must be replaced. We supply some of this need by drinking plain water. However, most of the body's water comes from the food we eat (including liquids). Practically all the foods we eat contain water, even those that seem to be dry.

Water is the only nutrient we can sense a need for. When the body needs water, we experience thirst.

CARBOHYDRATES

Carbohydrates include simple sugars, such as monosaccharides like glucose ($C_6H_{12}O_6$). Depending upon the number of simple sugars found in the carbohydrate, they are classified as monosaccharides, disaccharides, or polysaccharides. Only the monosaccharides are small enough to be absorbed and eventually taken into the cells. The other carbohydrates are broken down by digestion in the digestive tract into the smallest possible molecular subunits prior to absorption.

Carbohydrates are the main source of energy for the body. Excess carbohydrates are converted into fat and stored in fat tissue. Nutritionists recommend that carbohydrates comprise between 50 and 60% of the daily intake of calories.

A **calorie** is a unit that measures the amount of energy contained within the chemical bonds of different foods. The small calorie is defined as the amount of heat required to raise the temperature of one gram of water by one degree Celsius. A **kilocalorie** or large calorie is equal to 1000 small calories. The calorie content of food is determined by measuring the amount of heat released when food is burned. The energy content of fat (9 kilocalories per gram) is slightly more than twice that of carbohydrate (4 kilocalories per gram) or protein (4 kilocalories per gram).

A normal adult usually requires between 1600 and 3000 kilocalories a day depending on age, sex, body weight, and degree of physical activity. Newborn infants and young children have higher energy requirements per unit of body weight than adults because of the high energy expenditure of growth. See Table 18-1 for daily recommended energy intakes.

An excess of the wrong foods can cause an overweight condition called obesity. Obesity usually results when we take in more calories than we use. There are carbohydrates that should be avoided or minimized in the daily diet. These foods are candies, cakes, cookies, jams, sugar-coated cereals, and sugary soft drinks. All of these foods contain large amounts of highly refined carbohydrates as

TABLE 18-1 • *Median Heights and Weights and Recommended Energy Intake*

Category	Age (years) or Condition	WEIGHT		HEIGHT		REE[a] (Kcal/day)	AVERAGE ENERGY ALLOWANCE (kcal)[b]		
		(kg)	(lb)	(cm)	(in)		Multiples of REE	Per kg	Per day[c]
Infants	0.0-0.5	6	13	60	24	320		108	650
	0.5-1.0	9	20	71	28	500		98	850
Children	1-3	13	29	90	35	740		102	1,300
	4-6	20	44	112	44	950		90	1,800
	7-10	28	62	132	52	1,130		70	2,000
Males	11-14	45	99	157	62	1,440	1.70	55	2,500
	15-18	66	145	176	69	1,760	1.67	45	3,000
	19-24	72	160	177	70	1,780	1.67	40	2,900
	25-50	79	174	176	70	1,800	1.60	37	2,900
	51+	77	170	173	68	1,530	1.50	30	2,300
Females	11-14	46	101	157	62	1,310	1.67	47	2,200
	15-18	55	120	163	64	1,370	1.60	40	2,200
	19-24	58	128	164	65	1,350	1.60	38	2,200
	25-50	63	138	163	64	1,380	1.55	36	2,200
	51+	65	143	160	63	1,280	1.50	30	1,900
Pregnant	1st trimester								+0
	2nd trimester								+300
	3rd trimester								+500
Lactating	1st 6 months								+500
	2nd 6 months								+500

a. Calculation based on FAO equations, then rounded.
b. In the range of light to moderate activity, the coefficient of variation is ± 20%
c. Figure is rounded.
(Reprinted with permission from *Recommended Dietary Allowances, 10th Edition*, © 1989 by the National Academy of Sciences. Published by National Academy Press, Washington, D.C.)

sugar. They supply calories, but little else. Energy obtained from such foods is commonly referred to as "empty calories." Intake of these foods can also contribute to tooth decay. Foods containing starches and cellulose are a healthier source of carbohydrates. These foods, besides providing energy, can also provide needed minerals, roughage, and vitamins. **Roughage** is the undigestible part of food. Examples are whole grain breads and cereals, fruits, vegetables, macaroni, rice, and potatoes.

LIPIDS

Lipids are a group of compounds containing fatty acids combined with an alcohol. They can be subdivided into two groups: simple lipids (fats, oils, waxes) and compound lipids (phospholipids, glycolipids, sterols). Like carbohydrates, fats are a source of energy. The same amount of fats can release more than twice as many calories as the same amount of carbohydrate or protein. The human body stores reserves of energy as fat in fat cells. Likewise, any excess carbohydrate and protein in the diet is transformed into fat and stored along with any excess fat.

Fats are an essential nutrient to the maintenance of the human body. Stored fats provide a supply of energy during emergencies such as sickness or during deficient caloric intakes. Fats also cushion the internal organs and serve as an insulation against the cold. Fats are components of the cell membrane, and contribute to the formation of bile and steroid hormones, such as the sex hormones. Fats also contain certain kinds of vitamins called fat-soluble vitamins which are an important part of our daily diet. It is therefore essential to have a diet containing fats without exceeding the body's calorie needs. Total daily dietary fat intake should not exceed 25 to 30% of the daily caloric intake

CHOLESTEROL

Cholesterol is a fat found in animal products like meat, eggs, cheese and ice cream. Cholesterol is a white, wax-like substance used to build cells and make hormones. It is also manufactured by the liver. The cholesterol that you eat is not digested. There are no calories in cholesterol but once in the body it is difficult for your body to get rid of it. Fats and oils in food are called *triglycerides*. Your body turns excess calories into triglycerides which are stored throughout the body as adipose tissue.

Since oil and water do not mix, and blood is mostly water, triglycerides and cholesterol must be carried through blood cells by special proteins called *lipoprotein*: **HDL**, **LDL**, and **VLDL**. The lipoproteins LDL and VLDL carry fats to the cells; HDL or high density lipoprotein is sometimes referred to as the "heavenly" or "good" kind because it removes excess cholesterol from cells and carries it back to the liver to be broken down or eliminated.

Over the years, if more cholesterol is carried by the LDL than can be removed by HDL or used up in the cells, it will start to build up inside the artery walls, causing atherosclerosis.

A condition called *dyslipidemia* or disorder of fat in the blood (in other words, "high blood cholesterol") exists.

The recommended level of blood cholesterol for people age forty and over is under 200mg/dl; any level over 200 mg/dl is considered too high for the long term health of the heart.

The two most important steps you can take to lower your blood cholesterol are to reduce your intake of foods high in saturated fat and to lose weight if you are overweight. Fats are defined as:

- saturated fat—oil from animal products that are solid at room temperature, such as butter, cheese, and meat fat.

- polyunsaturated fat—oil from vegetable products, liquid at room temperature, used in moderation lowers blood cholesterol. These include safflower oil and sunflower oil.

- monosaturated fat—oil from other vegetable products, liquid at room temperature, lowers blood cholesterol. These include olive oil and peanut oil.

If a label says "cholesterol free" it does not necessarily mean it is good for you. Look carefully: Many products with no cholesterol have saturated fats in them.

Foods to substitute for saturated fat include skim milk, low fat cheese, poultry, margarine, and low fat ice cream. Some of the foods which help lower cholesterol include garlic, fresh fruit and vegetables, oat bran, wheat bran, and prunes. The FDA has recently approved the use of olestra as a fat substitute, which is currently being used in some snack foods.

PROTEINS

Proteins are structurally more complex than carbohydrates and lipids and contain an amino (NH_2) group. They are synthesized in the cell cytoplasm from constituent molecules called amino acids.

Proteins serve many different functions in the body. Some are enzymes and regulate the rate of chemical reactions; others are important in growth and repair of tissues. When necessary, proteins can also be used as a source of energy. In addition, contractile systems (muscles), hormonal systems, plasma transport systems, clotting and defense systems (antibodies) are all dependent upon proteins.

The body can synthesize some amino acids, but not all. The amino acids that cannot be made in the body are **"essential" amino acids**. Proteins that contain all of the essential amino acids are known as **complete proteins**. Sources of such complete proteins are eggs, meat, milk, and milk products. Proteins that do not contain all the essential amino acids are called **incomplete proteins**. Vegetables contain incomplete proteins. However, a varied diet including vegetables will supply all the necessary complete proteins. For example, beans and wheat eaten alone will not provide all of the necessary complete proteins. However, when eaten together, they will complement each other and supply the necessary complete proteins.

Unlike fats, the human body is unable to store excess amino acids. Any unused amino acids are broken down by the liver, and the amino group is excreted as a nitrogenous waste product called urea. The remainder of the amino acid may be burned for immediate energy or stored as fat or glycogen, a polysaccharide.

Protein synthesis cannot occur without all of the essential amino acids present at the same time. Therefore, it is important to include some source of complete protein throughout the various foods we eat during the day. The daily intake of calories from proteins should be no more than 15 to 20%.

Most adults in the United States eat a daily intake of protein in excess of the recommended dietary allowance. This practice puts an extra burden on the liver, and kidney, which must eliminate the urea from the body.

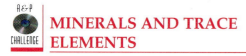

MINERALS AND TRACE ELEMENTS

A **mineral** is a chemical element that is obtained from inorganic compounds in food. Our knowledge of the role of the essential minerals and trace elements is incomplete. Many are notably necessary for normal human growth and maintenance.

Among the most important of these nutrients are sodium, potassium, calcium, iron, phosphorous, and zinc.

Trace elements are present in the body in very small amounts. These include zinc, copper, iodine, cobalt, manganese, selenium, chromium, molybdenum, and fluorine.

The toxic limits of some trace elements are extremely close to the required dosages. This means that there is a critical difference between toxicity, health, and deficiency. Most of the essential minerals and trace elements are already present in the average normal American diet in sufficient concentrations, and supplementation is only indicated for special conditions of disease, during pregnancy, and old age. However, governmental surveys indicate that females in the United States might be consuming less than optimal daily intakes of calcium and iron.

Age-related osteoporosis is one of the most severely debilitating diseases in the United States and the most prevalent bone disease in the world. While the question of whether osteoporosis is a nutritional disorder remains unanswered, there is much convincing evidence that calcium deficiency accelerates the age-related loss of bone. The hormonal consequences of female menopause result in diminished calcium absorption in the intestines. This physiological consequence of reduced estrogen, along with lower bone density in females than in males during young adulthood, requires that proper attention be paid to calcium intake throughout the life cycle to maximize peak bone density prior to menopause.

Women of child-bearing age have a tendency to be in low iron status because of blood loss during the menstrual flow. Fatigue and iron deficiency anemia in these women can usually be ameliorated by iron supplementation. Table 18-2 summarizes the most important minerals and trace elements in the human diet.

VITAMINS

A **vitamin** is defined as a biologically active organic compound, often functioning as a coenzyme, that is necessary for normal health and growth. Most enzymatic activity relies on the presence of coenzymes. A dietary deficiency of a vitamin results in a subclinical or obvious specific disorder. The term vitamin usually implies that the substance is not synthesized within the organism and, as a result, must be obtained from the diet. Vitamins are transported

TABLE 18-2 • *Summary of Essential Minerals and Trace Elements Needed for Health*

MINERAL	FOOD SOURCES	FUNCTION	DEFICIENCY DISEASES
Calcium	Milk, cheese, dark green vegetables, dried legumes, sardines, shellfish	Bone and tooth formation Blood clotting Nerve transmission	Stunted growth Rickets Osteoporosis Convulsions
Chlorine	Common table salt, seafood, milk, meat, eggs	Formation of gastric juices Acid-base balance	Muscle cramps Mental apathy Poor appetite
Chromium	Fats, vegetables oils, meats, clams, whole-grain cereals	Involved in energy and glucose metabolism	Impaired ability to metabolize glucose
Copper	Drinking water, liver, shellfish whole grains, cherries, legumes, kidney, poultry, oysters, nuts, chocolate	Constituent of enzymes Involved with iron transport	Anemia
Fluorine	Drinking water, tea, coffee, seafood, rice, spinach, onions, lettuce	Maintenance of bone and tooth structure	Higher frequency of tooth decay
Iodine	Marine fish and shellfish, dairy products, many vegetables, iodized salt	Constituent of thyroid hormones	Goiter (enlarged thyroid)
Iron	Liver, lean meats, legumes, whole grains, dark green vegetables, eggs, dark molasses, shrimp, oysters	Constituent of hemoglobin Involved in energy metabolism	Iron-deficiency anemia
Magnesium	Whole grains, green leafy vegetables, nuts, meats, milk, legumes	Involved in energy conversions and enzyme function	Growth failure Behavioral disturbances Weakness Spasms
Phosphorus	Milk, cheese, meat, fish, poultry, whole grains, legumes, nuts	Bone and tooth formation Acid-base balance Involved in energy metabolism	Weakness Demineralization of bone
Potassium	Meats, milk, fruits, legumes, vegetables	Acid-base balance Body water balance Nerve transmission	Muscular weakness Paralysis
Selenium	Fish, poultry, meats, grains milk, vegetables (depending on amount in soil)	Necessary for Vitamin E function	Anemia Increased mortality?
Sodium	Common table salt, seafood, most other foods except fruit	Acid-base balance Body water balance Nerve transmission	Muscle cramps Mental apathy
Sulfur	Meat, fish, poultry, eggs, milk, cheese, legumes, nuts	Constituent of certain tissue proteins	Related to deficiencies of sulfur-containing amino acids
Zinc	Milk, liver, shellfish, herring, wheat bran	Involved in many enzyme systems Necessary for Vitamin A metabolism	Growth failure Lack of sexual maturity Impaired wound healing Poor appetite

by the circulatory system to all the tissues of the body.

Recent evidence indicates that certain vitamins actually behave like hormones physiologically. For instance, both Vitamin D and niacin are synthesized in the human (in inadequate amounts) conferring on them hormonal qualities, since hormones are produced in the body. The fat-soluble vitamins A, D, E, and K are readily stored in the body, and within the cell they demonstrate many similarities to the steroid hormones (estrogen, testosterone, cortisol). The water-soluble vitamins are B_1, B_2, B_3, B_6, B_{12}, pantothenic acid, folic acid, biotin, and Vitamin C. An excessive intake of water soluble vitamins results in increased excretion rather than additional storage.

Certain conditions such as pregnancy, disease, emotional stress, old age, and vitamin destruction caused by methods of processing, storage, and preparing of foods must be considered when determining daily individual vitamin requirements. Table 18-3 summarizes the major vitamins needed in the human diet.

FIBER

Fiber is found only in plant foods like whole-grain breads, cereals, beans, and peas, and other vegetables and fruits. Eating a variety of fiber-containing plant foods is important for proper bowel function, reducing the symptoms of chronic constipation, diverticula disease, and hemorrhoids, and may lower the risk of heart diseases and some cancers. However, some of the health benefits associated with a high-fiber diet may come from other components present in these foods, not just from fiber itself. For this reason, fiber is best obtained from foods, rather than a supplement.

BIOCHEMICAL INDIVIDUALITY AND RECOMMENDED DAILY DIETARY ALLOWANCES

Developing universal "minimum daily requirements" that an apply to everyone is an extremely difficult task. Nutritional requirements among individuals might vary for several

CAREER PROFILES

DIETITIANS AND NUTRITIONISTS

Dietitians and nutritionists plan nutrition programs and supervise the preparation and serving of meals. They help prevent and treat illnesses by promoting healthy eating habits, scientifically evaluating client's diets, and suggesting modification such as reduced fat and sugar for those who are overweight.

Dietitians run food service systems for institutions such as hospitals and schools, and also promote sound eating habits through education and research.

Popular interest in nutrition has led to opportunities in food manufacturing, advertising, and marketing where dietitians analyze foods, prepare literature for distribution, or report on such issues as the nutritional content of recipes, dietary fiber, or vitamin supplements.

The basic education requirement is a bachelor's degree with a major in dietetics, food and nutrition, food service systems management, or a related area. The Commission on Dietetic Registration of the American Dietetic Association (ADA) awards the Registered Dietitian credential to those who pass a certification exam after completing their academic education and supervised experience.

Expectation of employment is expected to grow about as fast as the average for all occupations.

TABLE 18-3 • *Summary of Major Vitamins Needed in the Human Diet*

VITAMIN	FOOD SOURCES	FUNCTION	DEFICIENCY DISEASES
A (Fat-soluble)	Butter, fortified margarine, green and yellow vegetables milk, eggs, liver	Night vision Healthy Skin Proper growth and repair of body tissues	Night blindness Dry skin Slow growth Poor gums and teeth
B_1 (thiamine) (Water-soluble)	Chicken, fish, meat, eggs, enriched bread, whole grain cereals	Promotes normal appetite and digestion Needed by nervous system	Loss of appetite Nervous disorders Fatigue Severe deficiency causes beriberi
B_2 (riboflavin) (Water-soluble)	Cheese, eggs, fish, meat, liver, milk, cereals, enriched bread	Needed in cellular respiration	Eye problems Sores on skin and lips General fatigue
B_3 (niacin) (Water-soluble)	Eggs, fish, liver, meat, milk, potatoes, enriched bread	Needed for normal metabolism Growth Proper skin health	Indigestion Diarrhea Headaches Mental disturbances Skin disorders
B_{12} (Cyanocobalamin) (Water-soluble)	Milk, liver, brain, beef, egg yolk, clams, oysters, sardines, salmon	Red blood cell synthesis Nucleic acid synthesis Nerve cell maintenance	Pernicious anemia Nerve cell malfunction
Folic Acid (Water-soluble)	Liver, yeast, green vegetables, peanuts, mushrooms, beef, veal, egg yolk	Nucleic acid synthesis Needed for normal metabolism and growth	Anemia Growth retardation
C (ascorbic acid) (Water-soluble)	Citrus fruits, cabbage, green vegetables, tomatoes, potatoes	Needed for maintenance of normal bones, gums, teeth, and blood vessels	Weak bones Sore and bleeding gums Poor teeth Bleeding in skin Painful joints Severe deficiency results in scurvy
D (Fat-soluble)	Beef, butter, eggs, milk	Needed for normal bone and teeth development Controls calcium and phosphorus metabolism	Poor bone and teeth structure Soft bones Rickets
E (tocopherol) (Fat-soluble)	Margarine, nuts, leafy vegetables, vegetable oils, whole wheat	Used in cell respiration Protects red blood cells from destruction	Anemia in premature infants No known deficiency in adults
K (Fat-soluble)	Synthesized by colon bacteria Green leafy vegetables, cereal	Essential for normal blood clotting	Slow blood clotting

TABLE 18-4 • *Recommended Dietary Allowances*

FOOD AND NUTRITION BOARD, NATIONAL ACADEMY OF SCIENCES—NATIONAL RESEARCH COUNCIL RECOMMENDED DIETARY ALLOWANCES.[a] REVISED 1989. DESIGNED FOR THE MAINTENANCE OF GOOD NUTRITION OF PRACTICALLY ALL HEALTHY PEOPLE IN THE UNITED STATES

Age (years) or Condition	Weight (kg)	(lb)	Height[b] (cm)	(in)	Protein (g)	Vitamin A[c] (µg RE)	Vitamin D[d] (µg)	Vitamin E[e] (µg α-TE)	Vitamin K (µg)	Vitamin C (mg)	Thiamin (mg)	Riboflavin (mg)	Niacin[f] (mg NE)	Vitamin B6 (mg)	Folate (µg)	Vitamin B12 (µg)	Calcium (mg)	Phosphorus (mg)	Magnesium (mg)	Iron (mg)	Zinc (mg)	Iodine (µg)	Selenium (µg)
Infants																							
0.0-0.5	6	13	60	24	13	375	7.5	3	5	30	0.3	0.4	5	0.3	25	0.3	400	300	40	6	5	40	10
0.5-1.0	9	20	71	28	14	375	10	4	10	35	0.4	0.5	6	0.6	35	0.5	600	500	60	10	5	50	15
Children																							
1-3	13	29	90	35	16	400	10	6	15	40	0.7	0.8	9	1.0	50	0.7	800	800	80	10	10	70	20
4-6	20	44	112	44	24	500	10	7	20	45	0.9	1.1	12	1.1	75	1.0	800	800	120	10	10	90	20
7-10	28	62	132	52	28	700	10	7	30	45	1.0	1.2	13	1.4	100	1.4	800	800	170	10	10	120	30
Males																							
11-14	45	99	157	62	45	1,000	10	10	45	50	1.3	1.5	17	1.7	150	2.0	1,200	1,200	270	12	15	150	40
15-18	66	145	176	69	59	1,000	10	10	65	60	1.5	1.8	20	2.0	200	2.0	1,200	1,200	400	12	15	150	50
19-24	72	160	177	70	58	1,000	10	10	70	60	1.5	1.7	19	2.0	200	2.0	1,200	1,200	350	10	15	150	70
25-50	79	174	176	70	63	1,000	5	10	80	60	1.5	1.7	19	2.0	200	2.0	800	800	350	10	15	150	70
51+	77	170	173	8	63	1,000	5	10	80	60	1.2	1.4	15	2.0	200	2.0	800	800	350	10	15	150	70
Females																							
11-14	46	101	157	62	46	800	10	8	45	50	1.1	1.3	15	1.4	150	2.0	1,200	1,200	280	15	12	150	45
15-18	55	120	163	64	44	800	10	8	55	60	1.1	1.3	15	1.5	180	2.0	1,200	1,200	300	15	12	150	50
19-24	58	128	164	65	46	800	10	8	60	60	1.1	1.3	15	1.6	180	2.0	1,200	1,200	280	15	12	150	55
25-50	63	138	163	64	50	800	5	8	65	60	1.1	1.3	15	1.6	180	2.0	800	800	280	15	12	150	55
51+	65	143	160	63	50	800	5	8	65	60	1.0	1.2	13	1.6	180	2.0	800	800	280	10	12	150	55
Pregnant					60	800	10	10	65	70	1.5	1.6	17	2.2	400	2.2	1,200	1,200	320	30	15	175	65
Lactating																							
1st 6 months					65	1,300	10	12	65	95	1.6	1.8	20	2.1	280	2.6	1,200	1,200	355	15	19	200	75
2nd 6 months					62	1,200	10	11	65	90	1.6	1.7	20	2.1	260	2.6	1,200	1,200	340	15	16	200	75

a The allowances, expressed as average daily intakes over time, are intended to provide for individual variations among most normal persons as they live in the United States under usual environmental stresses. Diets should be based on a variety of common foods in order to provide other nutrients for which human requirements have been less well defined. See text for detailed discussion of allowances and of nutrients not tabulated.

b Weights and heights of Reference Adults are actual medians for the U.S. population of the designated age, as reported by NHANES II. The median weights and heights of those under 19 years of age were taken from Hamill et al. (1979) (see pages 16-17). The use of these figures does not imply that the height-to-weight ratios are ideal.

c Retinol equivalents. 1 retinol equivalent = 1 µg retinol or 6 µg β-carotene. See text for calculation of vitamin A activity of diets as retinol equivalents.

d As cholecalciferol. 10µg cholecalciferol = 400 IU of vitamin D.

e α-Tocopherol equivalents. 1 mg d-α tocopheral = 1 α-TE. See text for variation in allowances and calculation of Vitamin E activity of the diet as α-tocopherol equivalents.

f 1 NE (niacin equivalent) is equal to 1 mg of niacin or 60 mg of dietary tryptophan.

reasons. Malabsorption disorders sometimes require that an individual needs greater than the average daily dosage of certain nutrients. Differences in the microbial environment of the intestine, and genetic factors influencing biochemical reactions must also be considered. People experiencing psychological or physical stress often require a greater amount of certain nutrients to help the body maintain homeostasis or a relatively constant internal environment.

In recognition of individual variations in nutritional requirements, a table of **Recommended Dietary Allowances** (**RDA**) (see Table 18-4) has been approved by the Food and Nutrition Board, National Academy of Sciences. It contains the daily recommendations for protein, fat-soluble vitamins, water-soluble vitamins, and minerals. The allowances are intended to provide for individual variations among most normal persons as they live in the United States under usual environmental stresses.

DIETARY GUIDELINES FOR AMERICANS

In April of 1992, the United States Department of Agriculture unveiled the "Food Guide Pyramid" made up of six food groups, see Figure 18-1. This pyramid replaces the traditional pie chart with the basic four food groups. The recommended groups and amounts are as follows:

Bread, cereal, and pasta	— 6 to 11 servings
Vegetables	— 3 to 5 servings
Fruit	— 2 to 4 servings
Milk, yogurt, and cheese	— 2 to 3 servings
Meat, poultry, fish, dry beans, eggs, and nuts	— 2 to 3 servings
Fats, oils, sweets	— use sparingly

A Scientific Advisory Committee was appointed by the United States Government to develop Dietary Guidelines for the American public. The importance of consuming a diet of

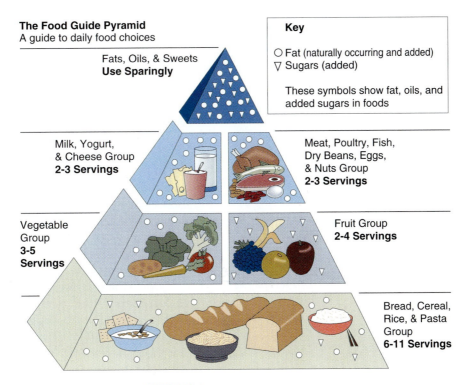

FIGURE 18-1 *Food guide pyramid*

a variety of foods to provide the essential nutrients at a caloric level to maintain desirable body weight is emphasized. The following specific guidelines are advocated by the Committee to help prevent the most prevalent and devastating diseases in our society: diabetes, cancer, hypertension, and heart disease.

1. Eat a variety of foods
2. Maintain desirable weight
3. Avoid too much fat, saturated fat (mostly animal fat), and cholesterol
4. Eat foods with adequate starch and fiber (roughage)
5. Avoid too much sugar
6. Avoid too much sodium
7. If you drink alcoholic beverages, do so in moderation.

Nutrition Facts

Serving Size: 1/2 Cup
Servings Per Container: 4

Amount Per Serving

Calories 100   Calories from Fat 30

	% Daily Value*
Total Fat 3g	**5%**
Saturated Fat 0g	**0%**
Cholesterol 0mg	**0%**
Sodium 340mg	**14%**
Total Carbohydrate 15g	**5%**
Dietary Fiber 1g	**4%**
Sugars 0g	
Protein 2g	

Vitamin A 0%	●	Vitamin C	0%
Calcium 0%	●	Iron	2%

*Percent Daily Values are based on a 2,000 calorie diet. Your daily values may be higher or lower depending on your calorie needs:

	Calories	2,000	2,500
Total Fat	Less than	65g	80g
Sat Fat	Less than	20g	25g
Cholesterol	Less than	300mg	300mg
Sodium	Less than	2,400mg	2,400mg
Total Carbohydrate		300g	375g
Dietary Fiber		25g	30g

Calories per gram:
Fat 9 ∞ Carbohydrate 4 ∞ Protein 4

Ingredients: Flour, Water, Yeast Vegetable Oil, Salt, Artificial Flavor and Color.

FIGURE 18-2 *A sample of nutrition labeling*

NUTRITION LABELING

Effective in May, 1994, the Food and Drug Administration requires nutrition labeling for most foods offered for sale and regulated by the FDA, Figure 18-2. The nutrition label is required to include information on total calories and on amounts of calories from fat, cholesterol, sodium, total carbohydrates, dietary fiber, sugars, protein, Vitamin A, Vitamin C, calcium and iron, in that order. The information on the package is to represent the packaged product prior to consumer preparation.

This final rule establishes a standard format for nutrition information on food labels consisting of:

1. the quantitative amount per serving of each nutrient except vitamins and minerals
2. the amount of each nutrient as a percent of the Daily Value for a 2,000 calorie diet
3. a footnote with reference values for selected nutrients based on 2,000 calories and 2,500 calorie diets
4. caloric conversion information

EATING DISORDERS

Obesity is one of the most common "nutritional diseases" in our society. An obese person is one who contains excess body fat and who weighs 15% more than the optimum body weight for gender, height, and bone structure.

Being obese can affect physical and mental health. Heart disease, high blood pressure, and non-insulin dependent diabetes mellitus are more common in significantly overweight people than in those closer to ideal body weight.

Since most cases of obesity are due to an excessive intake of calories in proportion to expenditure, a daily reduction of caloric intake along with an increase in exercise are recommended for most overweight individuals.

Unfortunately, the desire to be thin has resulted in a complex disorder, mostly seen in young women, called **anorexia nervosa**. In true anorexia nervosa, there is no real loss of appetite, but rather a refusal to eat because of a distorted body image and a fear of weight gain.

The criteria for diagnosis of anorexia nervosa are identified by the American Psychiatric Association as follows:

1. Intense fear of becoming obese that does not diminish as weight loss progresses

2. Disturbance of body image, such as claiming to feel fat even when emaciated

3. Weight loss of at least 25% of the original body weight

4. Refusal to maintain body weight over a minimal normal weight for age and height

5. No known physical illness that would account for the weight loss

6. Amenorrhea, or the cessation of menstruation

Another eating disorder associated with fear of weight gain is **bulimia**. It is characterized

MEDICAL HIGHLIGHT: HEALTH

Foods That Heal

How many people have family recipes that cure colds, hay fever, asthma, and arthritis? Today scientists are looking at antioxidants, nutrients found in plant foods (such as Vitamin C, carotenoids, Vitamin E, and certain minerals), because of their potentially beneficial role in reducing the risk of cancer and certain other chronic diseases. Most of this research is in its earliest stages but experts agree that certain food in moderation seem to boost healing.

Some foods believed to have healing power include:

- Barley—The soluble fiber in barley may be just as effective as oat bran in lowering cholesterol.[1]

- Carrots—Beta-carotene, a chemical found in carrots which offers an edge against cancer, may also protect against heart disease.

- Cheese—Identified in dental research as a food that fights, rather than creates, cavities. Tooth-friendly cheeses include cheddar, Monterey Jack, Edam, Gouda, Roquefort, mozzarella, and Stilton.

- Chili peppers—Eating chili peppers helps with a stuffed-up nose. The eye-watering, nose-running properties of peppers are good for people suffering from bronchitis, sinusitis, and colds.[2]

- Garlic—An all around healing food; it lowers blood pressure and cholesterol levels and fights infection.

- Persimmons—A more powerful source of Vitamin C than oranges, one persimmon is equal to 218mg of Vitamin C; one orange is equal to 70mg of Vitamin C.

- Prunes—Contain 60% of a fiber known as pectin which is known to reduce cholesterol. They are also high in iron, potassium, and beta-carotene.

- Dried beans—Help to lower cholesterol.

- Fish oil—Contains omega-3, a fatty acid currently being tested to help with inflammation from arthritis. Effective types of fish include mackerel, salmon, bluefish, oysters, mussels, crabs, and clams.

- Spinach and collard greens—Have two specific compounds which may be protective against the leading causes of irreversible blindness in older people, condition known as age-related macular degeneration.[3]

[1] Based on research conducted at Montana University.
[2] Based on research conducted by Dr. Irwin Zen at UCLA.
[3] According to the November 9, 1994 *Journal of the AMA*.

by episodic binge eating followed by purging behavior such as self-induced vomiting and laxative abuse. Bulimic patients are most often women somewhat older than those with anorexia nervosa. In some instances, a young woman alternates between the two disorders.

The treatment of anorexia nervosa and bulimia is difficult and lengthy. The goals are restitution of normal nutrition and resolution of the underlying psychological problems. Early intervention is essential; the starvation associated with anorexia can cause irreversible tissue damage and the purging associated with bulimia can cause homeostatic imbalances that lead to cardiac irregularities and, in extreme cases, to death.

● REVIEW QUESTIONS

Select the letter of the choice that best completes the statement.

1. Materials needed by the individual cells for proper cell function are:
   a. proteases
   b. enzymes
   c. amylases
   d. nutrients

2. A gram of fat contains:
   a. 9 calories
   b. 4 calories
   c. 5 calories
   d. 7 calories

3. The main source of energy for the body is provided by:
   a. fats
   b. carbohydrates
   c. proteins
   d. water

4. To build and repair body tissue you need:
   a. fats
   b. carbohydrates
   c. proteins
   d. water

5. The most common bone disease is:
   a. osteomyelitis
   b. fracture
   c. osteoporosis
   d. bone cancer

6. The minerals necessary to build bone and teeth are:
   a. iodine and calcium
   b. calcium and potassium
   c. calcium and phosphorus
   d. fluorine and calcium

7. Iodine is required for the formation of the:
    a. adrenal hormone
    b. thyroid hormone
    c. parathyroid hormone
    d. pituitary hormone

8. A vitamin needed to prevent night blindness is:
    a. Vitamin A
    b. Vitamin K
    c. Vitamin C
    d. Vitamin D

9. The vitamin essential for blood clotting is:
    a. Vitamin A
    b. Vitamin K
    c. Vitamin C
    d. Vitamin D

10. A food that has been identified to help lower cholesterol is:
    a. cheddar cheese
    b. garlic
    c. white bread
    d. broccoli

● APPLYING THEORY TO PRACTICE

1. In the spring of 1992, the USDA changed from the basic four food groups to the six group pyramid plan, the model for recommended dietary allowances. Compare your daily diet with the food pyramid plan. Should you consider changing your diet to meet these requirements?

2. Plan a three-day meal plan including between-meal snacks that will meet both recommended calorie intake and dietary allowances for yourself. Adjust this diet to meet the needs of a twelve-year old male, height 62". Adjust this diet to meet the needs of a seventy-year old female, height 60".

3. A patient has anemia. The doctor requests that you assist the patient in establishing a menu plan that will assist in the formation of red blood cells.

4. Nutritionists recommend 50-60% of carbohydrates daily in a 2,000 calorie diet. 60% would be what proportion of the diet? How many calories would be in carbohydrates?

5. A physician orders a diet of 20gm of protein, 300gm of carbohydrate, and 80gm of fat. What is the total calories, and how much caloric value is there in protein, carbohydrates, and fat? Calculate the percentage of protein, carbohydrates, and fat.

6. A sixty-year-old woman comes into the medical center. She informs you that she takes lots of calcium in foods like milk, cheese, and ice cream to prevent osteoporosis. You know she has a high blood cholesterol level. How would you counsel her regarding her diet?

CHAPTER

19

Urinary/Excretory System

KEY WORDS

acute kidney failure
afferent arteriole
aldosterone
anuria
Bowman's capsule
calyces
chronic renal
   failure
collecting tubule
cortex
cystitis
dialysis
dialyzer
distal convoluted
   tubule
dysuria
efferent arteriole
end stage renal dis-
   ease
filtrate

fistula
glomerulus
glomerulonephritis
graft
hematuria
hemodialysis
hilum
hydronephrosis
incontinence
kidney
kidney stones (renal
   calculi)
lithotripsy
loop of Henle
medulla
nephron
neurogenic bladder
oliguria
osmoreceptor
peritoneal dialysis

proximal
   convoluted
   tubule
pyelonephritis
pyuria
renal column
renal fascia
renal papilla
renal pelvis
renal pyramid
renin
retroperitoneal
threshold
uremia
ureter
urethra
urethritis
urinalysis
urinary bladder
urinary meatus

URINARY SYSTEM

Food is utilized through the process of digestion, absorption, and metabolism. The blood and lymph transport products of digestion to the tissues. After the cells of the tissues have used the food and oxygen needed for growth and repair, waste products formed by the process are taken away and excreted from the body. The excretory organs eliminate the metabolic wastes and undigested food residue.

The excretory organs through which elimination takes place include the kidneys, the skin, the intestines, and the lungs. The lungs, generally considered part of the respiratory system, serve an excretory function in that they give off carbon dioxide and water vapor during exhalation. The urinary system functions largely as an excretory agent of nitrogenous wastes, salts, and water, while the skin excretes dissolved wastes present in perspiration, mostly dissolved salts. The indigestible residue, water, and bacteria are excreted by the intestines. The excretion of waste products is described and summarized in Table 19-1.

The urinary system performs the main part of the excretory function in the body, see Figure 19-1. The most important excretory organs are the kidneys. Their primary excretory function is removal of the nitrogenous waste products. If the kidneys fail to function properly toxic wastes start to accumulate in the body. Toxic wastes accumulating in the cells cause them to "suffocate" and literally poison themselves.

The urinary system consists of two kidneys (that form the urine), two ureters, a bladder, and a urethra. Each kidney has a long, tubular ureter that carries urine to the urinary bladder. This is a temporary storage sac for urine, from which urine is excreted through the urethra.

FUNCTIONS OF THE URINARY SYSTEM

1. Excretion, which is the process of removing nitrogenous waste material, certain salts, and excess water from the blood.

2. Help to maintain acid-base balance by evaluating elements in the blood and selectively reabsorbing water and other substances to maintain the pH balance.

3. To secrete waste products in the form of urine.

4. To eliminate the urine from the bladder where it is stored.

KIDNEYS

The kidneys are bean-shaped organs resting high against the dorsal wall of the abdominal cavity; they lie on either side of the vertebral column, between the peritoneum and the back muscles. Because the kidneys are located behind the peritoneum, they are said to be retroperitoneal. They are positioned between the twelfth thoracic and the third lumbar vertebrae. The right kidney is situated slightly lower than the left due to the large area occupied by the liver.

TABLE 19-1 • *Elimination of Waste Products*

ORGAN	PRODUCT OF EXCRETION	PROCESS OF ELIMINATION
Lungs	carbon dioxide and water vapor	exhalation
Kidneys	nitrogenous wastes and salts dissolved in water to form urine	urination
Skin	dissolved salts	perspiration
Intestines	solid wastes and water	defecation

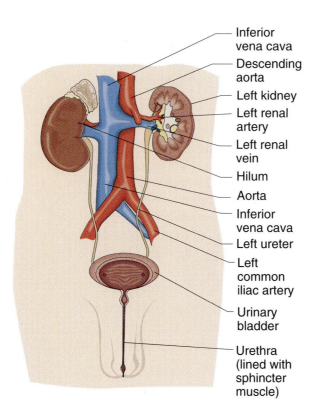

FIGURE 19-1 *The structures of the urinary system*

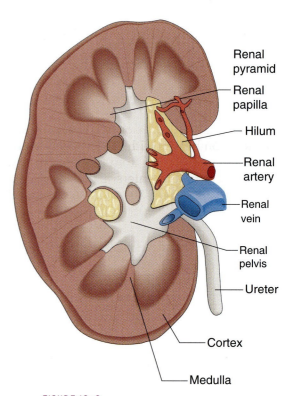

FIGURE 19-2 *The structures of the kidney*

Each kidney and its blood vessels is enclosed within a mass of fat tissue called the adipose capsule. In turn, each kidney and adipose capsule is covered by a tough, fibrous tissue called the **renal fascia**.

There is an indentation along the concave medial border of the kidney called the **hilum**. The hilum is a passageway for the lymph vessels, nerves, renal artery and vein, and the ureter. At the hilum the fibrous capsule continues downward, forming the outer layer of the ureter. Cutting the kidney in half lengthwise reveals its internal structure. The upper end of each ureter flares into a funnel-shaped structure known as the **renal pelvis**.

The kidneys have the potential to work harder than they actually do. Under ordinary circumstances, only a portion of the nephron are used. Should one kidney not function, or have to be removed, more nephrons and tubules open up in the second kidney to assume the work of the nonfunctioning or missing kidney.

Medulla and Cortex

The kidney is divided into two layers: an outer, granular layer called the **cortex**, and an inner, striated layer, the **medulla**. The medulla is red and consists of radially striated cones called the **renal pyramids**. The base of each renal pyramid faces the cortex, while its apex (**renal papilla**) empties into cuplike cavities called **calyces**. These, in turn, empty into the renal pelvis.

The cortex, reddish brown, is composed of millions of microscopic functional units of the kidney called nephrons. Cortical tissue is interspersed between renal pyramids, separating and supporting them. These interpyramidal cortical supports are the **renal columns**. The renal columns and the renal pyramids alternate with one another, see Figure 19-2.

NEPHRON

The **nephron** is the basic structural and functional unit of the kidney. Most of the nephron is located within the cortex, with only a small, tubular portion in the medulla. Each kidney has over one million nephrons which altogether comprise 140 miles of filters and tubes.

A nephron begins with the **afferent arteriole**, which carries blood from the renal artery. The afferent arteriole enters a double-walled hollow capsule, the **Bowman's capsule**.[1] Within the capsule the afferent arteriole finely divides, forming a knotty ball called the **glomerulus** which contains some fifty separate capillaries. The combination of the Bowman's capsule and the glomerulus is known as the renal corpuscle. The Bowman's capsule sends off a highly convoluted (twisted) tubular branch referred to as the **proximal convoluted tubule**.

The proximal convoluted tubule descends into the medulla to form the **loop of Henle**. In Figure 19-3, observe that the loop of Henle has a straight descending limb, a loop, and a straight ascending limb. When the ascending limb of Henle's loop returns to the cortex, it turns into the **distal convoluted tubule**. Eventually this convoluted tubule opens into a larger, straight vessel known as the **collecting tubule**. Several distal convoluted tubules join to form this single straight collection tubule. The collecting tubule empties into the renal pelvis, then into the ureter.

As Figure 19-3 shows, the walls of the renal tubules are surrounded by capillaries. After the afferent arteriole branches out to form the glomerulus, it leaves the Bowman's capsule as the **efferent arteriole**. The efferent arteriole branches to form the peritubular capillaries surrounding the renal tubules. All of these capillaries eventually join together to form a small branch of the renal vein which carries blood from the kidney.

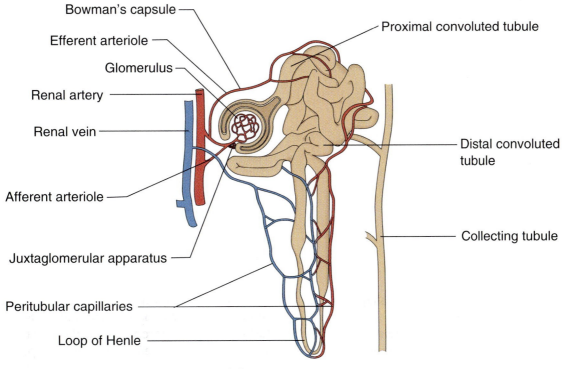

FIGURE 19-3 *Structure of the nephron*

[1] Sir William Bowman (1816-1892), English anatomist and ophthalmologist

The Path of the Formation of Urine

Blood enters the afferent arteriole → passes through the glomerulus → to Bowman's capsule → now it becomes filtrate (blood minus the red blood cells and plasma proteins) → continues through the proximal convoluted tubule → to the loop of Henle → to the distal convoluted tubule → to the collecting tubule (at this time about 99% of the filtrate has been reabsorbed) → approximately 1 ml or urine is formed per minute → the 1 ml of urine goes to the renal pelvis → to the ureter → to the bladder → to the urethra → to the urinary meatus.

URINE FORMATION IN THE NEPHRON

The kidney nephrons form urine by three processes: (1) filtration by the glomerulus, (2) reabsorption within the renal tubules, and (3) secretion by the tubular cells.

Filtration

The first step in urine formation is filtration. In this process, blood from the renal artery enters the smaller afferent arteriole, which in turn enters the even smaller capillaries of the glomerulus. As the blood from the renal artery travels this course, the blood vessels grow narrower and narrower. This results in an increase in blood pressure. In most of the capillaries throughout the body, blood pressure is about 25 millimeters of mercury; in the glomerulus, it is between 60 and 90 millimeters.

This high blood pressure forces a plasma-like fluid to filter from the blood in the glomerulus into the Bowman's capsule. This fluid is called the **filtrate**. It consists of water, glucose, amino acids, some salts, and urea. The filtrate does not contain plasma proteins or red blood cells because they are too large to pass through the pores of the capillary membrane. The Bowman's capsule filters out 125 milliliters of fluid from the blood in a single minute. In one hour, 7500 ml of filtrate leave the blood; this amounts to some 180 liters in a twenty-four period.

As the nephric filtrate continues along the tubules, 99% of this water is reabsorbed back into the bloodstream; therefore, only 1.–1.5 (1000 ml–1500 ml) liters of urine is excreted per day.

Reabsorption

This process includes the reabsorption of useful substances from the filtrate within the renal tubules into the capillaries around the tubules (peritubular capillaries). These include water, glucose, amino acids, vitamins, bicarbonate ions (HCO_3^-), and the chloride salts of calcium, magnesium, sodium and potassium. Reabsorption starts in the proximal convoluted tubules; it continues through the Henle's loop, the distal convoluted tubules, and the collecting tubules.

The proximal tubules reabsorb approximately 80% of the water filtered out of the blood in the glomerulus (180 liters). Water absorbed through the proximal tubules constitutes obligatory water absorption by osmosis. Simultaneously, glucose, amino acids, vitamins, and some sodium ions are actively transported back into the blood. However, when levels exceed normal limits, the selective cells lining the tubules no longer reabsorb substances such as glucose but allow it to remain in the tubule to be eliminated in the urine. The term used to describe the limit of reabsorption if the **threshold**. Passing this level is referred to as *spilling over the threshold*. For example, people who have diabetes spill sugar frequently and therefore sugar can be found in their urine (glycosuria). Another example is, when a person is taking medications the tubules will only reabsorb a certain amount of the drug; therefore, the medication may have to be taken every four to six hours to maintain a therapeutic dosage of the drug in the blood.

In the distal convoluted tubules about 10 to 15% of water is reabsorbed into the bloodstream, depending upon the needs of the body. This type of water absorption is called optional reabsorption. It is controlled by the antidiuretic

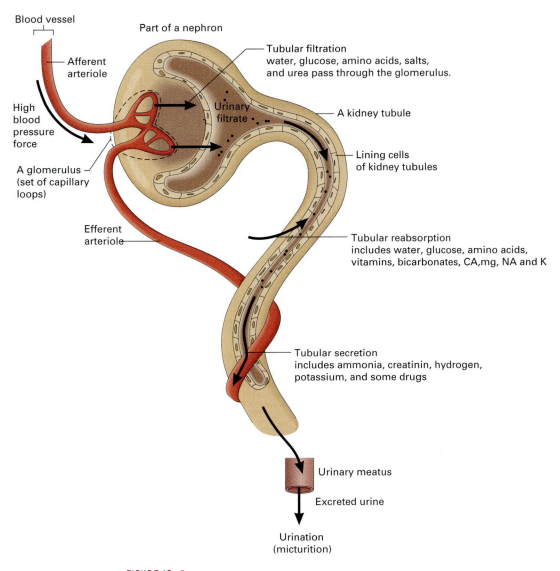

FIGURE 19-4 *Processes and structures of the nephron*

hormone (ADH) and aldosterone. ADH and aldosterone help maintain balance of body fluids, Figure 19-4.

Secretion

The process of secretion is the opposite of reabsorption. Some substances are actively secreted into the tubules. Secretion transports substances from the blood in the peritubular capillaries into the urine in the distal and collecting tubules. Substances secreted into the urine include ammonia creatinine, hydrogen ions (H^+), potassium ions (K^+), and some drugs. The electrolytes are selectively secreted to maintain the body's acid-base balance.

Urinary Output

The amount of urinary output is between 1000–2000 ml/24 hours with an average of 1500 ml per day. Volume will vary with diet, fluid intake, temperature, and physical activity. Another factor regulating secretion is the amount of solutes in the filtrate. Again considering the diabetic, when there is an increase in the amount of glucose, it spills over into the urine increasing the urine volume eliminated that day because more fluid is allowed to pass through to dilute the glucose content.

Urinalysis, an examination of the urine, can determine the presence of blood cells, bacteria, acidity level, specific gravity (weight), and physical characteristics such as color, clarity, and odor. A urinalysis is the most common non-invasive diagnostic test done. See Figure 19-5 for a lab report which shows normal values for a routine urinalysis.

URETERS

Urine passes from the kidneys out of the collecting tubules into the renal pelvis, down the ureter, into the urinary bladder. There are two ureters (one from each kidney) carrying urine from the kidneys to the urinary bladder. They are long, narrow tubes, less than 1/4" wide and 10 to 12" long. Mucous membrane lines both renal pelves and the ureters. Beneath the mucous membrane lining of the ureters are smooth muscle fibers. When these muscles contract, peristalsis is initiated, pushing urine down the ureter into the urinary bladder.

URINARY BLADDER

The urinary bladder, a hollow muscular organ, made of elastic fibers and involuntary muscle, acts like a reservoir. It stores the urine until about one pint (500 ml) is accumulated. The bladder then becomes uncomfortable and

---

PHYSICAL EXAMINATION:

Appearance _CLEAR, STRAW-COLORED_

pH _4.5 TO 7.5 (RANGE)_   Specific Gravity _1.010 TO 1.025 (RANGE)_

CHEMICAL ANALYSIS:

Albumin (protein) _NONE TO TRACE_   Urobilinogen _NEG._

Sugar (glucose, dextrose) _NONE_   Porphyrins _NEG._

Ketones (acetone) _NONE_   PKU _NEG._

Bilirubin _NONE_   Occult Blood _NEG._

MICROSCOPIC EXAMINATION:

Cells: Epithelial _FEW_

WBC's _0 TO 4_

RBC's _FEW TO OCCASIONAL_

Casts: Hyaline _NEG._

Epithelial _NEG._

Blood _NEG._   EA 1/20/97

Crystals: _FEW_

Other: _NEG._

FIGURE 19-5 *Lab report showing normal values for a routine urinalysis*

must be emptied. Emptying the bladder, or voiding, takes place by muscular contractions of the bladder which are involuntary, although they can be controlled to some extent through the nervous system. Contraction of the bladder muscles forces the urine through a narrow canal, the **urethra**, which extends to the outside opening, the **urinary meatus**.

CONTROL OF URINARY SECRETION

The control of the secretions of urine is under both chemical and nervous control.

Chemical Control

The reabsorption of water in the distal convoluted kidney tubules and the collecting ducts is influenced by the antidiuretic hormone ADH. ADH helps to increase the size of the cell membrane pores in the epithelial cells of the distal tubule and collecting ducts by increasing their permeability to water. The secretion and regulation of the ADH is under the control of the hypothalamus. In the hypothalamus, highly sensitive receptor cells, called **osmoreceptors**, are sensitive to the osmotic pressure of blood plasma. An increase in the osmotic blood pressure due to salt retention causes an increase in ADH secretion. This will inhibit normal urine formation, and water may also be held in the tissues. Figure 19-6 shows the effect of salt retention on human tissues.

There are other hormones involved in the reabsorption process. **Aldosterone** secreted by the adrenal cortex promotes the excretion of potassium and hydrogen ions and the reabsorption of sodium ions; chloride ions and water are also absorbed. As the blood passes through the glomerulus to Bowman's capsule, specialized cells are able to detect a drop in blood pressure. A hormone called **renin** is released by the kidneys into the bloodstream. Renin stimulates the release of aldosterone by the adrenal cortex and constricts the blood vessels. In the absence of aldosterone, sodium and water are excreted in large amounts, and potassium is retained. Any dysfunction to the adrenal cortex produces pronounced changes in the salt and water content of body fluids.

Diuretics increase urinary output by inhibiting the reabsorption of water. Alcohol and caffeine are examples of common diuretics. Alcohol inhibits the secretion of ADH from the pituitary gland. This increases urinary output and may cause dehydration. (This explains why after drinking alcohol the night before you may wake up feeling "parched" and dried out.) Caffeine increases the loss of sodium ion, thus increasing the loss of water.

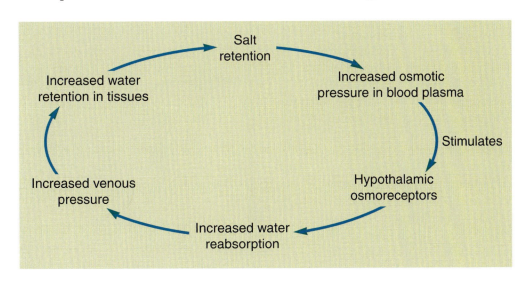

FIGURE 19-6 *How salt retention influences water retention in tissues*

Nervous Control

The nervous control of urine secretion is accomplished directly through the action of nerve impulses on the blood vessels leading to the kidney and on those within the kidney leading to the glomeruli. Indirect nerve control is achieved through the stimulation of certain endocrine glands, whose hormonal secretions will control urinary secretion.

DISORDERS OF THE URINARY SYSTEM

Acute kidney failure may be sudden in onset. Causes may be nephritis (inflammation of the nephron), shock, injury, bleeding, sudden heart failure, or poisoning. The symptoms of acute kidney failure include **oliguria** which is scanty or diminished production of the urine or **anuria** which is absence of urine formation. Suppression of urine formation is dangerous; unless anuria is relieved, **uremia** will develop. Uremia is a toxic condition which occurs when the blood retains urinary waste products. Symptoms resulting from uremia are headaches, dyspnea, nausea, vomiting, and in extreme cases, coma and death.

Chronic renal failure is the condition where there is a gradual loss of function of the nephrons.

Glomerulonephritis is an inflammation of the glomerulus of the nephron. The filtration process is affected. Plasma proteins are filtered through and protein is found in the urine as albumin (albuminuria). In addition, red blood cells are present (**hematuria**).

Acute glomerulonephritis occurs in some children about one to three weeks after a bacterial infection, usually a strep throat. The illness is treated with antibiotics and recovery takes place.

Chronic glomerulonephritis occurs when the filtration membrane may be permanently affected. There is diminished function of the kidney, which may result in kidney failure.

Hydronephrosis occurs when the renal pelvis and calyces become distended due to an accumulation of fluid. The urine "backs up" because of a blockage in the ureter or pressure on the outside of the ureter, which may narrow the passageway. The blockage may be caused by a kidney stone. Other conditions which may cause hydronephrosis are pregnancy or an enlarged prostate gland, which cause pressure on the ureters or bladder. The treatment for this condition is the removal of the obstruction.

Pyelonephritis is the inflammation of the kidney tissue and the renal pelvis. This condition generally results from an infection that has spread from the ureters. One of the symptoms is **pyuria**, the presence of pus in the urine. The course of treatment includes the administration of antibiotics.

Kidney stones or **renal calculi** are stones formed in the kidney. Some materials contained in urine are only slightly soluble in water. Therefore, when stagnation occurs, the microscopic crystals of calcium phosphate, along with uric acid and other substances, may clump together to form kidney stones. These kidney stones slowly grow in diameter. They eventually fill the renal pelvis and obstruct urine flow in the ureter. Usually, the first symptom of a kidney stone is extreme pain, which occurs suddenly in the kidney area or lower abdomen and moves to the groin. Other symptoms include nausea and vomiting, burning, frequent urge to void, chills, fever, and weakness. There may also be hematuria. Diagnosis is made by symptoms, ultrasound, and x-rays such as intravenous pyelogram (IVP) and kidney, ureter, and bladder (KUB). Treatment includes an increase in fluids which will increase urinary output. This may help to flush out the stone. Medications are given to help to dissolve the stone. If this is not successful, a urethroscope, or lithotripsy, may be done. (See medical highlight).

Cystitis is the inflammation of the mucous membrane lining of the urinary bladder. The most common cause of cystitis is from the bacteria E. Coli which is normally found in the rectum or from an urethritis usually leads to painful urination (**dysuria**) or frequent urination (polyuria). This condition is more common in the female. The length of the female urethra is about 1 1/4 to 2". Organisms can easily enter the urethra from the outside of the body. The treatment of cystitis involves antibiotics and

MEDICAL HIGHLIGHT: TREATMENT

Kidney Stone Removal

Extracorporeal Shockwave Lithotripsy

A surgical procedure called **Extracorporeal Shockwave Lithotripsy** (**ESWL**) may be done to remove kidney stones located high in the ureters or the renal pelvis. ESWL uses shockwaves created outside the body to travel through the skin and body tissues until the waves hit the dense stones. The stones become sand-like and are passed through the urinary tract. There are several devices used. One device positions the patient in the water bath while the shock waves are transmitted. Most devices use either x-ray or ultrasound to help the surgeon locate the stone during the treatment.

This procedure can be done on an outpatient basis. Recovery time is short and most people resume normal activities in a few days.

Some complications may occur such as hematuria, bruising, and minor discomfort on the back or abdomen. In addition, the shattered stone fragments may cause discomfort as they pass through the urinary tract. Previous treatment for kidney stones involved nephrolithotomy, an opening into the kidney, with a week's hospital stay and four to six weeks of recovery.

Uteroscopic Stone Removal

Ulteroscopic stone removal is done for mid and lower stones. A surgeon passes a small fiber-optic instrument called a urethroscope through the urethra and bladder into the ureter. The surgeon then locates the stone and either removes it with a cage-like device or shatters it with a special instrument that produces a form of shockwave.

---

urinary antiseptics with increased fluids. The patient should be taught proper wiping techniques after urination. The patient with cystitis must be reminded to complete the prescribed amount of medication to prevent reinfection.

Incontinence is also known as involuntary micturition (urination). Here, an individual loses voluntary control over urination. Incontinence occurs in babies prior to toilet training, since they lack control over the external sphincter muscle of the urethra. Thus, urination occurs whenever the bladder fills. Similarly, a person who has suffered a stroke, or one whose spinal cord has been severed may have no bladder control. In these conditions a patient may require an indwelling catheter. This is a tube inserted into the neck of the bladder through the urethra. It directs the urine into a sterile urinary drainage bag.

Neurogenic bladder is a condition caused by damaged nerves that control the urinary bladder. This results in dysuria, the inability to empty the bladder completely, and incontinence.

Dialysis

Dialysis is the type of treatment used for kidney failure. Dialysis involves the passage of blood through a device which has a semipermeable membrane to rid the blood of harmful wastes, extra salt, and water. Dialysis devices serve as a substitute kidney. The two forms of dialysis are hemodialysis and peritoneal dialysis.

Hemodialysis is a process for purifying blood by passing it through thin membranes and exposing it to a solution which continually circulates around the membrane. The solution is called a *dialysate*. Substances in the blood pass through the membranes into the lesser concentrated dialysate in response to the laws of diffusion. The part of the unit which actually substitutes for the kidney is a glass tube called a **dialyzer**, which is filled with thousands of minute hollow fibers attached firmly at both ends, Figure 19-7. Blood from the patient flows through the fibers, which are surrounded by circulating dialysate. The dialysate is individualized for each patient to provide the appropriate levels of sodium, bicarbonate, and other substances. These cross the membrane and enter the blood. At the same time, extra water and waste products leave the blood to enter the dialysate.

The patient is connected to the dialysis unit by means of needles and tubing that take blood from the patient to the machine and return it to the patient. A **fistula** (opening between an artery and a vein) or a **graft** (vein inserted between the artery and a vein) is surgically constructed to provide a site for inserting the needles. Artificial veins may last from three to five years. Most patients are assigned to a dialysis center for periodic treatment; however, treatment can also be done in the home if the patient and family are willing to assume responsibility. It is usually done two to three times a week and each treatment lasts from two to four hours. To avoid side effects, the patient is advised to follow special diet instructions and take medications as proscribed.

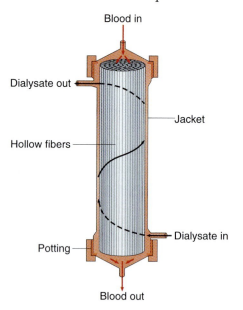

Blood in

Dialysate out

Jacket

Hollow fibers

Dialysate in

Potting

Blood out

FIGURE 19-7 *A dialyzer*

Peritoneal dialysis uses the patient's own peritoneal lining instead of a dialyzer to filter the blood. A cleansing solution called the dialysate travels through a catheter implanted into the abdomen. Fluid, wastes, electrolytes, and chemicals pass from tiny blood vessels in the peritoneal membrane into the dialysate. After several hours, the dialysate is drained from the abdomen, taking the wastes from the blood with it. The abdomen is filled with fresh dialysate and the cleaning procedure begins again. The most common types of peritoneal dialysis is continuous ambulatory peritoneal dialysis (CAPD). The dialysate stays in the abdomen for about four to six hours. The process of draining the dialysate and replacing it with fresh solution takes about thirty minutes. Most people change the solution four times a day, Figure 19-8.

Automated peritoneal dialysis, a type of peritoneal dialysis which can be done at night while the patient is asleep, takes six to eight hours.

The main complication of peritoneal dialysis is peritonitis, an inflammation of the peritoneal lining.

Kidney Transplants

Kidney transplants are done in cases of prolonged chronic debilitating diseases and renal failure involving both kidneys. Usually the patient has been on dialysis for a long period of time waiting for a compatible organ. The transplant requires a donor organ from an individual who has a similar immune system in order to prevent rejection. Blood and other cellular material must match to ensure the greatest potential for success in a transplant. The patient is usually in a state of relatively poor physical condition due to the effects of the extended illness. This status plus the tendency of the body to reject a "substance" that is foreign and not of the same cellular structure sometimes results in the organ not surviving in the new host. The use of drugs to control the body's natural defensive mechanism of rejection increases the rate of success.

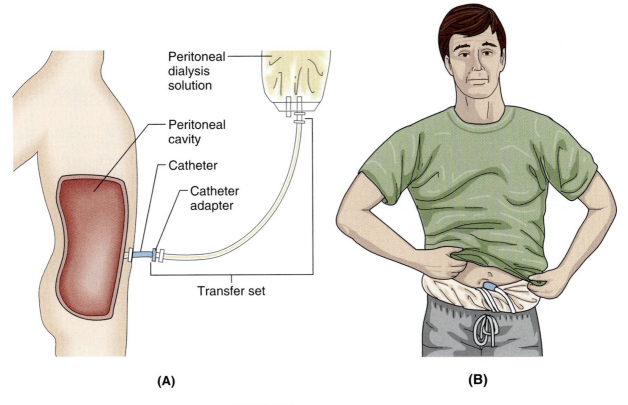

Peritoneal
dialysis
solution

Peritoneal
cavity

Catheter

Catheter
adapter

Transfer set

(A)

(B)

FIGURE 19-8 *Peritoneal dialysis*

● REVIEW QUESTIONS

Select the letter of choice that best completes the statement.

1. The kidneys are responsible for excreting:
   a. carbon dioxide and water
   b. solid wastes and water
   c. nitrogenous wastes and water
   d. perspiration

2. In addition to kidneys the organ responsible for excretion of carbon dioxide and water is:
   a. lungs
   b. kidneys
   c. skin
   d. large intestine

3. The kidneys are located in which area?
   a. abdominal
   b. pelvic
   c. peritoneal
   d. retroperitoneal

4. A ball of capillaries is called the:
   a. Bowman's capsule
   b. cortex
   c. glomerulus
   d. medulla

5. The process of plasma-like fluid passing through the glomerulus to Bowman's capsule is called:
   a. filtration
   b. reabsorption
   c. secretion
   d. excretion

6. The hormone ADH affects reabsorption in the:
   a. glomerulus
   b. proximal convoluted tubule
   c. loop of Henle
   d. dismal convoluted tubule

7. The pathway of urine formation is:
   a. kidney, ureter, urethra, bladder
   b. ureter, pelvis, urethra, bladder
   c. kidney, urethra, bladder, ureter
   d. kidney, ureter, bladder, urethra

8. The average normal daily urinary output is:
   a. 600 ml
   b. 1200 ml
   c. 1800 ml
   d. 2400 ml

9. Inflammation of the urinary bladder is called:
   a. nephritis
   b. cystitis
   c. pyelitis
   d. urethritis

10. Involuntary urination is known as:
    a. polyuria
    b. anuria
    c. incontinence
    d. frequency

● COMPLETION

If laboratory facilities and supervision are available, obtain and examine several specimens of fresh normal urine.

1. What is the color of the specimen?

2. Is it clear or cloudy?

3. Is the urine acid, alkaline or neutral? To test, dip blue litmus paper into the urine. If acid is present, it will turn red. Dip red litmus paper in. If urine is alkaline, it will turn paper blue. If neither paper changes color, the urine is neutral.

4. What is the specific gravity of a specimen? To test, use urinometer.

5. Using *Acetest* reagent tablets, examine the urine for acetone. Have the results and your interpretation checked by the instructor.

   Place the reagent tablet on a clean white sheet of paper. Place a drop of urine on the tablet. In thirty seconds, compare the resulting color with the color chart enclosed with the tablets. Record the result on the chart.

6. Using *Clinitest* tablets and/or Clinistix reagent strips, test for sugar. Have the results and your interpretation checked by the instructor.

   Clinitest tablets: Place five drops of urine and ten drops of water in a test tube. Add the Clinitest tablet. Observe the reaction. Then shake the test tube and compare the color of the solution with the color scale enclosed with the tablets. Record the result.

   Clinistix reagent strips: Dip the test end of the Clinistix in the urine and remove it. (Avoid contact with fingers or other objects because misleading results may occur.) If the moistened end turns blue, the result is *positive*. When sugar is present, the blue color will appear in less than one minute. Record the result.

● MATCHING

Match each term in Column I with its description in Column II.

Column I	Column II
_____ 1. nephron	a. tubes which connect the kidneys with the bladder
_____ 2. glomerulus	b. mass of capillaries
_____ 3. bladder	c. structure which absorbs filtrate from the capillary mass
_____ 4. urethra	d. one of millions of tiny filtering units
_____ 5. ureter	e. returns blood to the inferior vena cava
_____ 6. ADH	f. hormone which regulates water reabsorption
_____ 7. collecting tubules	g. contraction of bladder muscles
_____ 8. Bowman's capsule	h. canal which opens to the outside of the body
_____ 9. kidney	i. primarily acts as a reservoir
_____ 10. renal vein	j. allow urine to drain into the renal pelvis
_____ 11. anuria	k. bean-shaped organ
_____ 12. dysuria	l. scanty urine
_____ 13. pyuria	m. blood in the urine
_____ 14. hematuria	n. no urine
_____ 15. oliguria	o. pus in the urine
_____ 16. carbon dioxide	p. painful urination
_____ 17. calculi	q. helps regulate body temperature
_____ 18. urine	r. blood retains urinary waste products
_____ 19. cystitis	s. stones in the kidneys
_____ 20. uremia	t. waste product eliminated through the lungs
	u. inflammation of the mucous membranes lining the bladder
	v. water and nitrogenous wastes

● APPLYING THEORY TO PRACTICE

1. The amount of daily water loss is approximately 1500-1800 ml through urinary output, 500 ml through the skin, and 500 ml through the respiration. Keep a log for twenty-four hours. Measure your liquid intake and urinary output. Answer the question, "Are you taking enough fluid to maintain your body in good fluid balance?"

2. You have just run a mile and sweated profusely. When you urinate you notice there is only a small amount and it is concentrated. Explain what has happened.

3. You have to take an antibiotic. The instructions say to take it every six hours. Why is it necessary to maintain this over twenty-four hours?

4. A patient comes to the Emergency Health Center complaining of a severe back pain. After a patient examination and history, the diagnosis is kidney stones. The patient inquires "How did I get stones in my kidney?" Explain the cause and treatment.

5. In kidney failure, dialysis may be necessary. Define dialysis. What type do you think would be best for a vision-impaired seventy-year-old? What type do you think would be best for a mother with children ages two, six, and ten?

CHAPTER

20

Reproductive System

OBJECTIVES

- Compare somatic cell division (mitosis) with germ cell division (meiosis)
- Explain the process of fertilization
- Identify the organs of the female reproductive system and explain their functions
- Explain menopause and the changes which occur during this time
- Describe the stages and changes which occur during the menstrual cycle
- Identify the organs of the male reproductive system and explain their functions
- List some common disorders of the reproductive system
- Define the key words that relate to this chapter

KEY WORDS

amenorrhea
areola
artificial insemination
Bartholin's glands
BPH (benign prostatic hypertrophy)
breast
bulbourethral gland (Cowper's gland)
cervix
chlamydia
circumcision
clitoris
coitus
corona radiata
corpus luteum
cryptorchidism
ductus deferens
dysmenorrhea
ectopic pregnancy
ejaculatory duct
endometriosis
endometrium
epididymis
episiotomy
fallopian tube (oviduct)

fertilization
fibroid tumors
fimbriae
foreskin (prepuce)
fundus
gamete (germ cell)
genital warts
glans penis
gonorrhea
graafian follicle
hymen
hysterectomy
impotence
infertility
in-vitro fertilization
labia
laparoscopy
leukorrhea
mammogram
mastectomy
menarche
menopause
menstrual cycle
menstruation
myometrium
mons pubis
oogenesis

ova
ovary
ovulation
Pap smear (Papanicolaou)
penile shaft
penis
perineum
PID (pelvic inflammatory disease)
PMS (pre-menstrual syndrome)
prostate gland
prostatectomy
puberty
salpingitis
scrotum
seminal vesicle
seminiferous tubule
spermatogenesis
spermatozoa
sterile
syphilis
testes
uterus
vas deferens
yeast infection

All living organisms, whether unicellular or multicellular, small or large, must reproduce in order to continue their species. Humans and most multicellular animals reproduce new members of their species by sexual reproduction.

FUNCTIONS OF THE REPRODUCTIVE SYSTEM

1. Has the necessary organs capable of accomplishing reproduction, the creation of a new individual.

2. Manufacture hormones necessary for the development of the reproductive organs and secondary sex characteristics.

   • Females—estrogen and progesterone.

   • Male—testosterone.

Specialized sex cells or **germ cells** (**gametes**) must be produced by the gonads of both male and female sex organs before sexual reproduction can take place. The female gonads, called the ovaries, produce egg cells (ova). The male gonads, the testes, produce sperm. Normal cell division is known as mitosis. In the formation of the germ cells, a special process of cell division occurs called **meiosis**. In the female, the specific meiotic process is called **oogenesis**; in the male, **spermatogenesis**.

In humans, the somatic (body) cells, including skin, fat, muscle, nerve, bone cells, and so on contain 46 chromosomes in the nucleus. Forty-four of these are autosomes (nonsex chromosomes). The remaining two are sex chromosomes. Each chromosome has a partner of the same size and shape so that they can be paired, Figure 20-1. In the female, the somatic cells contain 22 pairs of autosomes, and a single pair of

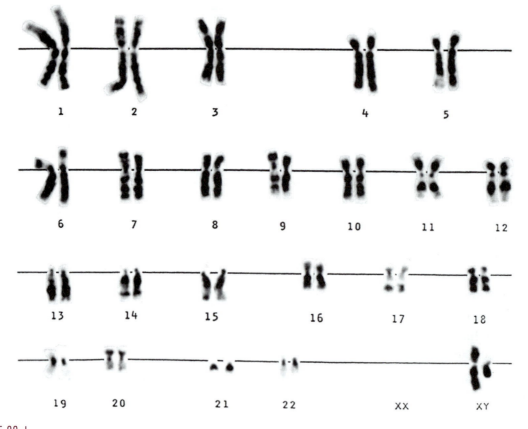

FIGURE 20-1 *Karyotype of human from a male somatic cell. A karyotype is the arrangement of chromosome pairs according to shape and size.*

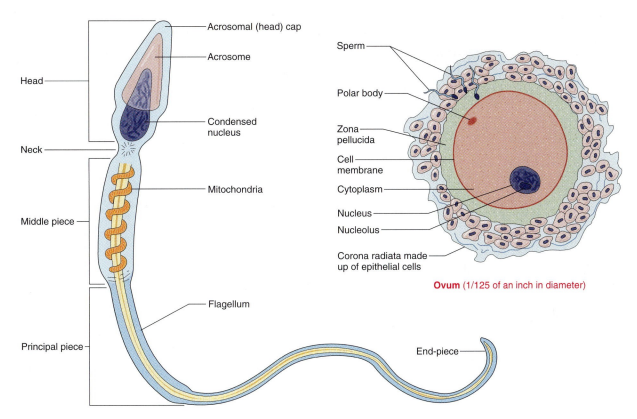

Head
- Acrosomal (head) cap
- Acrosome
- Condensed nucleus

Neck

Middle piece
- Mitochondria

Principal piece
- Flagellum

End-piece

Sperm
Polar body
Zona pellucida
Cell membrane
Cytoplasm
Nucleus
Nucleolus
Corona radiata made up of epithelial cells

Ovum (1/125 of an inch in diameter)

FIGURE 20-2 *Structures of the human sperm and ovum*

sex chromosomes (both are X chromosomes). In the male, the combination is also 22 autosomal pairs and a single pair of sex chromosomes. However, the male sex chromosomal pair consists of an X and Y chromosome.

Oogenesis and spermatogenesis reduces the chromosome number of 46 to 23 in the gametes or germ cells. All multicellular organisms start from the fusion of two gametes: the sperm (spermatozoon) from the male, and the ovum from the female. Figure 20-2 shows the structure of a spermatozoon and an ovum.

FERTILIZATION

During sexual intercourse, or coitus, sperm from the testes is deposited into the female vagina, Figure 20-3. Spermatozoa entering the female reproductive tract live for only a day or two at the most, though they may remain in the tract up to two weeks before degenerating.

Approximately 100 million spermatozoa are contained in 1 milliliter (1 cc) of ejaculated seminal fluid. They are fairly uniform in shape and size. If the count is less than 20 million per milliliter, the male is considered to be sterile. These millions of sperm cells swim towards the ovum that has been released from the ovary. The large quantity of sperm is necessary because a great number are destroyed before they even approach the ovum. Many die from the acidity of the secretions in the male urethra or the vagina. Some cannot withstand the high temperature of the female abdomen, while others lack the propulsion ability to progress from the vagina to the upper uterine (fallopian) tube.

In order for a sperm to penetrate and fertilize an ovum, the corona radiata must first be penetrated. This is the layer of epithelial cells surrounding the zona pellucida, see Figure 20-2. Eventually, only one sperm cell penetrates and fertilizes an ovum. To accomplish this success-

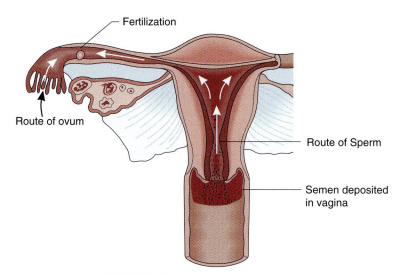

Fertilization

Route of ovum

Route of Sperm

Semen deposited
in vagina

FIGURE 20-3 *Route of the sperm and ovum*

fully, the sperm head produces an enzyme called hyaluronidase. Hyaluronidase acts upon hyaluronic acid, a chemical substance that holds together the epithelial cells of the corona radiata. As a result of the action of the hyaluronidase, the epithelial cells fall away from the ovum. This exposes an area of the plasma membrane for sperm penetration. Figure 20-3 illustrates the route of the ovum and the sperm.

True fertilization occurs when the sperm nucleus combines with the egg nucleus to form a fertilized egg cell, or zygote. The type of fertilization that occurs in humans is referred to as internal fertilization; fertilization takes place within the female's body.

Fertilization restores the full complement of 46 chromosomes possessed by every human cell, each parent contributing one chromosome to each of the 23 pairs.

Deoxyribonucleic acid (DNA) is found in the chromosomes. It contains the genetic code that is replicated and passed on to each cell as the zygote divides and redivides to form the embryo. The early process whereby the zygote repeatedly divides to form an early embryo is known as cleavage. After early cleavage, actual embryonic development occurs until the fetus is completely formed.

All of the inherited traits possessed by the offspring are established at the time of fertil-ization. This is a point to remember when working with parents. A young mother-to-be may hope that her baby will be a girl with curly hair, or a prospective father may insist that he wants a son. The health care provider can assure them that the sex, and physical characteristics such as eye color and curly hair, are determined at the time of fertilization. The sex chromosomes of the male parent determine the sex of the child but other characteristics are a combination of both parents.

FETAL DEVELOPMENT

If fertilization occurs, the zygote travels down the fallopian tube and is implanted in the endometrial wall of the uterus. The zygote rapidly grows into an embryo and then a fetus, see Figures 20-4 and 20-5.

DIFFERENTIATION OF REPRODUCTIVE ORGANS

Reproductive organs are the only organs in the human body which differ between the male and female and yet there is still a significant similarity. This likeness results from the fact that female and male organs develop from the same group of embryonic cells. For approximately

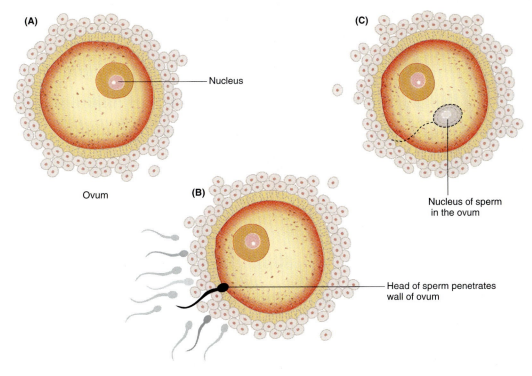

FIGURE 20-4 *Fertilization*

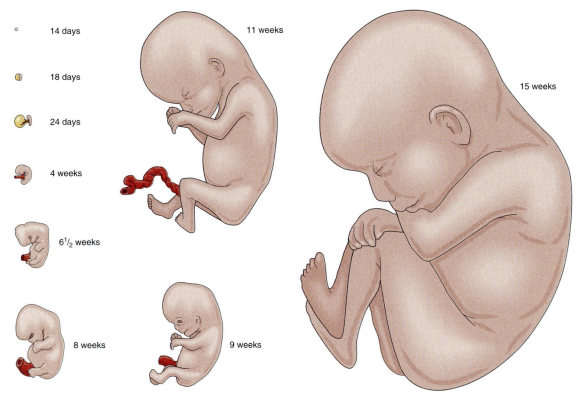

FIGURE 20-5 *Growth of an embryo into a fetus once fertilization has occured*

two months, the embryo develops without a sexual identity. Then the influence of the X or Y chromosome begins to make a difference.

The gonads (sexual organs) of the female begin to evolve at about the tenth or eleventh week of pregnancy. The ovaries of the female embryo develop from the same type of tissue as the testes of the male embryo. However, the testes evolve from the medulla of the gonad while the ovary develops from the cortex of the gonad. Figure 20-6 illustrates how the undiffer-

entiated external genitalia develop into fully differentiated structures. In the male, the tubercle becomes the **glans penis**, the folds become the **penile shaft**, and the swelling develops into the **scrotum**. In the female the tubercle becomes the **clitoris**, the folds the **labia minora**, and the swelling the **labia majora**. Internally there is also a differentiation from initially similar structures. The embryonic muellerian ducts degenerate and the wolffian ducts become the **epididymis**, **vas deferens**, and the **ejaculatory duct**

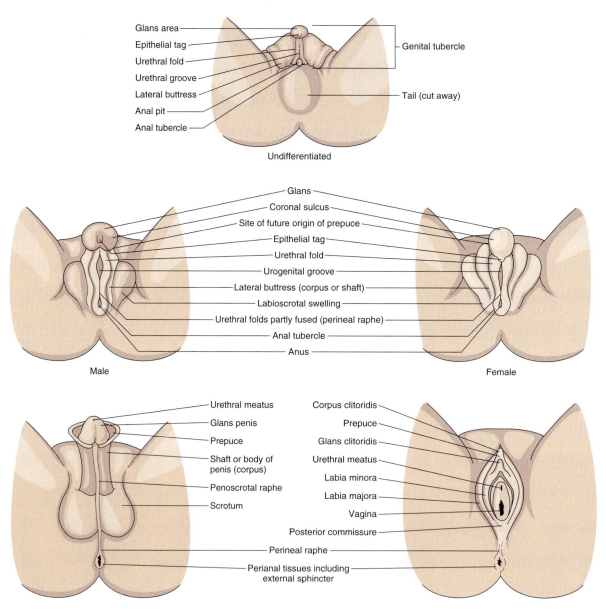

FIGURE 20-6 *Development of undifferentiated external genitalia into fully differentiated structures*

in the male. In the female, the wolffian ducts degenerate and the muellerian ducts develop into the **fallopian tubes**, the **uterus**, and the upper portion of the vagina. It is believed that the presence of the testes in the male is the differentiating factor in the development. Without the androgens (male hormones) from the testes, a female will develop. With the androgens, a male develops. Another substance called the muellerian inhibitor works in partnership with the androgen to produce the sex differentiation.

ORGANS OF REPRODUCTION

The function of the reproductive system is to provide for continuity of the species. In the human, the female reproductive system is composed of two ovaries, two fallopian tubes, the uterus, and the vagina. The male reproductive system is made up of two testes, seminal ducts, glands, and the penis. The principal male organs are located outside the body in contrast to the female organs which are largely located within the body.

FEMALE REPRODUCTIVE SYSTEM

Placement of the female reproductive organs in the pelvic cavity are shown in Figure 20-7. As shown in Figure 20-8, page 337, the female reproductive system consists of two ovaries, two fallopian tubes, the uterus, and the vagina. Accessory organs are the breasts.

Ovaries

The **ovaries** are the primary sex organs of the female. They are located on either side of the pelvis, lateral to the uterus, in the lower part of the abdominal cavity. Each ovary is about the shape and size of a large almond, measuring about 3 centimeters long and from 1.5 to 3 centimeters wide. An ovarian ligament, a short fibrous cord within the broad ligament, attaches each ovary to the upper lateral part of the uterus.

Ovaries perform two functions. They produce the female germ cells, or **ova**, and the

female sex hormones, **estrogen** and **progesterone**. Table 20-1 outlines the functions of the female sex hormones.

Each ovary contains thousands of microscopic hollow sacs called **graafian follicles** in varying stages of development. An ovum slowly develops inside each follicle. The process of development from an immature ova to a functional and mature ova inside the graafian follicle is called maturation. In addition, the graafian follicle produces the hormone estrogen.

Usually a single follicle matures every twenty-eight days through the reproductive years of a woman. The reproductive years begin at the time of **puberty** and the **menarche** (initial menstrual discharge of blood).

Occasionally two or more follicles may mature, releasing more than one ovum. As the follicle enlarges, it migrates to the outside surface of the ovary and breaks open, releasing the ovum from the ovary. This process is called **ovulation**; it occurs about two weeks before the menstrual period begins. The time of ovulation may vary depending on emotional and

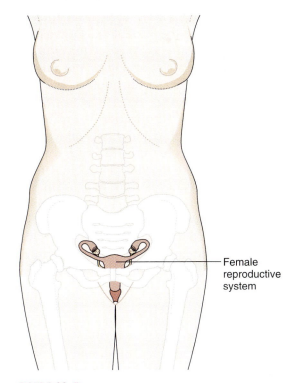

Female reproductive system

FIGURE 20-7 *Placement of the female reproductive system in the lower pelvic cavity*

TABLE 20-1 • *Functions of Estrogen and Progesterone*

HORMONE	FUNCTION
Estrogen	1. Affects the development of the fallopian tubes, ovaries, uterus, and the vagina. 2. Produces secondary sex characteristics: • broadening of the pelvis, making the outlet broad and oval to permit childbirth • the epiphysis (growth plate) becomes bone and growth ceases. • development of softer and smoother skin • development of pubic and axillary hair • deposits of fat in the breasts and development of the duct system • deposits of fat in the buttocks and thighs • sexual desire 3. Prepares the uterus for the fertilized egg.
Progesterone	1. Develops excretory portion of mammary glands. 2. Thickens the uterine lining so it can receive the developing embryo egg. 3. Decreases uterine contractions during pregnancy.

physical health, state of mind, and age. During a woman's reproductive years, she produces about 400 ova.

The ovum consists of cytoplasm and some yolk. This yolk is the initial food source for the growth of the early embryo. After ovulation, the ovum travels down one of the fallopian tubes, or oviducts. Fertilization of the ovum takes place only in the upper third of the oviduct. The time of fertilization is limited to a day or two following ovulation. Following fertilization, the zygote (fertilized egg) travels to the well-prepared uterus and implants itself in the wall of the endometrium (uterus lining).

The development of the follicle and release of the ovum occur under the influence of two hormones of the pituitary gland; the follicle-stimulating hormone (FSH) and the luteinizing hormone (LH). FSH also promotes the secretion of estrogen by the ovary.

Following ovulation the ruptured follicle enlarges, takes on a yellow fatty substance, and becomes the **corpus luteum** (yellow body). The corpus luteum secretes progesterone, which maintains the growth of the uterine lining. If the egg is not fertilized, the corpus luteum degenerates, progesterone production stops, and the thickened glandular endometrium sloughs off (see menstrual cycle).

Fallopian Tubes

The **fallopian tubes**, or **oviducts**, about 10 centimeters (4″) long, are not attached to the ovaries, see Figure 20-8. The outer end of each oviduct curves over the top edge of each ovary and opens into the abdominal cavity. This portion of the oviduct, nearest the ovary, is the infundibulum. Since the infundibulum is not attached directly to the ovary, it is possible for an ovum to accidentally slip into the abdominal cavity and be fertilized there. If the fertilized egg implants in the fallopian tube instead of the uterus it is called an **ectopic pregnancy**. An ectopic pregnancy can also occur outside the uterine cavity.

The area of the infundibulum over the ovary is surrounded by a number of fringelike folds called **fimbriae**. Each oviduct is lined with mucous membrane, smooth muscle, and ciliated epithelium. The combined action of the peristaltic contractions of the smooth muscles and the beating of the cilia helps to propel the ova down the oviduct into the uterus.

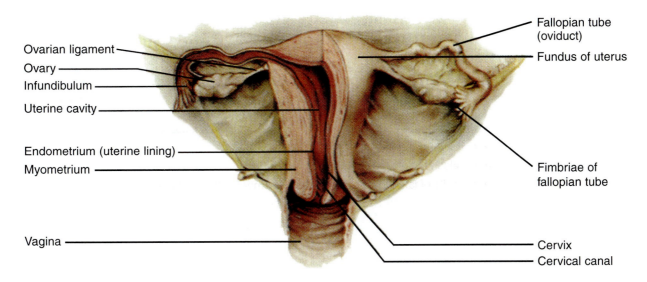

Ovarian ligament
Ovary
Infundibulum
Uterine cavity
Endometrium (uterine lining)
Myometrium
Vagina

Fallopian tube (oviduct)
Fundus of uterus
Fimbriae of fallopian tube
Cervix
Cervical canal

FIGURE 20-8 *Structures of the female reproductive system*

Conception (fertilization) takes place in the outer third of the fallopian tube.

Uterus

The **uterus** is a hollow, thick-walled, pear-shaped, and highly muscular organ. The non-gravid (non-pregnant) uterus measures about 7.5 centimeters in length, 5 cm wide, and 2.75 cm thick. This is about 3″ long, 2″ wide, and about 1″ thick. The uterus lies behind the urinary bladder and in front of the rectum. The uterine cavity is extremely small and narrow. During pregnancy, however, the uterine cavity greatly expands in order to accommodate the growing embryo and a large amount of fluid.

The uterus is divided into three parts: (1) the **fundus**, the bulging, rounded upper part above the entrance of the two oviducts into the uterus, (2) the body, or middle portion, and (3) the **cervix**, or cylindrical, lower narrow portion that extends into the vagina, see Figure 20-8. There is a short, cervical canal that extends from the lower uterine cavity (internal orifice, or os of the uterus) to the external os at the end of the cervix. The uterine wall is comprised of three layers:

1. the outer serous layer, or the visceral peritoneum

2. an extremely thick, smooth, muscular middle layer, the **myometrium**

3. an inner mucous layer, the **endometrium**

The endometrium, which lines the oviducts and the vagina, is also lined with ciliated epithelial cells, numerous uterine glands, and many capillaries.

During development of the embryo-fetus, the uterus gradually rises until the top part is high in the abdominal cavity, pushing on the diaphragm. This may cause the expectant mother some difficulty in breathing during the late stages of pregnancy.

Vagina

The **vagina** is the short canal which extends from the cervix of the uterus to the vulva. The vagina is composed of smooth muscle with a mucous membrane lining. This type of muscle tissue allows the vaginal canal to accommodate the penis during sexual intercourse; it also permits a baby to pass through the vaginal canal during the birthing process. A membrane called the **hymen** may be found at or near the entrance to the vagina. The hymen does have some openings which allow for the flow of blood during menstruation. During the first act of sexual intercourse, the openings in the hymen are enlarged and there may be slight bleeding. See Figures 20-9 and 20-10.

External Female Genitalia

The external female genitalia or vulva contains the external organs of the reproductive area, see Figure 20-10. The large pad of fat that is covered with coarse hair on the mature female and overlies the symphysis pubis is known as mons pubis. The area surrounding the openings of the urethra and vagina is called the vestibule. The urethra opening is superior to the vagina. Above the urethral opening is a small structure called the clitoris which contains many nerve endings. These receptors are stimulated during sexual intercourse.

The vagina is surrounded by folds of skin called the labia minora and the labia majora. At the entrance to the vagina are the Bartholin's glands which contain mucous.

The perineum is the area between the vaginal opening and the rectum. The perineal area is composed of muscles that form a sphincter for the vestibule. In childbirth, an incision called an episiotomy may be made from the vagina into perineal area to facilitate childbirth.

Breasts

The breasts are accessory organs to the female reproductive system, Figure 20-11. They are composed of numerous lobes arranged in a circular formation. Clusters of secreting cells surround tiny ducts. A single duct extends

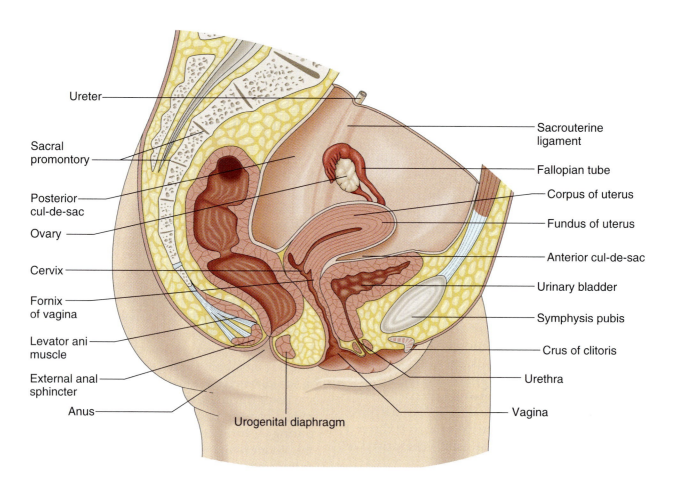

FIGURE 20-9 *Structures of the female reproductive system*

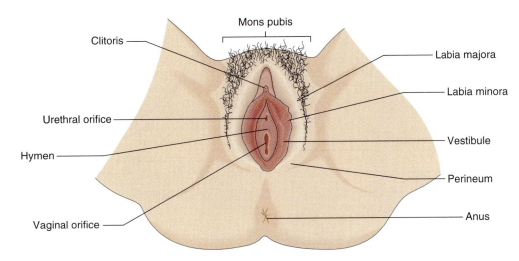

FIGURE 20-10 *External female genitalia*

from each lobe to an opening in the nipple. The areola, the darker area which surrounds the nipple, changes to a brownish color during pregnancy. Prolactin from the anterior lobe of the pituitary gland stimulates the mammary glands to secrete milk following childbirth.

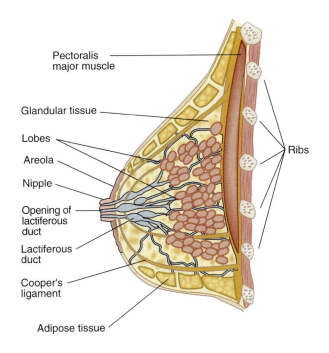

FIGURE 20-11 *Sagittal section of the female breast*

THE MENSTRUAL CYCLE

In the females, a mature egg develops and is ovulated from one of the two ovaries about once every twenty-eight days, through a complex series of action between the pituitary and the ovary. Before the mature egg is released from the ovary, a series of events occurs to thicken the uterine lining (endometrium). This is necessary to receive and hold a fertilized egg for embryonic development. If the egg is not fertilized, the endometrium starts to break down. Eventually the old unfertilized egg and the degenerated endometrium are discharged out of the female reproductive tract (menstruation). The cycle then starts all over again with the development of another ovum and the buildup of the endometrium.

This cycle is called the menstrual cycle. The menstrual cycle starts at puberty. It can start as early as nine years of age to as late as seventeen years of age. Generally, the age range is between twelve and fifteen. The changes that occur during the menstrual cycle involve hormones from the pituitary gland and the ovaries.

The menstrual cycle is divided into four stages: the follicle stage, the ovulation stage, the corpus luteum stage, and the menstruation stage. (See Figure 20-12 for a diagram of the menstrual cycle.)

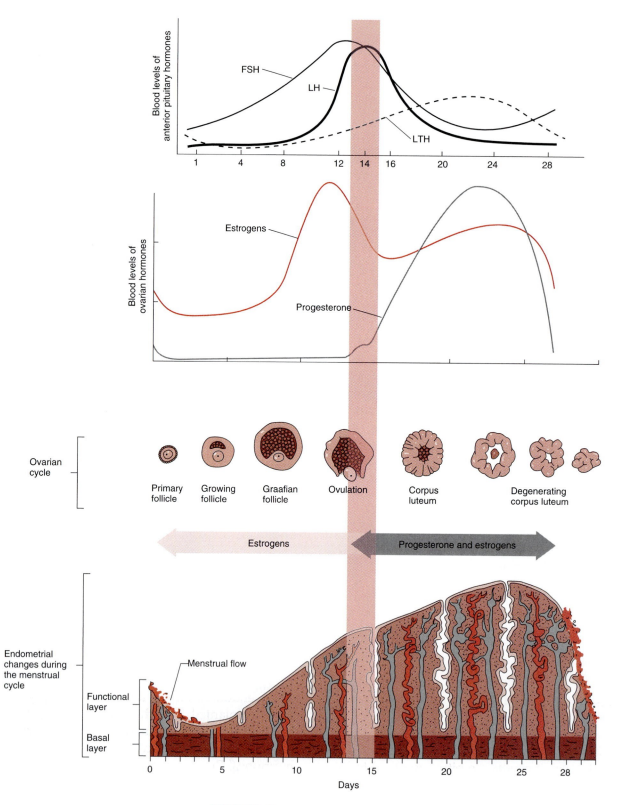

FIGURE 20-12 *The menstrual cycle*

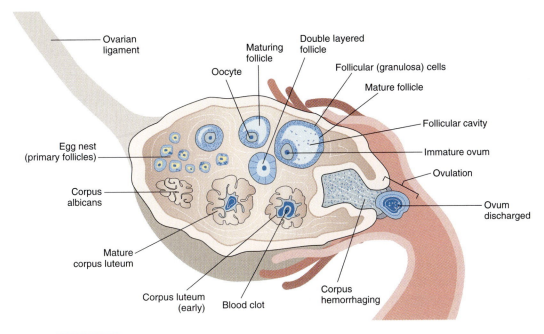

Ovarian ligament

Maturing follicle

Oocyte

Double layered follicle

Follicular (granulosa) cells

Mature follicle

Follicular cavity

Egg nest (primary follicles)

Immature ovum

Ovulation

Corpus albicans

Ovum discharged

Mature corpus luteum

Corpus luteum (early)

Blood clot

Corpus hemorrhaging

FIGURE 20-13 *An ovary showing the development of an ovum in a graafian follicle*

Stages of the Menstrual Cycle

Follicle Stage. Follicle-stimulating hormone (FSH) is secreted from the anterior lobe of the pituitary gland on day 5 of the menstrual cycle. FSH is then circulated to an ovary via the bloodstream. When FSH reaches an ovary, it will stimulate several follicles. However, only one matures. As the one follicle grows in size, an egg cell also begins to mature inside the follicle, Figure 20-13. As the follicle grows in size, it fills with a fluid containing estrogen. The estrogen stimulates the endometrium to thicken with mucous and a rich supply of blood vessels. These changes to the endometrium prepare the uterus for the implantation of an embryo. The follicle stage lasts about ten days.

Ovulation Stage. When the concentration of estrogen in the female bloodstream reaches a high level, it causes the pituitary gland to stop FSH secretion. As this occurs, the luteinizing hormone (LH) is secreted by the pituitary gland. At this point, there are three different

hormones circulating in the female bloodstream—estrogen, FSH, and LH. Each hormone is present in different concentrations. Around the fourteenth day of the menstrual cycle, this hormonal combination somehow stimulates the mature follicle to break. When the follicle ruptures, a mature egg cell is released into fallopian tube. This event is called ovulation.

Corpus Luteum Stage, or Luteal Phase. After ovulation, LH stimulates the cells of the ruptured follicle to divide quickly. This mass of reddish-yellow cells is called the corpus luteum. The corpus luteum, in turn, secrets a hormone called progesterone. Progesterone helps to maintain the continued growth and thickening of the endometrium, so if an embryo happens to be implanted into the uterine lining, the pregnancy can be maintained. That is why progesterone is often called the "pregnancy hormone." Progesterone also prevents the formation of new ovarian follicles by inhibiting the release of FSH. The corpus luteum stage lasts about fourteen days.

Menstruation Stage. If fertilization does not occur and an embryo is not implanted in the uterus, the progesterone reaches a level in the bloodstream that inhibits further LH secretion. With decreased LH secretion, the corpus luteum breaks down causing a decrease in progesterone secretion as well. As the progesterone level decreases, the lining of the endometrium becomes progressively thinner and eventually breaks down. The extra layers of the endometrium, the unfertilized egg, and a small quantity of blood that comes from the ruptured capillaries as the endometrium peels away from the uterus are discharged from the female's body through the vagina. This causes the characteristic menstrual blood flow, and the menstruation stage starts around the 28th day of the cycle. The menstruation stage lasts about four days. While menstruation is occurring, the estrogen level in the bloodstream is decreasing. The anterior lobe of the pituitary gland is now stimulated to secrete FSH, consequently a new follicle starts to grow and the menstrual cycle starts again.

The relationship between the pituitary gland hormones and the ovarian hormones is one of feedback. That means, pituitary hormones control the functioning of the ovaries; in turn, the ovaries secrete hormones that control pituitary functioning. This is another example of the automatic regulation of many of the body's processes.

MENOPAUSE

Menopause or "change in life" is the time in a female's life when the monthly menstrual cycle comes to an end. If frequently occurs between ages forty-five and fifty-five. Menopause signals the end of follicle growth and ovulation; consequently, it means the end of childbearing. However, a normal libido usually remains.

The menopausal female will experience the following anatomical changes:

1. Atrophy of the internal reproductive structures:
   - uterus
   - fallopian tubes
   - ovaries
2. Atrophy of the external genitalia
3. Vagina becomes conical shaped
4. Atrophy of the vaginal mucous membranes
5. Reduction of the secretory activity of the glands associated with the reproductive organs

These changes do not occur overnight, they happen gradually over a period of years. There are also pronounced physiological changes that occur. These are "hot flashes," dizziness, headaches, rheumatic pains in joints, sweating, and susceptibility to fatigue. Depending upon the menopausal female, sometimes these physiological changes are also accompanied by psychic changes. These include abnormal fears, depression, excessive irritability, and a tendency to worry. Many of these physiological and psychic symptoms can be alleviated by the careful administration of female hormones.

Menopause can be induced prematurely (artificial menopause) by either deactivation or removal of ovarian tissue.

MALE REPRODUCTIVE SYSTEM

The male reproductive organs, Figure 20-14, consist of the following structures:

1. The two testes produce the male gametes, **spermatozoa**, and the male sex hormone **testosterone**. They are suspended from the body wall by a spermatic cord and encased in a pouch called the scrotum.

2. A system of ducts carries the sperm cells out of the testes through the epididymis, two seminal ducts (ductus deferens or vas deferens), two ejaculatory ducts, and the urethra.

3. Accessory glands include the two seminal vesicles, two bulbourethral glands and a prostate gland. These glands add a viscous fluid to the sperm cells to form seminal fluid.

4. The penis is a copulatory structure that will transfer sperm cells to the female reproductive system.

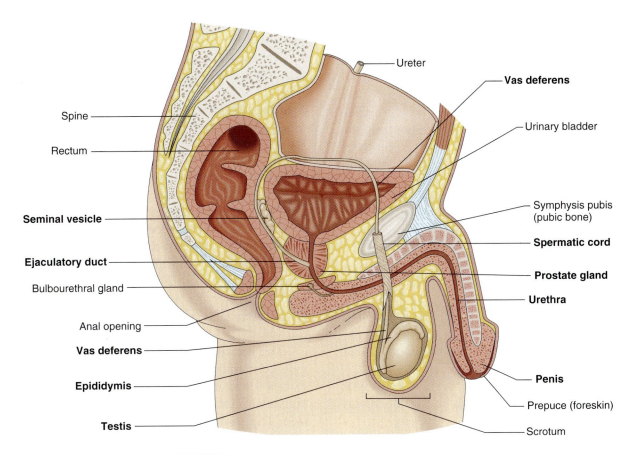

Ureter

Vas deferens

Spine

Urinary bladder

Rectum

Symphysis pubis
(pubic bone)

Seminal vesicle

Spermatic cord

Ejaculatory duct

Prostate gland

Bulbourethral gland

Urethra

Anal opening

Vas deferens

Penis

Epididymis

Prepuce (foreskin)

Testis

Scrotum

FIGURE 20-14 *Structures of the male reproductive system*

Testes and Epididymis

The two **testes** are the primary male reproductive organs, Figure 20-15. They are found in a pouch lying outside the male body called the scrotum. Each testis is about the size and shape of a small egg, approximately 4 centimeters long, 2.5 centimeters wide, and 2 centimers thick. The testes are attached to an overlying structure called the **epididymis**. A fibrous tissue called the tunica albuginea covers the testes and sends incomplete partitions into body of each testes. Each one of these partitions is called a lobule, and each testes contains 250 lobules.

Each testicular lobule contains one to four minute and highly convoluted (twisted) **seminiferous tubules**. FSH stimulates the production of sperm in the cells that line the tubules. As the sperm develop, they are released into the tubules. In males mature sperm formation

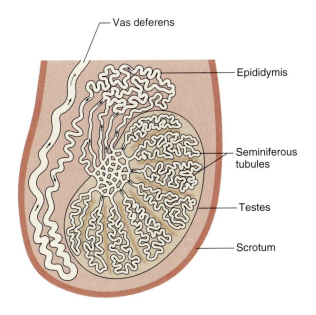

Vas deferens

Epididymis

Seminiferous
tubules

Testes

Scrotum

FIGURE 20-15 *Structures of the male reproductive system*

requires about seventy-four days. The function begins at about age twelve and the first mature sperm are ejaculated at about age fourteen. All of the seminiferous tubules intertwine and join together to form a small meshlike network of tubules called the rete testis. The rete testis unite to form the epididymis. The seminiferous tubules are supported by a type of tissue called interstitial tissue. The interstitial cells lining the interstitial tissue produce the male hormone testosterone. Testosterone is secreted in relatively steady amounts during the adult life of the male. Testosterone stimulates the growth and development of the male reproductive organs, underlies the sex drive, and is responsible for the secondary sex characteristics. These include the deepening of the voice, growth of hair (beard and body hair especially in the axillary and pubic area), increase in muscle mass, and thickening of the bones of the skeletal system.

The epididymides connect the testes with the ductus deferens and help in the final development of the sperm cells.

Descent of the Testes

In the embryo, the testes are formed and developed in the abdominal wall slightly below the kidneys. During the last three months of fetal development, the testes will migrate downward through the ventral abdominal wall into the scrotum. In its descent, each testis carries with it the ductus deferens, blood and lymphatic vessels, and autonomic nerve fibers. These structures and their fibrous tissue covering form the spermatic cord.

Occasionally, as in premature babies, the testes will not descend. If the testes do not descend, this condition is known as cryptorchidism. (If one testis does not descend, it is called unilateral cryptorchidism. For two testes, it is called bilateral cryptorchidism.) If the testes stay inside the abdomen after puberty, spermatogenesis will be affected. The increased body temperature will destroy any sperm cells. A simple surgical procedure done before puberty can correct this condition.

Scrotum

The scrotum is an external sac that contains the testes.

Ductus Deferens, Seminal Vesicles, and Ejaculatory Ducts

The right and left ductus deferens (vas deferens) are continuations of the epididymides. The ductus deferens has a dual function. It serves as a storage site for sperm cells and as the excretory duct of the testis. Each ductus runs from the epididymis up through the inguinal canal. It then runs downward and backward to the side of the urinary bladder. It then curves around the ureter and goes down to meet with the seminal vesicle duct on the posterior side of the bladder.

The seminal vesicles are two highly convoluted membranous tubes. A duct leads away from a seminal vesicle that joins to the ductus deferens to form the ejaculatory duct on either side. The seminal vesicles produce secretions which help to nourish and protect the sperm on its journey up the female reproductive system. At the precise moment of ejaculation, the seminal fluid is added to the sperm cells as they leave the ejaculatory ducts.

The ejaculatory ducts are short and very narrow. They begin where the ductus deferens and the seminal vesicle duct join. They then descend into the prostate gland to join with the urethra, into which they discharge their contents. See Figure 20-14.

Penis

A&P CHALLENGE

The external organs are the scrotum and the penis. Internally, the scrotum is divided into two sacs each containing a testis, epididymis, and lower part of the vas deferens. The penis contains erectile tissue that becomes enlarged and rigid during intercourse. Loose-fitting skin, called the foreskin or prepuce, cover the end of the penis. The foreskin can be removed in a simple operation known as circumcision.

Prostate Gland

The prostate gland is located in front of the rectum and just under the urinary bladder, and it surrounds the opening of the bladder leading into the urethra. It surrounds the beginning portion of the urethra that is called the prostatic urethra. The prostate gland is about the shape and size of a chestnut. It is covered by a dense fibrous capsule and contains glandular tissue surrounded by fibromuscular tissue that contracts during ejaculation. The contraction of the prostate gland closes off the prostatic urethra during ejaculation preventing the passage of urine through the urethra. This contraction of the muscular tissue also aids in the expulsion of semen during an ejaculation. The prostate gland secretes a thin, milk alkaline fluid that enhances sperm motility. It also gives semen its characteristic strong musky odor. Fluid in the ductus deferens is very acidic, and the female vaginal secretions are also quite acidic. Therefore, the alkaline prostatic fluid probably neutralizes the acidic semen and vaginal secretions. This enhances the viability and motility of the sperm cells.

Bulbourethral Glands

The bulbourethral glands, also known as Cowper's glands, are located on either side of the urethra below the prostate gland. They add an alkaline secretion to the semen that helps the sperm to live longer within the acid medium of the female reproductive tract.

Erection and Ejaculation

The urethra extends down the length of the penis, opening at the urinary meatus of the glans. The urethra serves two purposes: to empty urine from the bladder and to expel semen. Sexual intercourse becomes possible due to the columns of erectile tissue in the penis. When a male is sexually aroused, nerve impulses cause the erectile tissue to engorge with blood which makes the erectile increase in size and become firm. Blood entering the dilated arteries squeezes the veins against the penile structures prohibiting venous return.

Once stimulation of the glans results in maximum stimulation of the seminal vesicles, impulses are sent to the ejaculatory center and orgasm occurs. Orgasm is the result of muscular contractions from the vas deferens, ejaculatory ducs, and prostate glands. Secretions stored in these structures along with the sperm are forcibly expelled through the urethra after which the engorgement gradually subsides.

Impotence

Impotence is the inability to have or sustain an erection during intercourse. *Primary* impotence refers to the patient who has never had an erection. *Secondary* impotence refers to the patient who is currently impotent but has had intercourse in the past. Transient periods of impotence are not considered a dysfunction and probably occur in half the adult male population between the ages of forty and seventy; the incidence increases with age.

Impotence was thought to be 80% psychogenic until the mid-eighties. Doctors now know that the vast majority of cases involve organic causes, often multiple ones. Psychological factors such as anxiety and stress can also be causes of impotence.

The type of therapy chosen depends on the specific cause of the dysfunction. Treatment may be sexual therapy if the cause is thought to be related to psychological factors. At the present time, penile implants and injection therapy are being used to treat impotence. Many drug companies are in the process of clinical trials using oral medication to treat this worldwide problem.

CONTRACEPTION

Some religious and ethnic groups oppose birth control and this text does not ignore that issue. This subject matter is presented factually, from a clinical viewpoint, as information required for practice as a health care worker.

As the word implies, contraception is literally "against" conception. One choice in contraception is abstinence. Abstinence is the voluntary restraint of sexual intercourse. Abstinence is a positive, healthy choice many people make. Several reasons may be given to avoid pregnancy:

- Avoid health risks to the woman. A woman in poor health may not survive a pregnancy.

- Spacing pregnancies. Some women are very fertile and could conceive every year or less. The infant death rate is reported to be 50% higher at one-year intervals than at two or more years.

- Avoid having babies with birth defects. Some women have chromosome defects or are genetic disease carriers (or married to carriers) and choose not to risk pregnancy.

- Delay pregnancy early in marriage to allow a time for adjustment to avoid additional stress in the new relationship and establish a strong marriage.

- Limiting family size. It is sometimes a personal decision and other times a reality of limited resources.

- Avoid pregnancy among unmarried couples. Single parenthood is difficult.

- Curbing population growth. The concern over worldwide food supply and supportive environment prompts some to promote contraception.

Several methods to prevent conception and their relative percentage of effectiveness are listed in Table 20-2. Selection is usually made by the woman in consultation with her doctor. The cost, ease of use, degree of effectiveness, and likelihood of side effects, must be taken into consideration when selecting a method.

INFERTILITY

Infertility is when conception does not occur. Some causes of infertility may be damage to fallopian tubes, a low sperm count, hormonal imbalance, and other disorders. Recent medical advances have occurred in which a variety of different methods are used to increase fertility such as:

a) **Artificial insemination**—a procedure in which the semen is placed into the vaginal canal by means of canula and syringe, usually around the time of ovulation.

b) **In-vitro fertilization**—a procedure in which the female is given ovulation inducing drugs which stimulate the development of multiple ovarian follicles. A laparoscopy is done at a precise time to remove the ovarian follicles and extract the ova. The ova are then cultured in-vitro with the male's spermatozoa under careful laboratory conditions. If fertilization is successful, and when the zygote is at the four to eight cell stage, it is transferred to the uterus of the female.

ADVANCES IN MICROSURGERY FOR FEMALE INFERTILITY

Microsurgery is performed with the aid of magnification. The use of the operating microscope has produced better surgical results since it allows magnification from two to thirty fold. This procedure also allows the use of fine suture material and delicate handling.

Pelviscopy is a special type of operative laparoscopy in which extensive procedures are performed. This involves the use of magnification through lenses and frequently the use of a video camera which allows a surgical assistant to work with the surgeon. This procedure is used in the treatment of ectopic pregnancy, fibroids, ovarian cysts, tumors, endometriosis, and pelvic adhesions.

Gamete Intrafallopian Tube Transfer (GIFT)

In gamete intrafallopian transfer procedure the laparoscope is used to recover the eggs from the ovary, and to transfer the sperm and eggs back into the ends of the fallopian tube

TABLE 20-2 • *Different methods of preventing conception*

% EFFECTIVE	METHOD	DESCRIPTION/COMMENTS
100%	Abstinence	Refraining from sexual intercourse; absolutely most effective.
100%	Sterilization	Tubal/ligation (cutting of the fallopian tubes) in the female. The cut ends can be sewn back in opposite directions or cauterized. The surgical procedure is done through a laparoscope inserted into the abdomen. The procedure is considered permanent. A vasectomy in the male, with the ends being sewn in opposite directions. The surgery is performed through a small incision at the base of the scrotum. Vasectomies are usually not reversible; however, in some instances, reconstructive surgery has been successful, especially in cases of shorter duration; sperm production is usually significantly decreased in time. Usually a second marriage and the desire for another child prompt the attempt. The method is relatively expensive initially.
95%-99%	Birth control pills	Many different kinds are available. They are a combination of hormones that prevent ovulation; no ovum, therefore no pregnancy. Failure occurs when pills are not taken as prescribed. Side effects can be prohibitive for some women. Available only by prescription and requires regular visits to a physician. Cost is a factor to consider.
93%-99%	IUD	The intrauterine device is a small piece of plastic or coiled material inserted into the uterus to prevent implantation of a fertilized egg, presumably by providing irritation to the endometrium. Failure can occur if the device is expelled and during the first few months after being inserted. Initial insertion costs involved, and cost of removal. Side effects bother some women.
90%-99%	Diaphragm	A thin piece of dome-shaped rubber with a firm ring, which is inserted into the vagina to cover the cervix and provide a barrier to sperm. It is most effective when used in combination with a contraceptive cream placed into the dome before inserting. Failure usually results from improper insertion, a defect in the rubber, such as a hole, failure to insert before any penile penetration, or failure to maintain in place at least six hours following intercourse. Initial cost to examine and fit and purchase. No side effects. Requires cleaning and inspection after each use.
85%-97%	Condom	A thin sheath of rubber or latex that fits over an erect penis to catch the semen. A properly used condom is very effective. It must be unrolled onto an erect penis *before* any penetration occurs. It is important to leave about 1/2" of free air space at the tip (unless the condom is constructed with a tip) to catch the semen; otherwise, the force of the ejaculation may burst the condom. It must also remain in place throughout intercourse. After ejaculation has occurred, care must be taken to withdraw with the condom in place. It may require grasping with the fingers. This is the only contraceptive that also provides a level of protection against sexually transmitted diseases. It is relatively inexpensive, easy to use, and readily available. Remember, only a latex condom is also effective against the AIDS virus.
70%-75%	Spermicides	Contraceptive foams, jellies, and creams with *sperm-killing* ingredients, inserted by applicator, deep into the vagina before intercourse. It must remain for a least six to eight hours afterward. Each application is good for only one act of intercourse. They should not be relied on alone as an effective contraceptive. Combined with diaphragm or condom, they are effective. Few side effects (some report allergic reactions), easily used, and readily available. Must not be confused with lubricants such as K-Y or Lubafax, which contain NO spermicide.
?%	Douching	Absolutely not reliable. It only takes a couple of minutes for sperm to enter the cervix. In all reality, douching cannot be accomplished quickly enough. In fact, it may even assist sperm towards the cervix.
70%-80%	Withdrawal	This method has been practiced since ancient times. It simply requires that the penis be withdrawn and ejaculation occur outside the vagina. It is not very effective because some sperm are deposited in the vagina before ejaculation occurs. In addition, the man may not be able to withdraw in time. It requires a lot of concentration to control. It is also not advised because it may lead to a sexual dysfunction if practiced for a prolonged period of time.
65%-85%	Rhythm	Is the practice of abstinence during an eight-day period from day ten to seventeen of the menstrual cycle when conception is theoretically possible. The method works fairly well for women who are extremely regular in their cycles and couples who can practice strong self-control. However, it requires a careful assessment of at least six months of cycles to establish ovulation days. If cycles vary in length, the period of abstinence must be increased to cover the longest possible period of time.

after fertilization. In one of the newer areas of in-vitro fertilization, tubal embryo transfer, the laparoscope is used to place the embryo into the ends of the tubes with excellent pregnancy rates.

DISORDERS OF THE REPRODUCTIVE SYSTEM

Female Reproductive Disorders

Amenorrhea is a term used to define absence of the menstrual cycle. This is normal if the female is pregnant. Psychological factors, anorexia, and hormonal imbalance are other causes of this condition.

PMS or **Pre-menstrual syndrome** is a group of symptoms which are exhibited just prior to the menstrual cycle, caused by water retention in the body tissue. Irritability, nervousness, mood swings, and weight gain are some of the symptoms which are seen. PMS is no longer considered just a myth and is treated with medication and diet to reduce water retention.

Dysmenorrhea is a term used to describe painful menstruation. Dysmenorrhea is characterized by cramps, which may be caused by excessive production of an inflammatory substance such as prostaglandin. Aspirin-like substances which block the action of prostaglandin are helpful.

Endometriosis, a word that comes from endometrium, is a disease which affects women during their reproductive years. In this condition, endometrial tissue is found outside the uterus. It is found around the ovaries and other organs in the abdomino-pelvic cavity.

Every month, like the lining of the uterus, the tissue responds to hormonal changes. The tissue gets bigger, breaks down, and causes bleeding. Endometrial tissue outside the uterus allows no way for the blood to leave the body. The result is internal bleeding, inflammation of the surrounding areas, and formation of scar tissue. This condition causes pain before and during menstruation, during or after sexual activity, infertility, and heavy or irregular bleeding. The cause is unknown, but different theo-

MEDICAL HIGHLIGHT: TECHNOLOGY

Fertility Tests

Routine fertility tests may include the following:

- Transvaginal ultrasound is able to detect ovulation and the release of ova. This procedure is also able to assess the thickness of the endometrium.

- Lab tests for semen testing.

- Cervical mucous tests to see that sperm can penetrate and survive in the cervical mucous.

- Hormone tests to measure the levels of LH, FSH, Estradiol, and progesterone. In addi-

tion, other tests may include TSH, free testosterone, and prolactin hormone levels.

- Hysterosalpinogram is an x-ray procedure in which a radio-opaque dye is injected through the cervix into the uterus and fallopian tubes. The dye appears white on the x-ray and allows the radiologist to check for abnormalities.

- Hysteroscopy is when a fiber optic light is inserted through the cervix into the uterus to check for abnormalities.

- Laparoscopy may be done to check the reproductive organs.

ries exist. One theory is that during menstruation some of the tissue backs up through the fallopian tubes, implants in the abdomen, and grows. Some experts feel it is related to an autoimmune problem. Others suggest that endometrial is distributed from the uterus to other parts of the body through the lymph system.

Diagnosis is made by **laparoscopy**. Laparoscopy is a minor surgical procedure done under anesthesia in which the patient's abdomen is distended with carbon dioxide gas to make the organs easier to see. Then, a laparoscope (a tube with a light on it) is inserted through a tiny incision in the abdomen. By moving the instrument around the abdomen, the surgeon can check the condition of the organs and see the endometrial implants if they are present. The surgeon can also remove endometrial tissue through this method. In addition to laparoscopic surgery, another treatment is the use of hormonal drugs to stop ovulation and force endometriosis into remission during the time of treatment. Menopause generally ends the activity of mild or moderate endometriosis.

Fibroid tumors are usually benign growths which occur in the uterine wall. Fibroids may enlarge to cause pressure on other organs or may cause excessive bleeding. To treat fibroids, a **hysterectomy** (removal of the uterus) may be done.

Breast tumors are either benign or malignant. Benign tumors are usually fluid filled cysts which enlarge during the premenstrual cycle. Women are taught to do periodic breast examinations to detect any developing lumps. Breast examinations are done by palpating the breasts in a circular fashion. Any suspected lump should be reported to the doctor immediately.

Breast cancer or malignant tumor is the most common cancer in women. Early detection and treatment is vital to ones survival. Surgical treatment consists of a **lumpectomy** (removal of tumor only) or **mastectomy** (removal of the breast). Other types of treatments include radiation and chemotherapy (anti-cancer drugs). Benefits are associated with all types of treatment; the patient and physician select the most appropriate treatment. **Mammogram** is a special type of x-ray which can detect tumors of the breast before they can be palpated. This test is recommended on an annual basis for all women over the age of forty.

Endometrial cancer is the most common type of uterine cancer. It usually affects women after menopause. Women are instructed to immediately report to their physician any vaginal bleeding which occurs after menopause. Hysterectomy and irradiation are the usual types of treatment.

Ovarian cancer is a leading cause of cancer death in women. It usually occurs between the ages of forty and sixty-five. Early diagnosis is difficult and treatment is aggressive surgery to remove all reproductive organs.

Cervical cancer is frequently seen in women between the ages of thirty and fifty. The test to detect cancer of the cervix is called the **Pap smear** (**Papanicolaou**), where a sample of cell scrapings is taken from the cervix and cervical canal for microscopic study. Once a female is sexually active, this test should be done on an annual basis. Early detection and treatment are vital to the prognosis of the disease.

Infections of Female Reproductive Organs

Pelvic Inflammatory Disease (**PID**) may be due to infections which occur in the reproductive organs and spread to the fallopian tubes and peritoneal cavity. This disease may also be secondary to another infection such as gonorrhea. The inflammation causes pain, high temperature, and possible scarring of the fallopian tubes. Treatment consists of medications such as antibiotics and analgesics.

Salpingitis is an inflammation of the fallopian tubes which may result in permanent damage.

Toxic shock syndrome is a bacterial infection caused by a staphylococcus organism. Symptoms are fever, rash, and hypotension which may result in shock. The patient is treated with antibiotics.

Vaginal yeast infections are generally caused by an organism called *candida albincans*.

This fungus is part of the body's natural organisms. A problem arises when the environment of the vagina is altered. A yeast infection develops when the vagina becomes less acidic. This change results in an overgrowth of candida organisms, causing an infection.

Symptoms include itching, burning, and redness in the vagina and vulva. There may also be an odorless, thick, white discharge (leukorrhea) resembling cottage cheese. Treatment with an antibiotic (for another illness) which alters the normal bacteria of the vagina may cause a yeast infection to occur. Yeast infections are more common in people with diabetes, pregnant women, and those with other causes of hormonal changes. Treatment is the use of a fungicidal agent that destroys the organism. This may be used as a vaginal cream or vaginal insert.

Male Reproductive Disorders

Epididymitis is a painful swelling in the groin and scrotum due to infection of the epididymis. This is treated with antibiotic therapy.

Orchitis is an inflammation of the testes. It may be a complication of mumps, flu, or another infection. Symptoms are swelling of the scrotum, fever, and pain. This disease is treated with antibiotic therapy, pain relievers, and cold compresses.

Prostatitis is an infection of the prostate gland. The prostate gland lies below the urinary bladder and the prostatic urethra passes through the gland. Urinary symptoms are often the first indication there is a prostatic problem. The patient will complain of difficulty in urination. Treatment with antibiotic is effective.

Benign prostatic hypertrophy (**BPH**) indicates an enlarged prostate. The prostate gland continues to grow during most of a man's life; the enlargement usually does not cause problems until late in life. More than half of men in their sixties and as many as 90% in their seventies have some symptoms of BPH. As the prostate enlarges, the capsule around the prostate does not, which causes the prostate to press up against the urethra like a clamp

around a tube. The bladder becomes thick and irritable. Then the bladder begins to contract even when it contains only small amounts of urine, causing frequent urination. As the bladder weakens it loses the ability to empty itself and urine remains in the bladder. The narrowing of the urethra may cause retention of urine and an infection may occur.

Diagnosis is made by rectal exam, ultrasound, and *cystoscopy*. A cystoscopy is a flexible tube with lens and a light system which is inserted into the urethra. This enables the physician to see the inside of the urethra and the bladder.

Treatment may depend on the extent of the symptoms. At the present time a prostatectomy is the usual treatment.

Prostate cancer is the most common cancer in males over the age of fifty. Males over the age of forty should start to have annual rectal examinations which can detect enlargement of the prostate. A Prostate Specific Antigen Blood Screening Test detects an abnormal substance released by cancer cells. Symptoms include frequency of urination, dysuria (painful urination), urgency, nocturia (night voiding), and in some cases hematuria (blood in the urine). The most common treatment is a **prostatectomy** (removal of the prostate gland). This procedure is called a transurethral resection of the prostate (TURP). An instrument is inserted into the penis and resects or cuts away the prostate gland which is then removed through the penis. There is no abdominal incision made and recovery time is short.

SEXUALLY TRANSMITTED DISEASE

Sexually transmitted diseases (STD's) also known as venereal diseases, are transmitted through the exchange of body fluids such as semen, vaginal fluid, and blood. STD's can be serious, painful, and cause long term complications including sterility, chronic infection, scarring of the fallopian tubes, ectopic pregnancy, cancer, and death. The most common of these diseases are *chlamydia*, *genital herpes*, and *genital warts*.

MEDICAL HIGHLIGHT: TECHNOLOGY

Treatment for Cancer

Benign Prostatic Hypertrophy

A number of recent studies have questioned the need for early treatment for benign prostatic hypertrophy (BPH) when the prostate gland is just mildly enlarged. These studies report that early treatment may not be needed because the symptoms of BPH clear up without any treatment in as many as one-third of all mild cases. Instead of immediate treatment the study suggests regular checkups to watch for early problems. If the condition poses a threat to the health or is a major inconvenience, treatment is then recommended.

Some researchers are exploring the use of laser surgery to vaporize obstructing prostate tissue. Early studies suggest that this method may be as effective as conventional surgery.

Prostate Cancer

Since the advent of the Prostate Screening Antigen Blood Test to detect prostate cancer, there has been an increase in the number of people with positive results. This has led to more discussion on the type of treatment. In some patients the antigen level did not rise over a period of time; therefore, the question remains as to whether surgical removal should be done immediately or a "wait and see" period should occur.

The best therapy should be determined by the physician and then decided based on the individual circumstance of each case. In some cases surgery is the best choice. However, radiation also has been effective in reducing the tumor. Radiation is performed on an outpatient basis and given daily over a period of six to seven weeks. In cases where there has been extensive spread of the cancer, hormonal therapy is the method of treatment.

Hormonal therapy works by depriving the tumor cells of testosterone used for the maintenance and growth of the malignant cells. The treatment puts the cancer in remission and relieves pain.

NOTE: Early detection is still the key to fighting prostate cancer.

Some of these diseases have no symptoms. Several of the more common symptoms include:

- In females, an unusual discharge from the vagina, pain in the pelvic area, burning or itching around the vagina, unusual bleeding, and vaginal pain during intercourse.

- In males, a discharge from the penis.

- In both females and males, sores or blisters near the mouth or genitalia, burning and pain during urination or a bowel movement, flu-like symptoms, and swelling in the groin area.

The patient who is at a physician's office or a health care center to be checked for an STD may feel some embarrassment. It is critical that the health care worker treat the person in a non-judgmental manner since every day that the disease is untreated it causes more severe health problems. Some STD's are diagnosed by physical examination while others require blood or other laboratory tests. For bacterial diseases such as gonorrhea, chlamydia, and syphilis, treatment is with antibiotics. Viral infections usually cannot be cured but the symptoms can be relieved.

Protection from STD's includes abstinence and practicing safe sexual behavior. Abstinence is the voluntary refraining from sexual activity. Abstinence is a positive, healthy choice many people make. Safe sex means using condoms and looking for any signs of venereal disease *before* sexual activity occurs. Once a person is aware of the disease, he or she must notify their sexual partner(s) so he or she can also be checked for the disease. It is often necessary for previous sexual partners to also be notified. All sexually transmitted diseases need to be treated. A high incidence of STD is leading to an increase in sterility in young females.

Chlamydia is caused by the Chlamydia Trachomatous organism and is the most common curable sexually transmitted disease in the United States. It is the major cause of nongonococcal urethritis, bacterial vaginitis, and pelvic inflammatory disease. Up to 80% women and 25% of men have no symptoms. If symptoms do occur they are the usual symptoms of STD's. A screening test called a DNA probe assay may be done for this disease. The test examines secretion from the cervix, urethra, or rectum. Treatment is with antibiotics; however, immunity does not develop after being infected.

Genital warts, or human papillomavirus, is another commonly sexually transmitted disease. The wart can appear on the shaft of the penis or on the vagina. It is usually asymptomatic. In many cases the warts are not visible to the naked eye. In other cases they look like small, hard, round spots resembling a cauliflower. Although genital warts are usually painless, they become sore, itchy, and may burn if hit, rubbed, irritated, or ignored for a longer period of time. Diagnosis is made primarily by examination. To find very small warts the genital area may be examined with a magnifying instrument. Treatment involves the use of an acid to destroy wart tissue or *cryosurgery*. This procedure uses liquid nitrogen which is placed on the wart and a small area of the surrounding skin. The liquid nitrogen freezes the skin causing ice crystals which results in the sloughing off of the wart.

Gonorrhea is a bacterial infection caused by Neisseria gonorrhea. This condition is a sexually transmitted disease (STD). The symptoms in the male may be painful urination and the discharge of pus from the penis. In the female, the early stages of the disease may be asymptomatic (no symptoms). This disease is treated with antibiotic therapy. There is a problem with some strains of the organism which have become resistant to the usual treatment.

Complications may occur if the inflammation spreads to the epididymis of the male or the fallopian tube of the female. The tubes may become scarred and blocked, which will result in sterility. In addition, if a pregnant woman contracts the disease and it is untreated, her baby may be born with gonorrheal eye infection.

Genital herpes is a viral infection that is sexually transmitted. The herpes lesion may cause a burning sensation and small blister-like areas may appear in the genitalia. Other symptoms may be painful irritation and discomfort while sitting or standing. Herpes symptoms may simply disappear after two weeks, however the symptoms will continue to reappear throughout the lifetime of the individual. Females who are diagnosed with herpes must consult with their physician whether or not to have a Cesarean section to prevent herpes infection of the newborn during childbirth.

Syphilis is a bacterial sexually transmitted disease. This disease prevalent at one time, is once again on the increase in association with the AIDS epidemic.

This disease exists in four stages. In the first stage, a sore (chancre) appears at the site of infection. A chancre will heal whether or not a person gets treatment. The second stage occurs six to twelve weeks after the initial infection. Symptoms include discolored spots or patches on the hands and the soles of the feet, moist, raised or elevated skin lesions, mucous patches in the mouth, throat and cervix, rash over the body, and flu-like symptoms. The discolored spots disappear with or without treatment. In the early stage, there are no symptoms. In the tertiary stage or final stage, which occurs ten to forty years after the first stage, tissue and liver damage occur which may cause heart disease, brain damage, paralysis, and death. Syphilis is diagnosed by recognition of the signs and symptoms, examination of the lesion under a microscope, and a blood test. Syphilis is treated with penicillin or another antibiotic.

● REVIEW QUESTIONS

Select the letter of choice that best completes the statement.

1. One of the male hormones is:
   a. progesterone
   b. luteinizing hormone
   c. follicle-stimulating hormone
   d. testosterone

2. Ovulation usually occurs:
   a. the day before the menstrual period begins
   b. one week before the menstrual period begins
   c. three weeks before the menstrual period begins
   d. two weeks before the menstrual period begins

3. The ovaries contain:
   a. thirty graafian follicles
   b. thousands of graafian follicles
   c. hundreds of graafian follicles
   d. six graafian follicles

4. The development of the follicle and release of the ovum are under the influence of:
   a. the follicle-stimulating hormone and the luteinizing hormone
   b. estrogen and corpus luteum
   c. progesterone and the follicle-stimulating hormone
   d. estrogen and the luteinizing hormone

5. Which one of the following statements is *not* correct?
   a. The fallopian tubes are about four inches long.
   b. The fallopian tubes serve as ducts for the ovum on its way to the uterus.
   c. The fallopian tubes are also called oviducts.
   d. The fallopian tubes are attached to the ovaries.

● MATCHING

Match each term in Column I with its correct description in Column II.

Column I	Column II
_____ 1. scrotum	a. secondary sex characteristics
_____ 2. testosterone	b. external sac which holds the testes
_____ 3. facial and pubic hair	c. excreted from the pituitary gland
_____ 4. epididymis and penis	d. formed in the seminiferous tubules
_____ 5. spermatozoa	e. male gamete
	f. secondary reproductive organs
	g. male hormone produced in the testes

● COMPLETION

Fill in the blanks.

1. Painful or difficulty in menstruation is known as _____.

2. Amenorrhea is normal when a person is _____.

3. Gonorrhea is a sexually transmitted disease. The male complains of _____ and the female complains of _____.

4. The test done to detect breast tumors is called _____.

5. Sterility results from inflammation of the fallopian tube which can be caused by _____ and _____.

6. A group of symptoms which occur before the menstrual cycle is called _____.

7. The onset of ovulation is known as _____ and the cessation of ovulation is known as _____.

8. A sexually transmitted disease which has small blister-like areas is known as _____.

9. An enlarged prostate may cause problems with _____.

10. The best methods of preventing sexually transmitted diseases are _____ and _____.

● LABELING

Label the structures of the male reproductive system on the following diagram.

1. _____
2. _____
3. _____
4. _____
5. _____
6. _____
7. _____
8. _____
9. _____
10. _____
11. _____
12. _____
13. _____
14. _____
15. _____
16. _____
17. _____
18. _____
19. _____
20. _____
21. _____
22. _____

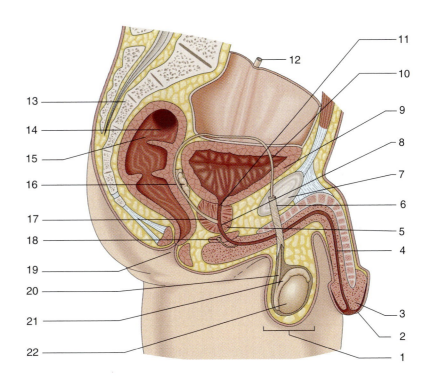

● APPLYING THEORY TO PRACTICE

1. A young pregnant woman comes into the doctor's office and states, "I told my husband I will give him a son, because in my family I was the only girl and I have four brothers." Is this a valid statement? Explain to the expectant mother how the sex of the newborn is determined.

2. If a person has a sperm count of 16 million, he would be considered sterile. Fertilization only requires the union of one egg and one sperm; why then are so many sperm necessary for fertilization to occur?

3. You are asked to describe the fertilization process. Explain how the sperm travels from the testes and arrives at the fallopian tube in time to meet the ova.

4. You are invited to a middle school to address eleven to fourteen year old adolescents and discuss puberty. Plan a program to describe how females are affected by estrogen and progesterone and how males are affected by testosterone.

5. A fifty year old female patient tells you it has gotten very hot in the waiting room and requests that you put on the air conditioner. The temperature outdoors is 30°F. She further states that the doctor told her about changes which usually occur at mid-life. Explain to the patient the physiological and psychological changes which are attributed to menopause.

CHAPTER

21

Genetics and Genetically Linked Diseases

OBJECTIVES

- ● Define mutation
- ● Differentiate between the two basic types of mutations
- ● Name three human genetic disorders and describe the cause and symptoms of each
- ● Explain genetic counseling
- ● Define the key words that relate to this chapter

KEY WORDS

amniocentesis
chorionic villi sampling
chromosomal mutation
chromosome
congenital disorder
cystic fibrosis
Duchenne's muscular dystrophy
gene
gene mutation

genetic counseling
genetic disorder
genetics
hemophilia
Huntington's Disease
interferon
lethal gene
mutagenic agent
mutation
phenylketonuria (PKU)

recombinant DNA
sickle-cell anemia
somatic cell mutation
Tay-Sachs Disease
Thalassemia (Cooley's anemia)
trisomy 21 or Down's Syndrome (Mongoloidism)

GENETICS

In sexual reproduction, a new individual is created from the union of the sperm cell and the egg cell. This process is called fertilization. Contained in the nucleus of each gamete are structures called **chromosomes**. The chromosomes contain DNA (deoxyribonucleic acid), the hereditary material referred to in Chapter 2. The DNA is packaged in small functional units found along the length of a chromosome, called **genes**. A gene is an area of DNA which carries information for the cellular synthesis of a specific protein. These genes are transmitted to the zygote, and will then control the development and characteristics of the embryo as it grows and matures. Eventually, due to the combined influence of all of the genes on all of the chromosomes, a new individual is formed. The new individual possesses all the necessary characteristics or traits needed for survival. Additionally, because the genes come from two parents, the offspring resemble both parents in some ways. However, it is also different from each parent. It has, for instance, all the characteristics of its species. Concurrently, it possesses its own unique traits that set it apart from all other members of its species.

Genetics is the branch of biology that studies how the genes are transmitted from parents to offspring. Occasionally, a gene or chromosome is changed, or mutated, in a gamete, and this mutated gene or chromosome is inherited by the offspring. The inheritance of such a mutated gene or chromosome will cause the appearance of a new and different trait, called a **mutation**. Sometimes the mutation is beneficial or harmless to an organism. Unfortunately, most inherited mutations are not beneficial. Still, it must be emphasized, that mutations in the genetic material are responsible for biological evolution on this planet.

TYPES OF MUTATIONS

There are two types of mutations. One type is called a **gene mutation**. When this mutation occurs, a new or altered gene is produced to replace a normal pre-existing gene. The other type is a **chromosomal mutation**. This mutation involves a change in the number of chromosomes found in the nucleus or a change in the structure of a whole chromosome.

Somatic Cell Mutation

Gene mutations occur occasionally at random in all cells of the human body. For instance, skin cells often undergo mutation as an individual ages. Mutations that occur in individual body (somatic) cells will not be transmitted to the offspring. This specific type of mutation is called a **somatic cell mutation**. A somatic cell mutation is not likely to affect other cells or the function of the organism as a whole. As an example, a single cell may lose the ability to make a certain protein and die without having an impact on the total organism.

Gametic Cell Mutation

Mutations that occur in the nucleus of the gametes (sperm and egg cell) will be passed on to the next generation. If either a gene or chromosomal mutation is present in a gamete at the moment of fertilization, all the cells of the embryo and the developed organism will have the mutation in at least half of their DNA.

LETHAL GENES

On the whole, inherited mutations are generally negative happenings to the individual. At times, they might even result in the formation of lethal genes. A **lethal gene** is a gene that results in death.

The time at which lethal genes exert their deadly influence varies. Some genes interfere with mitosis of the zygote and life ends before the zygote divides. Some lethal genes interfere with implantation of the fertilized egg in the uterus. Death would occur so early that a woman would never know that conception had even occurred. A lethal gene that prevents normal formation of the heart or normal blood production causes death at about three weeks after fertilization because this is the time when circulating blood becomes vital for continued existence. Others may kill at various times during development, depending on the time their products become vital for survival. Other lethal genes causing neonatal deaths involve abnormalities of the lungs and shifts in the circulatory system which must channel blood from the heart to the lungs instead of to the umbilical cord.

Some lethal genes do not exert their effects until later in life. Tay-Sachs Disease causes death several years after birth. Duchenne's muscular-dystrophy causes death in the teens and early childhood. Huntington's Disease usually brings about death at about forty to fifty years of age.

It is estimated that each person carries two or three different recessive lethal genes. Two similar recessive genes must be present in an individual in order for the gene to be expressed. Since there are so many kinds of lethal genes, one's chance of marrying someone with even one matching lethal is small. Statistically, should this happen, the lethal would be expressed in only one-fourth of the offspring.

When close relatives marry, the chance of the offspring inheriting two similar lethal genes increases. Persons with a common ancestry are more likely to share many genes than non-relatives. As a result, spontaneous abortions, still-births, neonatal deaths, and congenital deformities are higher among progeny of people sharing similar gene pools.

HUMAN GENETIC DISORDERS

Some diseases caused by gene mutations in humans are phenylketonuria (PKU), sickle-cell anemia, Tay-Sachs Disease, Duchenne's muscular dystrophy, Huntington's Disease, and cystic fibrosis.

It is important to note, there is a difference between genetic disorders and congenital disorders. A hereditary or **genetic disorder** is caused by a variation in the genetic pattern; a **congenital disorder** is something which evolves during fetal development and is not related to genetic malfunction.

Phenylketonuria

Phenylketonuria (**PKU**) is a human metabolic disorder caused by an enzyme deficiency. The individual with the trait cannot break down the amino acid phenylalanine and, consequently, there is a buildup of this substance in the body. Excess phenylalanine disrupts the normal development of the brain. If a child born with the defect eats proteins containing phenylalanine during childhood, mental retardation results. A newborn infant is tested for this defect, and, if the test is positive, a phenylalanine-restricted diet is prescribed. In most cases, this diet can be liberalized as the child grows older and brain development and maturation are completed.

Sickle-Cell Anemia

Sickle-cell anemia is a blood disorder common in individuals of African descent. It is caused by a gene mutation resulting in an abnormal hemoglobin molecule in a red blood cell. Refer to Figure 21-1. Especially in times of low oxygen availability, the shape of a red blood cell changes from that of a biconcave disc to a crescent shape. This is referred to as sickling. The sickle shape causes the cells to clump together, thus clogging small blood vessels and capillaries. Since a sickle cell has an abnormal hemoglobin (the pigment that combines with oxygen), it also carries less oxygen to the tissues, resulting in fatigue and listlessness. Breakage of these cells is also very common since their membranes are excessively fragile. See Figure 21-2 for tissue damage and physiological effects caused by sickle-cell anemia.

Tay-Sachs Disease

Tay-Sachs Disease is a genetic disorder caused by a mutation resulting in a deficiency of a lysosomal enzyme. The missing enzyme functions in breaking down lipid molecules in the brain. Without the enzyme, lipids accumulate in the brain cells and destroy them. This results in severe mental and motor deterioration leading to death several years after birth.

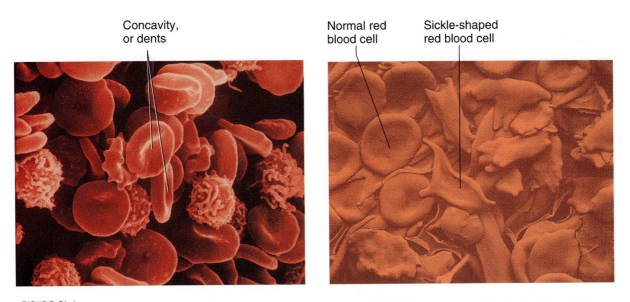

Concavity, or dents

Normal red blood cell

Sickle-shaped red blood cell

FIGURE 21-1 *(a) Normal red blood cells; seen from the side, normal RBC's have a concavity (or dent) on the two sides. (b) Sickle-shaped red blood cells (crescent-shaped).*

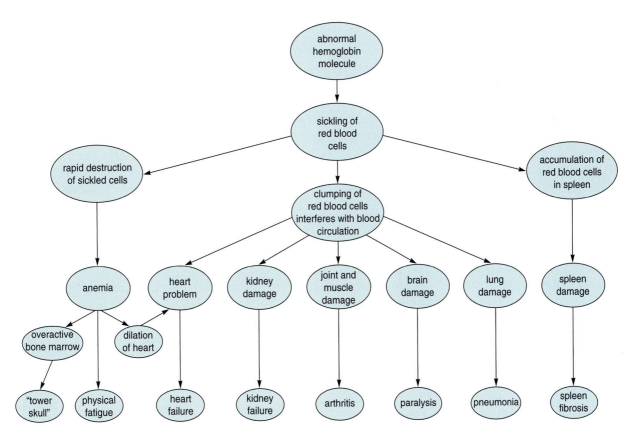

FIGURE 21-2 *A series of damages and effects caused by sickle-cell anemia*

This disorder is found most frequently among Jewish people or central European ancestry.

Huntington's Disease

Huntington's Disease is characterized by the degeneration of the central nervous system, which ultimately results in abnormal movements and mental deterioration. In this disorder, the product of an abnormal gene interferes with normal metabolism in nerve tissue.

Duchenne's Muscular Dystrophy

In Duchenne's muscular dystrophy, the muscles suffer a loss of protein and the contractile fibers are eventually replaced by fat and connective tissue, rendering skeletal muscle useless. As the weakening process of the disease continues, the teen or young adult is confined to a wheelchair. In many cases, the victim dies before the age of twenty from respiratory or heart failure.

Cystic Fibrosis

Cystic fibrosis is a disease of the exocrine gland. The lining of the digestive tract, the ducts of the pancreas, and the respiratory tract produce thick mucous which blocks the passageways. The blockage of the respiratory passages causes chronic bronchitis and pneumonia. Pulmonary therapy consists of a procedure called "cupping and clapping," which helps to dislodge the thick mucous from the respiratory tract. These treatments have helped to prolong the life span of patients with cystic fibrosis; however, only one half of the patients live to the age of twenty-five. Science has discovered the gene which transmits this disease and may soon be able to treat and prevent this illness. The involvement of the lungs is why this is one of the most fatal heriditary disorders.

Thalassemia

Thalassemia (Cooley's anemia) is a blood disease found among people of Mediterranean descent. Symptoms are the same as those associated with any anemia; there is also enlargement of the spleen and possible congestive heart disease. This disease is treated with blood transfusions to replace the defective hemoglobin molecules.

Hemophilia

Hemophilia is a sex-linked genetic disorder which means it is only transmitted on the X chromosome. In this disease the person is unable to produce the factor VIII which is necessary for blood clotting. Persistent bleeding may occur as a result of an injury or spontaneously. Treatment consists of giving the person factor VIII.

Chromosomal Aberrations

Some mutations are caused by chromosomal aberrations. Some involve entire chromosomes and others involve parts of chromosomes. During meiosis (the cell division occurring during the formation of the gametes) a pair of chromosomes may adhere to each other and not pull apart at metaphase. As a result of this nondisjunction, duplicate chromosomes go to one daughter cell and none of this type of chromosome to the other. Nondisjunction of certain chromosomes referred to as sex chromosomes causes various abnormalities of sexual development such as Turner's Syndrome in females and Klinefelter's Syndrome in males.

One of the most common chromosomal abnormalities involves an extra chromosome designated as chromosome 21. In fact, this disorder is referred to as trisomy 21 or Down's Syndrome (Mongoloidism). The risk of bearing a child with Down's Syndrome significantly increases with the age of the mother. Many physicians therefore recommend amniocentesis for all women who become pregnant after age thirty-five. Cells from the amniotic fluid will show trisomy 21 (as well as other chromosomal defects) if it is present. If a serious defect is detected prospective parents have the option of therapeutic abortion.

Mutagenic Agents

Although most gene or chromosomal mutations occur spontaneously, the rate or speed of mutations can be increased. This happens when a cell, a group of cells, or an entire organism is exposed to certain chemicals or radiations. Agents that speed up the occurrence of mutations are called **mutagenic agents**. Mutagenic agents can be radiations like cosmic rays, ultraviolet rays from the sun, x-rays, and radiation from radioactive elements. Some mutagenic chemicals are benzene, formaldehyde, phenol, and nitrous acid.

In recent times, the accelerated use of various chemical and physical agents with mutagenic properties has caused concern among some geneticists who fear possible significant alterations to genes and chromosomes that will be passed onto future generations. The increased use of ionizing radiation in medical diagnosis and the problem of the disposal of nuclear waste from reactors are examples. Certain chemical pollutants in the environment, such as herbicides and insecticides, are also suspect as causing genetic defects.

Since people are being exposed to more and more new substances, and since changes in genes are irreversible, caution should be the rule with regard to any unnecessary exposure to those suspected of being mutagens.

A&P CHALLENGE
GENETIC COUNSELING

Genetic counseling involves talking to parents or prospective parents about the possibility of genetic disorders. The counseling team usually is made up of members of the health care team, a genealogist, a nurse, laboratory personnel, and social service professionals. In genetic counseling a family history is obtained which is called a pedigree. Any and all facts which pertain to the parents or prospective parents and family members are considered. After careful analysis a genotype is determined; this analysis will be able to predict the possibility of a genetic disorder.

The prospective parents are made aware of what diagnostic tests are available during pregnancy which may indicate a problem. **Chorionic villi sampling** is a test which may be done as early as eight to ten weeks into the pregnancy. A sample of fetal cells is removed from the fetal side of the placenta and is examined. **Amniocentesis** is withdrawal of amniotic fluid during the 16th week of pregnancy. An examination of the fluid is able to pick up as many as 200 possible genetic disorders. Prior to performing an amniocentesis, a sonogram is done to determine where the fetal structures are located so as to prevent any problems.

Genetic counseling helps prospective parents make informed decisions regarding having children.

GENETIC ENGINEERING

Recent advances in the methods of gene transfer from the cell of one species to another offer exciting possibilities for the treatment of genetic deficiencies. Human insulin, human growth hormone, and human **interferons** (proteins that interfere with virus replication) are now being produced using the sophisticated technology of **recombinant DNA**. We can isolate a desired gene (to correct for a defective one) and grow millions of copies of it in the cells of bacteria and yeast which in turn produce the gene product on a commercial scale.

Some scientists even envision a time when we will have the ability to introduce copies of normal genes into humans whose genes are defective, thus alleviating a large segment of human suffering.

MEDICAL HIGHLIGHT: TECHNOLOGY AND ETHICS
Gene Therapy

Every day there are more scientific discoveries about genetic disorders. Scientists now know which genes cause muscular dystrophy, types of deafness, mental retardation, and cancer. Identifying these genes can be the first step toward treatment. Gene therapy could eventually free mankind from dozens of birth defects, diseases, and untold amounts of human suffering. People who may be especially interested in genetic counseling or testing include

- those who think they may have a birth defect or genetic disorder.
- women who are pregnant after age thirty-four.
- couples who have had one child born with a genetic defect.
- women who have had two or more miscarriages or whose babies died in infancy.

- couples who need information about genetic disorders that occur frequently in their ethnic group.
- couples who are first cousins or other blood relatives.

Gene therapy is a procedure that treats a disorder by replacing or counteracting a faulty gene. There are some trial studies being done which are producing promising results.

Many people are concerned about ethics and possible misuse of the therapy. The purpose of this treatment is to help with serious medical problems. All gene therapy trials in this country are strictly regulated by the federal government and national review panels.

Gene therapy may provide the answer to many health problems.

● REVIEW QUESTIONS

Select the letter of the choice that best completes the statement.

1. The branch of science that deals with how human traits are passed down is called:
   a. genetic engineering
   b. biology
   c. genetics
   d. genetic counseling

2. When a change takes place in a gene, what has occurred?
   a. a mutation
   b. lethal gene
   c. congenital defect
   d. mutant

3. A deficiency in breaking down fat molecules is characteristic of:
   a. sickle-cell
   b. Tay-Sach's
   c. PKU
   d. Down's Syndrome

4. An extra chromosome can cause a defect known as trisomy 21 or:
   a. Cooley's anemia
   b. Huntington's Disease
   c. Down's Syndrome
   d. PKU

5. A disease that produces thick mucous is called:
   a. PKU
   b. sickle-cell
   c. Huntington's Disease
   d. cystic fibrosis

● APPLYING THEORY TO PRACTICE

1. A young couple comes to the doctor's office and states that they have heard about genetic counseling. There is a family history of Tay-Sach's disease. Explain to them about genetic counseling and the probability of having a child with Tay-Sach's disease.

2. A friend tells you she has been advised to have an amniocentesis; she is 16 weeks pregnant. The thought of having someone stick a needle in her belly and what may happen to her baby is frightening. Explain the test to her.

3. PKU is a genetic disorder which can be detected in the nursery. Explain the disease and the special dietary restrictions.

4. Sickle-cell anemia trait can be diagnosed with a simple blood test. People are afraid to have this test done. List some of the factors which influence people's opinions regarding this test.

5. You are going to participate in a debate on the issue of genetic engineering. One side must present legal, scientific, and moral issues for the limited use of this science, while the other side will support unrestricted use of the technology.

GLOSSARY

abdomen (ab'-do-mun): portion of body lying between thorax and pelvis

abdominal hernia (ab-dom'-i-nul hur'-nee-uh): abnormal protrusion of an organ, or part of an organ, through abdominal wall

abdominopelvic (ab-do'-man-o pel'-vic): area below diaphragm, with no separation between the abdomen and pelvis

abduction (ab-duck'-shun): movement away from midline or axis of body

abscess (ab'-sess): pus-filled cavity

absolute zero (ab'-suh-lewt zee'-row): complete absence of heat or about –273.2°C (–459.8°F)

absorption (ub-sorp'-shun): passing of a substance into body fluids and tissues

accessory digestive organs (ack-sez'-uh-ree di-jes'-tiv or'-gunz): structures helping in mechanical digestion of food; glands producing secretion to assist chemical digestion in mouth, stomach, small intestine. Accessory organs include teeth, tongue, salivary glands, pancreas, liver, and gallbladder

acetabulum (as"-e-tab'-you-lum): a cup-shaped cavity in the innominate bone receiving the head of the femur

acetylcholine (as'-e-til-ko-len): chemical released when a nerve impulse is transmitted

Achilles tendon (ack-i'-leez ten'-dun): cord at rear of the heel

acid (as'-id): chemical compound that ionizes to form hydrogen ions (H+) in aqueous solution

acidosis (as"-i-do'-sis): disturbance in the acid-base balance from excess acid, or excessive loss of bicarbonate; depletion of alkaline reserve

acne (ak'-ne): chronic disorder of sebaceous gland

acquired immunity (a-kwir'-ed im-yu'-net-e): immunity as a result of exposure to a disease

acromegaly (ak'-ro-meg'a-le): excess of growth hormone in adults, overdevelopment of bones of hand, face, feet.

action potential (ak'-shan po-ten'-shal): the electric change occurring across the membrane of a nerve or muscle cell during transmission of a nerve impulse

active acquired immunity (ack'-tiv a-kwir'-ed im-yu'-net-e): two types natural and artificial acquired immunity

active transport (ack'-tiv tranz'-port): process by which solute molecules are transported across a membrane against a concentration gradient, from an area of low concentration to one of high concentration

Addison's disease (Ad'-e-sen di-zez): hypofunction of adrenal gland

adduction (a-duck'-shun): movement of part of body or limb toward the midline of body; opposite of abduction

adenitis (ad'-n-i'-tis): inflammation of a lymph gland

adrenal gland (a-dre'-nal gland): endocrine gland that sits on top of kidney; consists of cortex and medulla

adenoids (ad'-e-noydz): pair of glands composed of lymphoid tissue, found in nasopharynx; also called *pharyngeal tonsils*

adenosine triphosphate (ATP) (a-den'-o-seen try-fos'-fate): chemical compound consisting of one molecule of adenine, one of ribose, three of phosphoric acid

adipose (ad'-i-pose): fatty or fat-like

afferent arteriole (af'-ur-unt ahr-teer'-ee-ole): takes blood from the renal artery to the Bowman's capsule of kidney

afferent nerve (af'-ur-unt nurv): a nerve that carries nerve impulses from the periphery to the central nervous system; also known as *sensory nerve*

agglutinin (a-gloo'-ti-nin): antibody found in normal or immune serum, causing antigen and cellular clumping

agglutinogen (a-gloo'-tin-o-jen): chemical substance (antigen) which stimulates the formation of a specific agglutinin

agranulocyte (ay-gran'-yoo-lo-site): nongranular, white blood cell; known as *agranular leukocyte*

albinism (al'-bi-nizm): partial or total absence of melanin pigment from eyes, hair, and skin

albumin (al-bew'-min): plasma protein, maintains osmotic pressure

albuminuria (al-bew'-mi-new'-ree-uh): excess of albumin protein in urine

aldosterone (al-dos'-ta-ron'): hormone secreted by adrenal cortex, regulates salt and water balance in the kidney

alimentary canal (al''-i-men'-tuh-ree kuh-nal'): entire digestive tube from mouth (ingestion) to anus (excretion)

alkali (al'-kuh-li'): a substance when dissolved in water ionizes into negatively charged hydroxide(OH) ions and positively charged ions of a metal

alkalosis (al''-kuh-lo'-sis): excessive alkali; disturbance in acid-base balance from excess loss of acid

allergen (al'-er-jen'): substance causes an allergic reaction

alopecia (al'-e-pe'-she): loss of hair, baldness

alveoli (al-vee'-o-li): air cells found in the lung

Alzheimer's disease (alts'-hi'-merz di-zez): progressive disease with degeneration of nerve endings in the cortex of the brain

amenorrhea (a-men''-o-ree'-uh): absence of menstruation

amino acid (a-me'-no as'id): small molecular units that make up protein molecules

amblyopia (am'-ble-o'-pe-a): dimness of vision

amniocentesis (am'ne-osen-te'-sis): withdrawal of amniotic fluid for testing

amphiarthrosis (am-phi-är-thro'-sis): partially moveable joint, e.g. symphyis pubis

ampulla of Vater (am-pul'-uh of vah-ter): a junction or common passageway formed from the common bile duct of the liver and the pancreatic duct. It helps to empty bile into the duodenum.

amylase (am'-e-layz): enzyme that converts starch or glycogen to glucose

amylopsin (am'-e-lop'-sin) pancreatic amylase

anabolism (anab'-o-lizm): building up of complex materials in metabolism

analgesic (an'-el-je'-zik) drug that reduces pain

anal sphincter (ay'-nul sfink'-tur): muscles surrounding anal opening

anaphase (an'-e-fayz'): phase four in mitosis

anatomical position (an-a-tom'-i-kel): body standing erect, face forward, arms at side and palms forward

anatomy (a-nat'-a-me): the study of the structure of an organism

anaphylactic shock (an-a-fa-lac'-tic shok): or anaphylaxis; severe and sometimes fatal allergic reaction

androgen (an'-dro-jen): male hormones

anemia (uh-nee'-mee-uh): blood disorder characterized by reduction in number of red blood cells or hemoglobin

aneurysm (an'-you-rism): a widening, or sac, formed by dilation of a blood vessel

angina pectoris (anji'-nuh peck'-to-ris): severe chest pain caused by lack of blood supply to heart

angioplasty (an'-je-o-plas-te) balloon surgery to open blocked blood vessels

ankylosis (ank''-i-lo'-sis): abnormal immobility and consolidation of a joint

anorexia (an''-o-rek'-see-uh): loss of appetite

anorexia nervosa (an''-o-rek'-see-uh nur-vo'-suh): an illness in which a person refuses to eat

antagonist (an-tag'-a-nist): a muscle whose action opposes the action of another muscle

anterior (an-teer'-ee-ur): front or ventral

anterior chamber (an-teer'-ee-ur chame'-bur): space between cornea and iris

antibody (an'-tih-bod''-ee): substance produced by the body, that inactivates a specific foreign substance which has entered the body

anticoagulant (an''-tih-ko-ag'-yoo-lunt): chemical substance that prevents or slows down blood clotting (like heparin)

anticonvulsant (an''-tih-kun-vul'-sunt): therapeutic agent that stops or prevents convulsions

antidiuretic hormone (an''-tih-dye-yoo-ret'-ik hor'-mone): hormone secreted by the posterior pituitary gland, which prevents or suppresses urine excretion

antigen (an'-tih-jin): substance stimulating formation of antibodies against itself

antiprothrombin (an''-tih-pro-throm'-bin): chemical substance that directly or indirectly reduces or retards action of prothrombin (such as heparin)

antithromboplastin (an''-tih-throm-bo-plas'-tin): chemical substance inhibiting clot-accelerating effect of thromboplastins

anuria (a-noor'-e-a): absence of urine

anus (ay'-nus): outlet from rectum

anvil (an'-vil): middle ear bone, or ossicle, in a chain of three ossicles of the middle ear

aorta (ay-or'-tuh): largest artery in body, rising from left ventricle of the heart

aortic-semilunar valve (ay-or'-tik sem''-ee-loo-nur valv): made up of three half-moon-shaped cups, located between junction of aorta and left ventricle of heart

apex (ay'-peks): top of object; point or extremity of a cone

apex of the lung (ay'-pecks of the lung): upper extremity of lung, behind border of the first rib

aphasia (a-fay'-zhuh): loss of ability to speak, may be accompanied by loss of verbal comprehension

aplastic anemia (a-plas'-tik uh-nee'-mee-uh): anemia caused by a suppression of the bone marrow

apnea (ap'-nee-uh): temporary stoppage of breathing movements

aponeurosis (ap"-o-new-ro'-sis): flattened sheet of white, fibrous connective tissue; serves as attachment for flat muscles, or as sheet enclosing/binding muscle groups

appendicitis (a-pen"-di-si'-tis): inflammation of the appendix

appendicular skeleton (ap"-en-dik'-yoo-lur skel'-uh-tun): part of skeleton consisting of pectoral and pelvic girdles, and limbs

aqueous humor (a'-kwe-as hyoo'-mar): watery fluid found in anterior chamber of the eye

arachnoid (uh-rak'-noyd): weblike middle membrane of meninges

areola (a-ree-o'-luh): pigmented ring around nipple; any small space in tissue

arrhythmia (a-rith'-mee-uh): absence of a normal rhythm in heartbeat

arteriole (ahr-teer'-ee-ole): small branch of artery

arteriosclerosis (ahr-teer"-ee-o-skleh-ro'-sis): hardening of arteries, resulting in thickening of walls and loss of elasticity

artery (ahr'-tur-ee): blood vessel which carries blood away from heart

arthritis (ahr-thry'-tis): inflammation of a joint

articular cartilage (ar-tik'-ye-lar kar'-ta-lij): thin layer of cartilage over the ends of long bones

artificial acquired immunity (ar'-ta-fish'-el a-kwir-ed im-yu-net-e): immunity from injection of vaccine, antigen or toxoid

artificial insemination (ar'-ta-fish'-el in-sem'-a-na'-shun): procedure in which semen is placed in vagina by means of cannula or syringe

ascites (a-si'-teez): accumulation of fluid in the peritoneal cavity

assimilation (a-sim"-i-lay'-shun): process of changing food into form suitable for absorption by the circulatory system

associative neuron (a-so'-she-a'-tiv noor'-on): carries messages from sensory neuron to motor neuron

asthma (az'-ma): airways obstructed because of inflammatory reaction to a stimulus

astigmatism (a-stig'-ma-tiz'-em): irregular curvature of cornea or lens

ataxia (ay-tak'-see-uh): muscle incoordination, particularly of muscle groups involved in walking or reaching for objects

atelectasis (a-te-lec'-ta-sis): lungs fail to expand normally

atheriosclerosis (ath"-er-o-scle-ro'-sis): hardening of arteries due to deposits of fat-like material in lining of the arteries

athlete's foot (ath'-leets foot): fungal infection of the foot

atlas (at'-lus): first cervical vertebra; articulates with axis and occipital skull bone

atom (at-om): smallest piece of an element

atrial fibrillation (ay'-tree-ul fib"-ri-lay'-shun): cardiac arrhythmia, characterized by rapid, irregular atrial impulses and ineffective atrial contractions

atrioventricular or A-V node (ay"-tree-o-ven-trik'-yoo-lur node): small mass of interwoven conducting tissue

atrioventricular valves (ay"-tree-o-ven-trik'-yoo-lur valvz): tricuspid and mitral (bicuspid) valves of heart

atrium (ay'-tree-um): upper chamber of heart

atrophy (a'-truh-fee): wasting away of tissue

auricle (aw'-ri-kul): (1) pinna, or ear flap of external ear; (2) atrium of the heart

autoimmunity (aw"-to-im-yu'-net-e): action of antibodies against one's own body

autonomic (aw"-tuh-nom'-ik): independent or self-regulating

autonomic nervous system (aw"-tuh-nom'-ik nur'vus sis'tum): collection of nerves, ganglia, and plexuses through which visceral organs, heart, blood vessels, glands, and smooth (involuntary) muscles receive their innervation

autosome (aw'-to-sohm): non-sex determining chromosome

axial muscle group (ack'see-ul mus'-ul groop): muscles of the head, face, neck, and trunk

axial skeleton (ack'see-ul skel'-e-tun): skeleton of head and trunk

axilla (ak-sil'-uh): armpit

axis (ack'-sis): (1) imaginary line passing through center of the body, (2) second cervical vertebra

axon (acks'-on): nerve-cell structure which carries impulses away from cell body to dendrites

avascular (a-vas'-ku-lar): without blood vessels

B

bactericidal (bak-teer"-i-sigh'-dul): bacterial destruction

ball and socket (bol and sok'-it): diarthroses joint allows the greatest freedom of movement

Bartholin's gland (Bar-thol'-inz gland): mucous glands at opening of vagina

basal cell cancer (bay'-sal sel kan'-ser): most common and least malignant type of skin cancer

base (bays): (1) lowest part of a body, (2) main ingredient of a substance, (3) chemical compound yielding hydroxyl ions (OH$^-$) in an aqueous solution which will react with acid to form a salt and water

basophil (bay'-suh-fil): leukocyte cell, substance, or tissue that shows an attraction for basic dyes

Bell's palsy (Belz pol'-zee): disorder which affects the facial nerve

belly (bel'-ee): the central part of a muscle

benign (be-nine'): non-malignant

bicarbonate ion (by-kahr'-buh-nate eye'-on): salt of carbonic acid characterized by ion HCO_3-

biceps (bye'-seps): muscle on front part of upper arm

bicuspid (bye-kus'-pid): having two cusps

bicuspid or mitral valve (bye-kus'-pid [my'-trul] valv): atrioventricular valve of left side of heart

bifurcation (bye"-fur-kay'-shun): division into two branches

bilateral symmetry (bye-lat'-ur-ul sim'-e-tree): relating to both sides of body

bile (biyl): substance produced by liver, emulsifies fat

bilirubin (bil"-ee-roo'-bin): one of two pigments that determines the color of bile. Bilirubin is reddish in color

biochemistry (bye-o-kem'-is-tree): study of chemical reactions of living things

biology (bye-ol'-ah-jee): the study of all forms of life

biopsy (bye'-op-see): excision of a piece of tissue from a living body for diagnostic study

bipedal (bye-ped'-ul): having two feet

blood brain barrier (blud brayn bar'-ee-ur): substance cannot penetrate the brain tissue

blood pressure (blud presh'-ur): pressure of blood in arterial walls as heart contracts and relaxes

boil (boyl): bacterial infection of sebaceous gland

bolus (boh'-lus): rounded mass; food prepared by mouth for swallowing

Bowman's capsule (boh-manz kap'-sel): double walled capsule around the glomerulus of nephron

bowel (bow'-ul): intestine

brachial (bray'-kee-ul): pertaining to the upper arm

brachiocephalic artery (bray'-kee-o-se-fal'-ik ahr'-tur-ee): artery rising from right side of aortic arch; it divides into right subclavian and right common carotid arteries

bradycardia (brad"-ee-cahr'-dee-uh): abnormally slow heartbeat, less than 60 beats per minute

brainstem (brayn'-stem): portion of brain other than cerebral hemispheres and cerebellum

breast (brest): mammary gland, secretes milk after childbirth

bronchiectasis (bran"-kee-ek'-tah-sis): chronic dilatation of the bronchial tubes

bronchiole (bran'-kee-ole): one of small subdivisions of a bronchus (1 mm or less)

bronchitis (bran-kiy'-tis): inflammation of the bronchial tubes

bronchoscopy (bran-kas'-koh-pee): tubular instrument with light to inspect the interior of the bronchial tubes

bronchus (bran'-kus): one of two primary branches of trachea

buffer (buf'-er): a compound that maintains the balance in a living organism

buccal (buk'-ul): pertaining to the cheek or mouth

buccal cavity (buk'-ul kav'-i-tee): mouth cavity bounded by the inner surface of the cheek

bulbourethral gland (bul"-bo-yoo-re'-thral gland): located on either side of urethra in male, adds alkaline substance to semen

bulimia (bul-ee'-mee-a): episodic binge eating

bunion (bun'-yun): swelling of bursa of foot

burn (burn): a result of destruction of the skin by fire, boiling water, steam, sun, chemicals or electricity, classified as: first degree, only epidermal layer affected; second degree, epidermis and some dermis is affected, third degree, complete destruction of epidermis, dermis and subcutaneous layers.

bursa (bur'-suh): small sac interposed between parts that move on one another

bursitis (bur-sigh'-tis): inflammation of a bursa

C

calcaneus (kal-kay'-nee-us): heel bone

calciferol (kal"-sif'ur-ol): vitamin D_2

calcify (kal'-si-fiy): to deposit mineral salts

calcitonin (kal-si-to'-nin): hormone secreted by thyroid gland that controls calcium ion concentration in body

calculus (kal'-kew-lus): stone-like formation in any part of the body, usually composed of mineral salts

callus (kal'-us): area of hardened and thickened skin

calorie (kal'-or-ee): a unit that measures the amount of energy

calyx (kay'-liks): cup-shaped part of the renal pelvis

canine (kay'-nine): sharp teeth of mammals, between incisors and premolars

capillary (kap'-i-lair-ee): microscopic blood vessel which connects arterioles with venules

carbohydrate (kar"-boh-high'-drayt): an organic compound composed of carbon, hydrogen and oxygen as sugar or starch

carboxyhemoglobin (kahr-bock"-see-hee'-moh-gloh-bin): compound of carbon monoxide and hemoglobin formed when carbon monoxide is present in blood

carcinoma (kahr"-si-noh'-muh): a malignant tumor

cardiac (kahr'-dee-ak): relating to the heart

cardiac arrest (kahr'-dee-ak uh-rest'): syndrome resulting from failure of heart as a pump

cardiac arrhythmia (kahr'-dee-ak a-rith'-mee-uh): any change or abnormality in the normal heart rhythm or beat

cardiac muscle (kahr'-dee-ak mus'-ul): muscle of the heart

cardiac sphincter (kahr'-dee-ak sfink'-tur): circular muscle fibers around cardiac end of esophagus

cardiopulmonary resuscitation (kahr"-dee-oh-puhl'-mun-nair-ee ree-sus"-i-tay'-shun): prevention of asphyxial death by artificial respiration

caries (kair'-eez): decay of tooth or bone

cardiotonic (kar"-dee-oh-ton'-ic): drug to slow and strengthen the heart

carotid (kah-ro'-tid): an artery which supplies blood to the neck and head

carpal (kahr'-pul): bones of the wrist

cartilage (kahr'-ti-lidj): white, semi-opaque, nonvascular connective tissue

casein (kay'-see-in): protein obtained from milk

catabolism (ca-tab'-oh-lizm): the breaking down and changing of complex materials with the release of energy—process in metabolism

catalyst (kat'-uh-list): chemical substance which alters a chemical process but does not enter into the process

cataract (kat'-uh-rakt): condition in which the eye lens becomes opaque

caudal (kod'-el): refers to direction, near the tail end of the body

cecum (see'-kum): pouch at the proximal end of the large intestine

cell (sel): basic unit of structure and function of all living things

cell membrane (sel mem'-brayn): structure which encloses the cell

cellular respiration (sel'-yu-lar res'-pa-ra'-shun) or oxidation: use of oxygen to release energy from the cell

centrioles (sen'-tree-olz): two cylindrical organelles found near the muscles in a tiny-body called the centrosome. They are perpendicular to each other

centrosome (sen'-tro-sohm): tiny area near the nucleus of an animal cell; it contains two cylindrical structures called centrioles

cerebral hemorrhage (ser-ee'-bral hem'-ar-ij): bleeding from blood vessels in brain

cerebral vascular accident (CVA) (ser'-ee-bral vas'-cu-lar ak'-su-dent) or stroke: sudden interruption of blood flow to brain

cerumen (see-roo'-men): ear wax

cervical vertebrae (sur'-vi-kul vur'-tuh-bray): first seven bones of the spinal column

cervix (sur'-viks): narrow end of the uterus

chemistry (kem'-is-tree): the study of structure of matter, composition of substances, their properties and their chemical reactions

chemotaxis (kem"-o-tack'-sis): a response of an organism or a cell to a chemical stimulus by either moving towards or away from the chemical stimulus

cholecystectomy (kol-ah-sis-tek'-tuh-mee): removal of the gallbladder

cholecystitis (kol"-ah-sis-ti'-tis): inflammation of the gallbladder

cholecystokinin (kol"-ah-sis"-tih-kigh'-nen): hormone secreted by the duodenum and jejunum which stimulates pancreatic juice secretion.

cholesterol (koh-les'-tur-ol): a steroid normally synthesized in the liver and also ingested in egg yolks, animal fats and tissues

chromatid (kroh'-muh-tid): each strand of a replicable chromosome

chromatin (kroh'-mah-ten): DNA and protein material in a loose and diffuse state. During mitosis chromatin condenses to form the chromosomes

chromosomal mutation (kroh"-muh-soh"-mul mew-tay'-shun): a mutation that involves change in the number of chromosomes in the organism's nucleus or a change in the structure of a whole chromosome

chromosome (kroh'-muh-sohm): nuclear material which determines hereditary characteristics

chronic obstructive pulmonary disease (COPD) (kron'-ik ub-struk'-tiv pul'-mun-ar-ee di-zeez'): indicates chronic lung condition such as emphysema or bronchitis

chyme (kime): food which has undergone gastric digestion

chymotrypsin (kigh"-mo-trip'-sen): enzyme that digests proteins or incompletely digested proteins turning them into peptides, proteases, polypeptides, peptides, and finally into amino acids

cicatrix (sik'-a-triks): scar tissue

cilia (sil'-ee-uh): tiny lashlike processes of protoplasm

circumcision (sur"-kum-si'-shun): removal of the foreskin of the penis

circumduction (sur"-kum-duk-shun): circular movement at a joint

cirrhosis (sa-ro'-sis): chronic, progressive inflammatory disease of the liver characterized by the formation of fibrous connective tissue

claudication (klo"-di-kay'-shun): pain in legs or buttocks when walking

clavicle (kla'-vi-kul): collar bone

clean wound (kleen woond): a wound where infection is not present

clitoris (kli-tor'-is): small structure over female urethra, has many nerve endings

coagulation (ko-ag"-yu-lay'-shun): process of blood clotting

coccyx (kok'-siks): tailbone

cochlea (kock'-lee-uh): spiral cavity of the internal ear containing the organ of Corti

cochlear duct (kock'-lee-ur dukt): an endolymph-filled triangular canal containing the spiral organ of Corti

coitus (ko-oi'-tus): act of intercourse

collagen (kol'-uh-jen): fibrous protein occurring in bone and cartilage

collecting tubule (ko-lek'-ting too'-byool): structure in nephron which collects urine from distal convoluted tubule

colitis (ko-liy'-tis): inflammation of the colon

colon (ko'-lun): known as the large intestine about five feet in length and two inches in diameter, divided into ascending, transverse, descending and sigmoid colon

colostomy (ko-los'-tah-mee): artificial opening from the colon onto the surface of the skin

common bile duct (kah'-mun biyl dukt): formed by the union of the hepatic duct and cystic duct which brings bile to the duodenum

complete proteins (kum-pleet' pro'-teenz): proteins that contain all the essential amino acids; they enable an animal to grow and carry on fundamental life activities

compound (kom'-pownd): elements combined together in definite proportion by weight to form new substance

conduction defect (kon-duk'-shun de'-fekt): a defect in the electrical impulse system of the heart muscle

congenital (kun-jen'-i-tul): present at birth

congestive heart failure (kon-jes'-tive hart fayl'-yer): heart failure with edema of lower extremities

connective tissue (ka-nek'-tiv tish'-yu): cells whose intercellular secretions (matrix) support and connect the organs and tissues of the body

Cooley's anemia (koo'-leez a-nee'-mee-uh) or Thallesemia minor: anemia caused by defect in hemoglobin formation

coronal (kor'-en-l): frontal plane at a right angle to sagittal, divides the body into anterior and posterior

corona radiata (kor-oh'-nah ra-dee-ay'-tah): layer of epithelial cells around ova

coronary (kor'-o-nair"-ee): referring to the blood vessels of the heart

coronary bypass (kor'-o-nair"-ee biy'-pas): a shunt to go around   area of blockage in the coronary arteries, to provide blood supply to myocardium

coronary circulation (kor'-o-nair"-ee sur"-kyu-la'-shun): brings blood from aorta to myocardium and back to right atrium

coronary sinus (kor'-o-nair"-ee siy'-nus): pocket in posterior of right atrium into which the coronary vein empties

corpus (kor'-pus): body

corpus luteum (kor'-pus lut'-ee-um): yellow body formed from ruptured graafian follicle and produces progesterone

cortex (kor'-teks): outer part of an internal organ

costal (kos'-tul): pertaining to the ribs

coughing (kof'-ing): deep breath followed by forceful exhalation from mouth

cranial (kray'-nee-al): refers to brain or direction towards the head of the body

cretinism (kree'-tin-izm): congenital and chronic condition due to the lack of thyroid hormone

crown (krown): pertains to part of tooth that is visible

cryptorchidism (krip-tor-kih'-dizm): failure of testes to descend into the scrotal sac

Cushing's disease (koosh'-ings di-zeez'): disorder of hyperfunction of adrenal cortex

cutaneous (kew-tay'-nee-us): pertaining to the skin

cyanosis (si"-uh-noh'-sis): bluish color of the skin due to nsufficient oxygen in the blood

cystic duct (sis'-tik dukt): duct from gallbladder to common bile duct

cystitis (sis-ti'-tis): inflammation of the mucous membrane of the urinary bladder

cytology (siy-tol'-uh-jee): study of cells

cytoplasm (sigh'-toh-plazm): protoplasm of the cell body, excluding the nucleus

cytoskeleton (si"-to-skel'-ah-tin): internal framework of the cell which is made up of microtubule, intermediate filaments and microfilaments

D

deciduous teeth (de-sid'-yoo-us teeth): temporary teeth usually lost by six years of age

defecation (def"-eh-kay'-shun): elimination of waste material from the rectum

defibrillator (de-fib'-rul-ay-tor): an electrical device used to discharge an electrical current to shock the pacemaker of the heart back to a normal rhythm

dementia (di-men'-sha): loss in at least two areas of complex behavior

deglutition (dee"-gloo-ti'-shun): act of swallowing

deltoid (del'-toyd): triangular-shaped muscle which covers the shoulder prominence; used for intramuscular injections in adults

dendrite (den'-drite): nerve cell process that carries nervous impulses toward the cell body

dentin (den'-tin): main part of the tooth located under the enamel

dentition (den-tish'-un): number, shape, and arrangement of teeth

deoxygenate (dee-ock'-si-jen-ate): process of removing oxygen from a compound

deoxyribonucleic acid (DNA) (dee-ok"-see-ri-boh-nu-klay'-ik as-id): a nucleic acid containing the elements of carbon, hydrogen, oxygen, nitrogen and phosphorous; it is the genetic material

deoxyribose sugar (dee-ock-see-ri'-bos shuh'-gar): a sugar that has one less oxygen atom than the ribose sugar

dermatitis (dur"-muh-tiy'-tus): inflammation of the skin

dermatology (dur"-mah-tol'-ah-jee): study of the physiology and pathology of the skin

dermis (dur'-mis): true skin; lying immediately beneath the epidermis

dextrose (deks'-trose): glucose, monosaccharide

diabetic insipidus (dye'-a-be'-tik in-sip'-ah-dus): decrease of ADH of pituitary causing excessive loss of water

diabetic mellitus (dye"-a-be'-tik ma-liy'-tus): pancreas is unable to produce insulin or is unable to produce enough insulin for the cells to use glucose

dialysis (dye-al'-i-sis): the separation of smaller molecules from larger molecules in a solution by selective diffusion through a semi-permeable membrane

dialyzer (dye'-al-i-zer): a device to perform dialysis; a kidney machine

diapedesis (dye"-ih-peh'-dee'-sis): passage of blood cells through unruptured vessel wall into tissues

diaphragm (dye'-uh-fram): muscular partition between the thorax and the abdomen

diaphysis (dye-af'-i-sis): shaft of long bone

diarrhea (dye"-ah-ree'-uh): excessive elimination of watery feces

diarthrosis (dye-ar-throh'-sis): moveable joints, e.g. elbow, knee

diastole (dye-as'-tuh-lee): dilation state of the heart; the rest between systoles

diencephalon (dye"-en-sef'-ah-lon): posterior part of the brain; contains the thalamus, hypothalamus and pituitary gland

diffusion (dif-yu'-szen): molecules move from higher concentration to lower

digestion (dye-jes'-chun): the complex process of the breaking down of food to be utilized by the body

dilator (dye'-la-tor): a muscle which opens or closes an orifice

diplopia (di-ploh'-pee-uh): double vision

diphtheria (dif-theer'-i-uh): infectious disease of respiratory system. Because of DPT vaccine it is rarely seen.

disaccharide (dye-sak'-a-ride): double sugar

dislocation (dis"-loh-kay'-shun): displacement of one or more bones of a joint or of any organ from original position

distal (dis'-tul): farthest from point of origin of a structure; opposite of proximal

diuretic (dye-yoo-re'-tik): drug to reduce the amount of fluid in the body

diverticulosis (dye-vur-tik"-yul-o'-sis): numerous diverticula in the colon

dorsal cavity (dor'-sul kav'-eh-tee): or posterior cavity of the body which houses the brain and spinal column

dorsal (dor'-sul): pertaining to the back

ductus arteriosus (duk'-tus ar-teer'-ee-oh-sus): fetal structure which permits blood to flow from pulmonary artery to aorta

ductus deferens or **vas deferens** (duk'-tus def'-uh-renz or vas def'-uh-renz): the part of the excretory duct system of the testes which runs from the epididymus to the ejaculatory duct

duodenum (dew"-o-dee'-num): first part of small intestine, beginning at pylorus

dura mater (dew'-ruh may'-tur): fibrous membrane forming outermost covering of brain and spinal cord

dwarfism (dworf'-izm): caused by hypofunction of growth hormone; growth of long bone is decreased

dysmenorrhea (dis-men"-o-ree'-uh): difficult or painful menstruation

dyspareunia (dis"-puh-roo'-nee-uh): difficult or painful sexual intercourse

dysphasia (dis-fa'-zya): impairment of speech and verbal comprehension

dyspnea (disp-nee'-uh): labored breathing or difficult breathing

dysuria (dis-yoor'-ee-a): painful urination

E

ectopic (ek-top'-ik): in an abnormal position; said of an extrauterine pregnancy or cardiac beats

eczema (ek'-se-mah): acute or chronic non-contagious inflammation of the skin edema (eh-dee'-muh): excessive fluid in tissues

efferent arteriole (ef'-er-ant ar-teer'-ee-ul): carries blood from glomerulus

efferent neuron *see* motor neuron

ejaculatory ducts (e-jak'-yoo-luh-tor"-ee dukts): short and narrow ducts that begin where the ductus deferens and the seminal duct join

elastic (e-las'-tik): capable of returning to original form after being compressed or stretched

electrocardiogram (ECG or EKG) (e-lek"-tro-kar'-dee-u-gram): device used to measure the electric conduction system of the heart

electrolytes (e-lek'-tro-lights): electrically-charged particles which help determine fluid and acid-base balance

electromyograph (e-lek"-troh-miy'-oh-graf): device used to measure electrical muscle activity

element (el'-e-ment): made up of like atoms, substance which can neither be created nor destroyed

embolism (em'-bo-lizm): obstruction of a blood vessel by a circulating blood clot, fat globule, air bubble, or piece of tissue

embryo (em'-bree-oh): the human young up to the first three months after conception; the young of any organism in early development stage

embryology (em-bree-ol'-u-jee): study of the formation of an organism from fertilized egg to birth

emesis (em'-eh-sis): vomitus

emphysema (em-fi-see'-muh): lung disorder in which inspired air becomes trapped and is difficult to expire

empyema (em-pye-ee'-muh): pus in a cavity

emulsify (e-mul'-si-fye): to make into an *emulsion*, a product consisting of small globules of one liquid intermixed throughout the body of a second liquid

enamel (e-nam'-ul): hard calcium substance which covers the teeth

encephalitis (en-sef-u-liy'-tis): inflammation of the brain

endocardium (en"-do-kahr'-dee-um): membrane lining interior of heart

endocrine (en'-doh-krin): pertaining to a gland which secretes into the blood or tissue fluid instead of into a duct

endocrinology (en"-doh-krah-nol'-u-jee): study of physiology and pathology of hormonal system

endometrioses (en"-doh-mee-tree-o'-sis): the presence of endometrium which is normally confined to the uterine cavity in other areas of the pelvic cavity

endometrium (en"-do-mee'-tree-um): mucous membrane lining uterus

endoplasmic reticulum (en-do-theel'-ee-um re-tik'-u-lum): transport system of the cell

endosteum (en-dos'-tee-um): lining of the medullary cavity in the long bone

endothelium (en"-do-theel'-ee-um): epithelial cells lining the blood vessels, heart, and lymph vessels or any closed cavity in the body

energy (en'-er-jee): ability to do work

enteritis (en-ter-i'-tis): inflammation of the small intestine

enzyme (en'-zime): organic catalyst that initiates and accelerates a chemical reaction

eosinophil (ee"-o-sin'-uh-fil): white blood cell whose granules stain red with eosin or other acid dyes

epidermis (ep"-i-dur'-mis): outermost layer of skin

epididymitis (ep"-i-did'-i-miy-tis): inflammation of epididymis

epididymus (ep"-i-did'-i-mis): portion of the seminal duct lying posterior to the testes; connected by the efferent ductulis of each testis

epigastric (ep-i-gas'-trik) upper region of the abdominal cavity, located just below the sternum

epiglottis (ep-i-glot'-is): elastic cartilage which prevents food from entering the trachea

epilepsy (ep-ul-ep'-see): seizure disorder

epiphysis (ee-pif'-ah-sis): the end of the long bone

epinephrine (ep"-i-nef'-rin): adrenalin; secretion of the adrenal medulla, which prepares the body for energetic action

episiotomy (e-peez-e-ot'-um-ee): a surgical incision into the perineum

epithelial cells (e-pi-thee'-lee-al selz): cover body's external and internal surfaces

equilibrium (ee-kwuh-lib'-ree-um): a state of balance

ergonomics (er-ga-nom'-iks): the application of biology and engineering to the relationship between the worker and their environment; also called "biotechnology"

erythroblastosis fetalis (e-rith"-ra-blast-o'-sus fetal'-es): hemolytic disease of the newborn

erythrocyte (e-rith'-ro-sight): red blood cell

erythropoiesis (e-rith"-ro-poy-ee'-sis): formation or development of red blood cells

esophagus (e-sof'-uh-gus): a muscular tube; takes food from pharynx to the stomach

essential amino acids (e-sen'-chul a'-mee'-noh as'-ids): amino acids that are necessary for normal growth and development and are not made in the human body

estrogen (es'-tra-jen): secretion of the ovary, female hormone

ethmoid (eth'-moyd): bone of the cranium located between the eyes eupnea (yoop'-nee-uh): normal or easy breathing with usual quiet inhalations and exhalations

eustachian tube (yoo-sta'-shen tube): passageway from throat to middle ear, equalizes pressure

excitability (ek-sih'-tah-bil'-eh-tee): ability to respond to stimuli

exocrine (ex'-o-krin): pertaining to a gland which secretes into a duct

exophthalmos (ek"-sof-thal'-mus): abnormal protrusion of the eyes

expiration (ek"-spir-ay'-shun): act of breathing forth or expelling air from lungs

extensor (ek-sten'-sur): muscle which extends or stretches a limb or part

external (ek-ster'-nul): superficial at or near the surface of the skin

external respiration (ek-ster'-nul res-pih-ray'-shun): breathing; act of inspiration and expiration

extension (ek-sten'-shun): act of increasing the angle between two bones

extracellular fluid (ek-stra-sel'-u-lar floo'-id): fluid outside the cell

F

fallopian tube (fa-lo'-pee-un tewb): uterine tube or oviduct which carries egg from ovary to uterus

fascia (fay'-shuh): band or sheet of fibrous membranes covering or binding and supporting muscles

fat (fat): sometimes called triglyceride; organic compound composed of carbon, hydrogen, and oxygen; made of glycerol and fatty acids

feces (fee'-seez): waste material from the digestive system

femur (fee'-mur): thighbone

fertilization (fur-til-ah-zay'-shun): the process of the union of the egg and sperm

fetal circulation (fet'-ul ser-kyul-a'-shun): brings blood to the fetus

fetus (fee'-tus): the human young the third month of the intrauterine period until birth

fiber (fiy'-ber): compound found in plant foods

fibrillation (fi-bre-lay'-shun): heart muscle fibers contract at random without coordination

fibrin (fih'-brin): an insoluble protein necessary for the clotting of blood

fibrinogen (fi-brin'-o-jen): a protein which is converted into fibrin by the action of thrombin

fibroid (fye'-broyd): a benign tumor of smooth muscle especially in the uterus

fibromyalagia (fi-broh-mi-al'-gee-uh): chronic muscle pain

first degree burn *see* burns

fibula (fib'-yoo-luh): slender bone at outer edge of lower leg

filtration (fil-tray'-shun): movement of water and particles across a semipermeable membrane by a mechanical force such as blood pressure

fistula (fis'-choo-luh): an abnormal duct from an abscess, cavity or hollow organ to the body surface or to another hollow organ

flat feet (flat feet): weakening of the leg muscles that support the arch of the foot

flatulence (flach'-uh-lenz): the presence of excessive gas in the digestive tract

flexion (fleks'-ee-on): the act of bending a limb or decreasing the angle between two bones

flexor (fleks'-or): a muscle that bends a joint

follicle stage (fol'-i-kul stayj): first stage of the female menstrual cycle during which follicle-stimulating hormone (FSH) secreted from the anterior lobe of the pituitary gland is circulated via the bloodstream. FSH reaches an ovary, it stimulates several follicles; however, only one matures. As the one follicle grows in size, an egg cell begins to grow inside the follicle

follicle-stimulating hormone (FSH) (fol'-i-kul stim'-yoo-lay-ting hor'-mone): an adenohypophyseal hormone which stimulates follicular growth in the ovary

fontanel (fon"-tuh-nel'): unossified areas in the infant skull; soft spot

foramen (fo-ray'-men): an opening in a bone

foramen ovale (fo-ray'-men o-val'): an opening in the septum between the right and left atrium of the fetus

foreskin (for'-skin): loose fitting skin around the end of the penis

fracture (frak'-chur): a break in a bone

frontal (frunt'-el): pertaining to the forehead

frontal lobe (frunt'-el lobe): in cerebral cortex, controls the motor function

fundus (fun'-dus): part farthest from opening of an organ

G

gallbladder (gol'-blad-er): a small pear shaped organ under the right lobe of the liver, it stores bile

gamma globulin (gam'-uh glob'-ye-lin): fractionated part of globulin used to treat infectious diseases

ganglion (gang'-glee-un): a mass of nerve cell bodies outside the central nervous system

gangrene (gang-green'): death of body tissue due to insufficient blood supply gastric (gas'-trik): pertaining to the stomach

gastric glands (gas'-trik glands): glands lining stomach

gastritis (gas-tri'-tis): inflammation of the stomach

gastrocnemius (gas-trok-nem'-ee-us): calf muscle

gastroenteritis (gas-troh-en"-tur-i'-tis): inflammation of stomach and small intestines

gastroesophageal reflux (gas-tro-ee-sof'-u-jeel re'-fluks): stomach contents flow back into the esophagus

gene (jene): part of the chromosome that transmits a specific hereditary trait

genetics (je-net'-iks): the branch of biology that studies the science of heredity and the difference and similarities between parents and offspring

genitals (jen-i-tuls): reproductive organs, also called genitalia

gestation (jes-tay'-shun): development period of the human young from conception to birth

genital herpes (jen'-i-tul hur'-peez): a sexually transmitted recurrent disease caused by a virus

genital warts (jen'-i-tul wortz): or human papillomavirus, sexually transmitted disease

gigantism (ji-gan'-tizm): hypersecretion of the growth hormone, overgrowth of long bones

gingiva (jin'-jeh-vae): gums

glans penis (glanz pe'-nis): the head or tip of the penis

glaucoma (gloh-koh'-muh): increase in interocular eye pressure

glenoid fossa (glee'-noyd fos'-uh): articular surface on scapula for articulation with head of humerus

gliding joint (glid'-ing joynt): the nearly flat surfaces of the bone glide across each other, i.e.: vertebra

globin (glo'-bin): protein molecule of hemoglobin

globulin (glob'-yeh-len): plasma protein made in liver, helps in synthesis of antibodies

glomerulonephritis (gla-mer-yul-o-ne-fri'-tis): an inflammation of the glomerulus of the kidney

glomerulus (gla-mer'-yah-lus): part of the nephron, tuft of capillaries situated within Bowman's capsule

glottis (glot'-is): space within the vocal cords of the larynx

glucocorticoid (gloo-koh-kor'-ti-koyd): hormones of the adrenal cortex, namely cortisone and cortisol

glucose (gloo'-kos): a monosaccharide or simple sugar; the principal blood sugar

gluteal (gloo'-tee-ul): pertaining to the area near the buttocks

glycerin or glycerol (glis'-ur-in or glis'-ur-ole): product of fat digestion

glycogen (glye'-kuh-jin): polysaccharide formed and stored largely in the liver

goiter (goy'-ter): enlargement of the thyroid gland

Golgi apparatus (gol'-jee ap-ah-ra'-tus): a membranous network looks like a stack of pancakes, that stores and packages secretions to be secreted by the cell

gonads (goh'-nads): sex glands (ovaries or testes)

gonorrhea (gon-eh-ree'-uh): an infectious disease of the genitourinary tract caused by gonococcus, transmitted mainly by sexual contact

gout (gowt): increase in uric acid crystals in bloodstream which are deposited in joint cavities, especially the great toe

graafian follicle (graf'-ee-an fol'-e-kel): a follicle in the ovary which stores the immature ova

graft (graft): to transplant tissue into a body part to replace damaged tissue

granulation (gran"-yoo-lay'-shun): tiny red granules that are visible in the base of a healing wound; consists of newly formed capillaries and fibroblasts

granulocyte (gran'-ye-loh-site): granular white blood cell

greater omentum (grat'-er o-men'-tum): double fold of peritoneum which hangs down over the abdominal organs like an apron

greenstick fracture (green'-stik frak'-chur): incomplete fracture of long bone; seen in children; bone is bent but splintered only on convex side

gyri (ji'-ree): convolutions in the brain

H

hair follicle (hayr fol'-i-kul): in pocketing of the epidermis which holds the hair root

heart block (hart blok): interruption of the SA node message to the AV node, there is a lack of coordination between the atria and the ventricles

heart failure (hart fayl'-yur): heart ventricles do not contract effectively

heartburn (hart'-burn): a burning sensation in the esophagus and stomach

hematoma (hee"-muh-toh'-muh): localized clotted mass of blood formed in an organ, tissue, or space

hematuria (heem-ah-toor'-ee-ah): blood in the urine

heme (heem): iron compound part of the hemoglobin

hemiplegia (hem"-i-plee'-jee-uh): paralysis of one side of the body

hemoccult (heem'-o-kult): hidden blood

hemodialysis (heem"-oh-di-al'-i-sis): a procedure for removing waste products in the circulating blood of patients with kidney failure

hemoglobin (heem'-uh-gloh-bin): oxygen-carrying pigment of the blood hemolysis (heem-ol'-ah-sis): the bursting of red blood cells

hemophilia (heem"-oh-fil'-ee-uh): sex-linked, hereditary bleeding disorder occurring only in males but transmitted by females; characterized by a prolonged clotting time and abnormal bleeding

hemorrhoids (hem'-uh-roydz): enlarged and varicose condition of the veins in the lower part of the anus or rectum and the tissues of the anus

heparin (hep'-uh-rin): substance obtained from the liver, which slows blood clotting

hepatic duct (he-pat'-ik dukt): structure from the liver to the common bile duct, carries bile

hepatic vein (he-pat'-ik vayn): vein which drains blood from liver into inferior vena cava

hepatitis (hep-ah-tit'-is): inflammation of the liver

hepatomegaly (hep"-ah-toh-meg'-ah-lee): enlargement of the liver

hereditary (he-red'-i-tayr-ee): of or pertaining to inheritance; inborn; inherited

herpes (hur'-peez): a contagious viral infection in which small blisters appear

hernia (hur'-nee-uh): protrusion of a loop of an organ through abnormal opening

hiccough (hik'-up): spasm of diaphragm and spasmodic closure of glottis

high density lipoprotein (HDL) (high den'-si-tee li'-poh-proh-teen) removes excess cholesterol from walls of the artery

hilum (high'-lem): indentation along the medial border of the kidney hinge joint; joint movement in one direction such as the elbow

histology (his-tol'-uh-jee): microscopic study of living tissues

Hodgkin's disease (Hoj'-kinz di-zeez'): specific type of cancer of the lymph nodes

homeostasis (ho-me-oh-stay'-ses): state of balance

hormone (hor'-mone): chemical secretion, usually from an endocrine gland

Huntington's disease (hunt'-ing-tunz di-zeez'): genetic disorder characterized by degeneration of the central nervous system

hyaline (hi'-a-line): type of cartilage which forms the skeleton of the embryo

hydrocephalus (hi-dro-sef'-a-lus): increase in the volume of cerebral spinal fluid within the cerebral ventricles, may occur in fetal development

hydronephrosis (high-droh-nef-roh'-sis): renal pelvis and calyces become distended due to the accumulation of fluid

hymen (high'-men): membrane at the opening of the vagina

hyoid bone (high'-oyd bone): bone between root of the tongue and larynx, supporting tongue and giving attachment to several muscles

hyperglycemia (high-per-gligh-see'-mee-ya): high concentration of glucose in the blood

hypernea (high-pur'-nee-uh): increase in the depth and rate of breathing accompanied by abnormal exaggeration of respiratory movements

hyperopia (high"-pur-oh'-pee-uh): farsightedness

hypersensitivity (high-per-sen-sah-tiv'-i-tee) an abnormal response to a drug or allergen

hypertension (high-pur-ten'-shun): abnormally high blood pressure

hypertrophy (high-per'-tra-fee): an increase in the size of the muscle cell

hyperventilation (high-per-ven-til-ay'-shun): rapid breathing, rapid loss of carbon dioxide; sometimes causes dizziness or fainting

hypogastric (hghi-poh-gas'-trik): lower region of the abdominal area

hypoglycemia (high"-poh-gliy-see'-mee-ya): low concentration of glucose in the blood

hypotension (high"-pho-ten'-shun): reduced or abnormally low blood pressure

hypothalamus (high"-poh-thal'-a-mus): part of the diencephalon, lies below the thalamus

hysterectomy (his"-tur-ek'-tuh-mee): partial or total surgical removal of the uterus

I

ileum (il'-ee-um): the lower part of the small intestine, extending from the jejunum to the large intestine

ilium (il'-ee-um): upper broad portion of the hipbone

immunization (im-yoo-nah-zay'-shun): process of increasing resistance to disease

immunoglobulin (im"-yoo-noh-glob'-ya-lin): protein that acts like an antibody

immunosuppressant (im'-yoo-noh-suh-press'-unt): an agent, such as a drug, chemical, or X-ray used to suppress the immune system of a patient

immunity (im-yoo'-neh-tee): ability to resist a disease

incisor (in-sigh'-zur): cutting tooth; one of four front teeth of either jaw

incomplete proteins (in"-kum-pleet' pro'-teens): proteins that lack some or most of the essential amino acids

impetigo (im-peh-tay'-goh): acute and contagious skin disease

impotence (im'-peh-tens): inability to sustain an erection

incontinent (in-kon'-tah-nent): unable to control excretory functions of the body

incus (ing'-kus): the middle ear bone, also called the anvil

infectious mononucleoses (in-fek'-shus mon"-oh-nuk-lee-oh'-sis): contagious disease caused by Epstein-Barr virus, sometimes called the "kissing disease"

inferior (in-feer'-ee-er): below another or lower

inferior concha (in-feer'-ee-er kon'-cha): bones which make up side walls of the nasal cavity

infertility (in-fer-til'-ah-tee): incapable of reproduction

inflammation (in"-flah-may'-shun): occurs when tissues are subjected to chemical or physical trauma (cut or heat); invasion by pathogenic microorganisms can cause inflammation. Pain, heat, redness, and swelling occur.

influenza (in-floo-en'-zah): inflammation of the mucous membrane of the respiratory tract

ingestion (in-jes'-chun): act of taking substances, especially food, into body

inguinal (ing'-gwi-nul): pertaining to the groin

inhalation (in-huh-lay'-shun): taking air into the lungs

innominate bone (in-om'-i-nut bone): hipbone

insertion of muscle (in-sur'-shun of mus'-ul):muscle is attached to the movable part of the bone

inspiration (in"-spih-ray'-shun): drawing in of air; inhalation

insulin (in'-sah-lin): hormone produced by the pancreas necessary for glucose metabolism

integument (in-teg'-yoo-munt): covering, especially the skin

intercostal muscles (in-tur-kos'-tul mus'-uls): muscles found between adjacent ribs

interneuron (in-ter-neur'-on): *see* associative neuron

interphase (in'-ter-faz): the resting phase in the process of mitosis

interstitial tissue (in"-tur-stish'-ul tish'-ew): intercellular connective tissue

intracellular fluid (in-tra-sel'-ya-ler flu'-id): fluid within the cell

intramuscular (in"-truh-mus'-kew-lur): into the muscle

intravenously (in'-truh-vee'-nus-lee): within, or into, the veins

intrinsic factor (in-trin'-sik fak'-tor): a protein secreted by the stomach which is essential for absorption of Vitamin B12

invitro fertilization (in-vee'-tro fer"-til-ih-zay'-shun): a process of fertilization outside the living organism

involuntary (in-vol'-un-tayr-ee): opposite of voluntary, not within the control of will

involution (in"-vo-lew'-shun): return of an organ to its normal size after enlargement; also the regressive change due to aging

ion (eye'-on): an electrically charged atom

iris (i'-ris): colored muscular layer surrounding the pupil of the eye

irradiation (ir-ay-dee-ay'-shun): exposure to radiation such as infrared, gamma, roentgen, and ultraviolet rays

irritability (ir"-ih-tuh-bil'-ih-tee): ability to react to a stimulus; excitability

ischium (is'-kee-um): lower part of hipbone

islets of Langerhans (i'-letz of lang'-er-hanz): specialized cells in pancreas which produce insulin

isometric (i-soh-meh'-trik): tension in muscle increases but muscle does not shorten

isotonic (i-soh-ton'-ik): muscle contracts and shortens

isotope (i'-soh-tope): atoms of a specific element which have the same number of protons but a different number of neutrons

J

joint (joynt): place where two bones meet

jaundice (jon'-dis): yellow

jejunum (je-joo'-num): section of small intestine between duodenum and ileum

K

kaposi (ka-poh'-si): sarcoma—blood vessel malignancy

keratin (ker'-uh-tin): chemical belonging to albuminoid or scleroprotein group found in horny tissue, hair, nails

kilogram (kil'-oh-gram): 1000 grams or approximately 2.2 pounds

kinetic (ki-neh'-tik): pertaining to motion

kyphosis (ki-fose'-is): hunch back, humped curvature in spinal column

L

labia (lay'-bee-uh): lips

lacrimal (lak'-ri-mul): pertaining to tears

lactation (lak-tay'-shun): secretion of milk from the breasts

lactose (lak'-tose): milk sugar; a disaccharide used in infant formulas

larynx (lar'-inks): voicebox, found between trachea and base of tongue; contain the vocal cords

lateral (lat'-ur-ul): toward the side

lateral ventricles *see* cerebral ventricles

laxative (laks'-uh-tiv): chemical substance that relieves constipation; a mild purgative

lens (lenz): crystal or glass for refraction of light rays

leukocyte (lew'-ko-sight): white blood cell

leukocytosis (lew"-ko-sigh-tow'-sis): an increase in the white blood cell count, above 10,000 cells per cubic millimeter (mm^3)

leukopenia (lew"-ko-pee'-nee-uh): a decrease in the normal number of white blood cells (leukocytes)

leukorrhea (lew"-ko-ree'-uh): whitish, mucopurulent discharge from vagina

ligament (lig'-uh-ment): a band of fibrous tissue connecting bones or supporting organs

lipase (lip'-ase): enzyme that changes fats into fatty acids and glycerol

lipid (lip'-id): fatty compound

lithotripsy (lith-oh-trip'-see): or extracorpeal shockwave, a procedure used to reduce kidney stones to sand to enable them to pass through the urinary tract

liver (liv'-ur): large organ of the digestive system, located in the upper right quadrant of the abdominal cavity

lobule (lob'-yool): small lobe or a small section of a lobe

locomotion (lo"-kuh-moh'-shun): act of moving from place to place

lordosis (lor-do'-sis): forward curvature of lumbar region of spine

lubb-dupp sound (lub dup sownd): sounds made by the heart valves when they close

lumbago (lum-bay'-goh): backache occurring in the lower lumbar or lumbosacral area of the spinal column

lumbar (lum'-bahr): pertaining to the loins; region between the posterior thorax and sacrum

lumbar vertebrae (lum'-bahr vur'-te-bray): five vertebrae associated with lower part of back

lumen (lew'-min): passageway or opening to a tubular structure such as a blood vessel

lymph (limf): watery fluid in the lymphatic vessels

lymphadenitis (lim-fa"-den-i'-tis): inflammation of the lymph nodes

lymphatic (lim-fat'-ik): vessel carrying lymph

lymphatic system (lim-fat'-ik sis'-tum): system of vessels and nodes supplemental to blood circulatory system, carrying lymph

lymphocyte (lim'-foh-sight): a type of white blood cell

lysosome (lye"-so-sohm): cytoplasmic organelle and containing digestive enzymes

M

macrophage (mak'-rah-faj): a large phagocytic cell, which can wall off and isolate an infected area

macular degeneration (mak'-yu-ler de-jen"-er-ay'-shun): thinning of retinal layer of eye or leakage may develop under retina disturbing sharp central vision

malignant (mah-lig'-nent): rapidly spreading; cancerous

malleus (mal'-ee-us): largest of three middle ear bones; also called the hammer

maltose (mawl'-tose): disaccharide formed by the hydrolysis of starch

mammary (mam'-ur-ree): pertaining to the breast

mammogram (mam'-e-gram): an X-ray of the breast

mandible (man'-dih-bul): lower jawbone

manubrium (mah-new'-bree-um): (1) handle-like process; (2) upper part of the sternum (breastbone)

mastectomy (mas-tek'-ta-mee): removal of a breast

mastication (mas"-ti-kay'-shun): process of chewing

matter (mat'-ur): anything that has weight and occupies space

maturation (match"-oo-ray'-shun): process of coming to full development

maxilla (mak-sil'-a): bone of the upper jaw

meatus (mee-ay'-tus): passageway or opening

medial (mee'-dee-ul): toward midline of body

mediastinum (mee"-dee-as'-tih-num): intrapleural space separating the sternum in front and the vertebral column behind

medulla (mah-dul'-uh): inner portion of an organ

medulla oblongata (mah-dul'-uh ob'-lon-gah'-tuh): part of the brainstem, contains the nuclei for vital functions

medullary canal (med'-ul-er-ee cuh-nal'): center of the shaft of long bone

meiosis (mi-yo'-sis): cell division of gamete or cells; there is a reduction in the number of chromosomes

melanin (mel'-a-nin): pigment which gives color to hair, skin and eyes

melanoma (mel-eh-noh'-muh): malignant tumor which occurs in the melanocytes

melatonin (mel-eh-toh'-nin): hormone produced by the pineal gland

membrane (mem'-brayn): a thin layer of tissue which covers a surface or divides an organ

memory (mem'-eh-ree): process by which we store information we have learned

menarche (me-nahr'-kee): time when menstruation begins

Meniere's disease (man-arz' di-zeez'): condition affecting semi-circular canals of inner ear

meninges (men-en'-jez): any of three linings enclosing the brain and spinal cord

menopause (men′-o-pawz): physiologic termination of menstruation, generally between fifty and fifty-five years

menstrual cycle (men′-stroo-ul sigh′-kul): recurring series of changes that take place in the ovaries, uterus, and accessory sexual structures during menstruation

menstruation (men″-stroo-ay′-shun): monthly shedding of endometrial lining if ova is not fertilized

mesentery (mez′-en-ter-ee): peritoneum attached to posterior wall of the abdominal cavity

metabolism (me-tab′-oh-lizm): sum total of processes of digestion, absorption, and the resulting release of energy

metacarp (met″-uh-kahrp): bones of wrist

metaphase (met′-uh-faze): phase three in the process of mitosis. Nuclear membrane disappears

metastasis (me-tas′-tuh-sis): transfer of malignant cells from an original site to a distant one through the circulatory system or lymph vessels

metatarsal (met″-uh-tahr′-sal): sole of foot, forms the arch

microbe (migh′-krobe): microscopic organisms, especially bacterium

microgram (migh′-kro-gram): one one-thousandth of a milligram, abbreviated as mcg and symbolized as μg

micturition (mich″-tew-rish′-un): voiding, or urinating

mid-sagittal plane (mid-saj′-eh-tel plane): an imaginary line dividing the body into equal right and left halves

miotic (miy-ot′-ik): causing contraction of pupil

milligram (mil′-ih-gram): one one-thousandth of a gram, abbreviated as mg

mineral (min′-ur-ul): an inorganic, solid chemical compound found in nature

mineral corticoids (min′-ur-ul cort′-ih-coydz): hormones of the adrenal cortex, namely aldosterone

mitochondria (miy-toh-kon′-dree-a): organelle which supplies energy to the cell

mitosis (migh-toe′-sis): cell division which is divided into two distinct processes: (1) mitosis—the exact duplication of the nucleus to form two identical nuclei. (2) cytoplasmic division—after nuclear division, the cytoplasm is divided into two approximately equal parts

mitral valve prolapse (miy′-tral valv proh′-laps): valve between the left atrium and the left ventricle does not close properly

mixed nerve (mikst nurv): nerve composed of both afferent (sensory) fibers and efferent (motor) fibers

molar (moh′-lar): teeth designed for crushing and tearing

molecule (mol′-uh-kyool): the smallest unit of the compound that still has the properties of the compound

monocyte (mon′-oh-sight): large mononuclear leukocyte with deeply indented nucleus, slate-gray cytoplasm, and fine bluish granulations

monorchidism (mon-or′-kid-izm): presence of only one testis

monosaccharide (mon″-oh-sack′-uh-ride): simple sugar; glucose

morphology (mor-fol′-ah-jee): the study of the shape of an organism

motor neuron (moh′-ter neur′-on): or efferent neuron, carries messages from brain and spinal cord to muscles and glands

motor unit (moh′-ter u′-nit): a motor nerve plus all the muscle fibers it stimulates

mucilaginous (mew″-si-ladj′-ih-nus): gumlike consistency

mucin (mew′-sin): mixture of glycoproteins forming basis of mucus

mucosa (mew-koh′-suh): mucous membrane

multicellular (mul-ti-sel′-u-lar): many-celled

multiple sclerosis (mul′-tih-pul skle-roh′-sis): chronic inflammatory disease in which the immune cells attack the myelin sheath of a nerve

murmur (mur′-mer): gurgling or hissing sound from heart valves failing to close properly

muscle fatigue (mus′-ul fah-teeg′): caused by an accumulation of lactic acid in the muscle

muscle spasm (mus′-ul spa′-zum): sustained muscle contraction

muscle tissue (mus′-ul tis′-ew): contains cell material that has the ability to contract and move the body

muscle tone (mus′-ul tone): muscles always in a state of partial contraction

muscular dystrophy (mus′-kew-ler dis′-tre-fee): muscle disease in which the muscle cells deteriorate

mutagenic agent (mew″-tuh-jen′-ik ay′-junt): any substance causing a genetic mutation

mutate (mew-tate′): to change or alter a characteristic which will make it different from that of the parental type

mutation (mew-tay′-shun): the appearance of a new and different organic trait caused by the inheritance of a mutated gene or chromosome

myalgia (migh-al′-juh): muscular pain

myasthenia gravis (migh-es-the′-nee-a gra′vis): disease in which there is abnormal weakness and eventual paralysis of muscles

myelin (migh'-e-lin): a lipoid substance found in the sheath around nerve fibers

myeloblast (migh'-eh-loh-blast): cells which synthesize granulocytes in bone marrow

myocarditis (migh"-o-kahr-dye'-tis): inflammation of muscular tissue of heart

myocardium (migh"-o-kahr'-dee-um): muscle of the heart

myometrium (migh"-o-mee'-tree-um): uterine muscular structure

myopia (migh-o'-pee-uh): nearsightedness

myositis (migh'-oh-sigh'-tis): inflammation of muscle tissue, generally voluntary muscle

myotonia (migh"-oh-toh'-nee-uh): condition where there is an abnormally slow muscle relaxation after voluntary muscle contraction

myringotomy (mir-en-got'-oh-mee): opening into the tympanic membrane

myxedema (mik-se-de'-ma): hypofunction of the thyroid gland, swelling around nose and lips.

N

nares (nair'-eez): pertaining to the nostrils

nasal (nay'-zul): nose

nasal cavity (nay'-zul kav'-ih-tee): one of the pair of cavitties between anterior nares and nasopharynx

nasal polyps (nay'-zul pol'-ips): growth which occurs in sinus cavity

nasal septum (nay'-zul sep'-tum): partition between the two nasal cavities

natural acquired immunity (na'-chur-al a-kwi'-erd i-mu'-ni-tee): immunity which is the result of having the disease and recovering.

natural immunity (na'-chur-al i-mu'-ni-tee): immunity a person is born with

neck of tooth (nek of tooth): that part of tooth at gum line

negative feedback (neg'-uh-tiv feed'-bak): the return of part of the output to the source or beginning; this leads to an adjustment in the system. Negative feedback may occur in hormonal or nervous control systems

neoplasm (nee'-o-plaz-em): a tumor; can be benign or malignant

nephron (nef'-ron): unit of structure of kidney, contains glomerulus, Bowman's capsule, proximal distal tubule, loop of Henle, and distal tubule

nervous tissue (nur'-vus tis'-yoo): contains cells that react to stimuli and conduct an impulse

neuralgia (noo-ral'-ja): severe, stabbing pain along the pathway of a nerve

neuritis (noo-rih'-tis): inflammation of a nerve

neurogenic bladder (noor-o-jen'-ik blad'-ur): condition caused by damaged nerves that control the bladder

neuroglia (noo-rog'-lee-ah): network of cells that insulate, support and protect the nerves of the central nervous system

neurohypophysis (new"-roh-high-pof'-ih-sis): posterior lobe of the pituitary gland; it stores two hormones produced by the hypothalamus: antidiuretic hormone and oxytocin

neurology (noo-rol'-ah-jee): the study of the physiology and pathology of the nervous system

neuromuscular junction (noor-oh-mus'-kya-lur junk'-shun): point between the motor nerve axon and the muscle cell membrane

neuron (new'-ron): nerve cell, including its processes

neurotransmitter (noor-o-trans'-mit-er): a chemical substance such as acetylcholine released from nerve endings and transmitting impulses across a synapse to nerve, muscle or other cells

neutralization (noo-tral-ah-zay'-shun): an acid and a base combine to form a salt and water

neutrophil (noo'-trah-fil): many-lobed white blood cell phagoytizes bacteria, sometimes called "polys"

nongravid (non"-grav'-id): not pregnant

nonpathogenic (non"-path-o-jen'-ik): incapable of producing disease

nuclear membrane (noo'-klee-er mem'-brayn): double-layered membrane that surrounds the nucleus

nucleic acid (noo-klay'-ik as'-id): organic compound containing carbon, hydrogen, oxygen, nitrogen, and phosphorous; i.e.: DNA, RNA

nucleolus (new-klee-uh'-lus): small spherical structure within cell nucleus

nucleoplasm (new'-klee-o-plazm): protoplasm of the nucleus, also called *nuclear sap* or *karyolymph*

nucleus (new'-klee-us): core or center of a cell containing large quantities of DNA

nutrient (new'-tree-unt): affording nutrition

nystagmus (ni-stag'-mis): rapid involuntary movement of the eyeball

O

obesity (oh-bee'-sih-tee): increase of body weight due to fat accumulation of 10 to 20% above normal range for the specific age, height, and sex

occipital lobe (ok-cip'-ih-tel lobe): part of the cerebrum that houses the visual area

occiput (ok'-sih-put): pertaining to the back of the head

olecranon process (oh-lek'-ruh-non pro'-ses): large projection at upper extremity of ulna olfactory (ol-fak'-tur-ee): pertaining to the sense of smell

oogenesis (o"-oh-jen'-e-sis): process of origin, growth, and formation of ovum in ovary during preparation for fertilization

ophthalmic (of-thal'-mik): referring to the eyes

opportunistic infection (op-er-toon-is'-tik in-fek'-shun): an infection which may occur because a person's immune system dysfunctions

oral cavity (or'-el ca'-vi-tee): encloses the teeth and tongue

orbital cavity (or'-bi-tel ca'-vi-tee): contains the eye and its external structures

orchitis (or-ki'-tis): inflammation of testis

organ (or'-gan): group of tissues organized according to structure and function

organ of Corti (or'-gan of kor'-tee): hearing organ

organic compound (or-gan'-ik kom'-pownd): compound which contains the element, carbon

organelle (or-guh-nel'): microscopic specialized structure within the cell having a special function or capacity

origin (or'-eh-jin): part of the skeletal muscle which is attached to the fixed part of the bone

oropharynx (or"-o-fayr'-inks): oral pharynx, found below level of lower border of soft palate and above larynx

orthopnea (or"-thup'-nee-uh): difficult or labored breathing

osmoreceptor (oz"-moh-ree-sep'-tur): structures found in the hypothalamus; sensitive to changes in the osmotic blood pressure and control the release of the antidiuretic hormone (ADH)

osmosis (oz-moh'-sis): passage of fluid through a membrane

osmotic pressure (oz-mot'-ik presh'-ur): pressure developed when two solutions of different concentrations of the solute are separated by a membrane permeable only to the solvent

ossa carpi (os'-sa kahr'-pye): the eight bones of the wrist

osseous (os'-ee-us): bony; composed of or resembling bone

ossicle (os'-ih-kul): a small bone; usually refers to the three small bones of the middle ear

ossification (os"-eh-fi-kay'-shun): process of bone formation

osteitis (os"-tee-eye'-tis): inflammation of bone tissue

osteoarthritis (os"-tee-oh-ahr-thry'-tis): degenerative joint disease

osteoblast (os'-tee-oh-blast): cells involved in formation of bony tissue

osteoclast (os'-tee-oh-klast): cells involved in resorption of bony tissue

osteocyte (os'-tee-oh-site): bone cell

osteomyelitis (os-tee-o-mi e-lit'-is): inflammation of the bone

osteoporosis (os"-tee-oh-pour-oh'-sis): loss of calcium in bone, causing brittleness, occurs mainly in females after menopause

osteosarcoma (os-tee-oh-sar-koh'-mah): bone cancer

otosclerosis (ah"-toh-skle-roh'-sis): chronic, progressive ear disorder in which the bone in the region of the oval window first becomes spongy and then hardened, causing the stirrup or stapes to become fixed or immobile.

ova (o'-va): female reproductive cell

ovary (o'-veh-ree): female reproductive organ produces ova, estrogen and progesterone

ovulation stage (ah"-vyoo-lay'-shun staydj): second stage of the menstrual cycle, when a ripe egg cell is released from an ovarian follicle cell

oxygenate (ok"-si-ji'-nate): to saturate a substance with oxygen, either by chemical combination or by mixture

oxyhemoglobin (ok"-see-hee'-muh-gloh"-bin): hemoglobin combined with oxygen

P

palate (pal'-ut): roof of the mouth

Pap or Papanicolaou (pap or pah"-peh-nik'-oh-low) smear: cytological, diagnostic cancer technique that studies exfoliated cells, especially those from the vagina

papilla (pa-pil'-uh): small, nipple-shaped elevations

palpitation (pal"-pah-tay'-shun): irregular, rapid, pulsation of the heart

pancreas (pan'-kree-as): organ of digestion lies behind the stomach, produces digestive juices, insulin, and glucagon

paralysis (pah-ral'-ih-sis): loss of power of motion or sensation

paraplegia (par"-eh-plee'-jee-a): complete paralysis of the lower body including both legs

parasympathetic nervous system (par'-ah-sim'-pah-thet'-ik nerv'-us sis'-tem): division of the autonomic nervous system inhibits or opposes the effects of the sympathetic nervous system

parathyroid gland (par"-uh-thiy'-royd gland): four small endocrine glands embedded in the thyroid gland; secretes parathormone

paresthesia (par"-es-theez'-shuh): preverted sensation of tingling, crawling, or burning of skin

parietal lobe (pah-ryi'ah-tel lobe): division of the cerebrum lies beneath the parietal bone

parietal membrane (pah-ryi'ah-tel mem'-brayn): the lining of a body cavity

Parkinson's disease (par'-kin-senz di-zeez'): marked tremors may be due to decrease of neurotransmitter dopamine

parotid gland (pah-rot'-id gland): largest of the salivary glands

passive acquired immunity (pas'-iv a-kwi'-erd i-mu'-ni-tee): borrowed immunity, has a temporary effect. i.e. gamma globulin

patella (pah-tel'-uh): kneecap

pathogenic (path"-uh-jen'-ik): disease-causing

pectoral (pek'-tuh-rul): pertaining to the chest

pelvis (pel'-vis): any basin-shaped structure or cavity

pericardium (per"-ih-kahr'-dee-um): closed membranous sac surrounding heart

peripheral (pe-rif'-eh-rul): outside surface, or the area away from the center

perineum (per'ah-nee-um): area between the vagina and the rectum

periodontal membrane (per-ee-o-dan'-tel mem'-brayn): membrane that anchors a tooth in place

periosteum (per-ee-os'-tee-um): fibrous tissue covering the bone

peripheral nervous system (pe-rif'-er-al): made up of 12 pairs of cranial nerves and 31 pairs of spinal nerves

peripheral vascular disease (pe-rif'-er-al vas'-kul-ar di-zeez'): blockage of arteries usually in the legs

peristalsis (per"-ih-stal'-sis): progressive wave of contraction in tubular structures provided with longitudinal and transverse muscular fibers, as in esophagus, stomach, small and large intestines

peritoneum (per-ih-toh'-nee-um): serous membrane lining of abdominal cavity

pernicious anemia (per-nish'-us a-nee'-mee-a): caused by decrease of B_{12} or lack of intrinsic factor in the stomach

pH: hydrogen ion concentration of solution or air mixture; potential of hydrogen

phagocyte (fag'-oh-sight): cell having property of engulfing and digesting foreign particles or cells harmful to body

phagocytosis (fag"-oh-si-toh'-sis): ingestion of foreign or other particles by certain cells

phalanges (fah-lan'-jez): bones of fingers and toes

pharynx (fair'-inks): throat

phase (faze): condition or stage of a disease or a biological, chemical, physiological, and psychological function at a given time

phenylketonuria (PKU) (fen"-il-kee-toh-new'-ree-uh): a metabolic disorder. The body cannot make an enzyme needed for normal metabolism or breakdown of the amino acid phenylalanine.

Excess phenylalanine will disrupt the normal development of neurons in the brain

phlebitis (fle-bye'-tis): inflammation of a vein, with or without infection and thrombus formation

phospholipids (fos'-foh-lip'-ids): fats which contain carbon, hydrogen, oxygen and phosphorous

phrenic nerve (fren'-ik nurv): stimulates the diaphragm

physiology (fiz"-ee-ol'-uh-jee): science that studies functions of living organisms and their parts

physiotherapy (fiz"-ee-oh-ther'-uh-pee): the treatment of disease and injury by physical means using light, heat, cold, water, electricity, massage, and exercise

pia mater (pee'-uh may'-tur): innermost vascular covering of brain and spinal cord

pigment (pig'-ment): (1) dye or coloring matter, (2) organic coloring matter of body

pineal gland (pin'-ee-al gland): located in the third ventricle of the brain produces melatonin

pinna (pin'-ah): outer ear

pinocytic vessel (pin"-oh-si'-tik ves'-el): formed by having the cell membrane fold inward to form a pocket

pinocytosis (pin"-oh-sye-toh'-sis): process of engulfing large molecules in solution and taking them into the cell

pituitary (pi-too'-e-tayr'-ee): a small gland located in the sphenoid bone in the cranium, its hormones effect all other glandular activity; it is called the master gland

pivot joint (piv'-et joynt): joint in which an extension of one bone rotates in a 2nd arch shaped bone

planes (planez): imaginary, anatomical dividing lines useful in separating body structures

plasma (plaz'-muh): liquid part of blood containing corpuscles

pleura (ploor'-uh): serous membrane enclosing lung and lining internal surface of thoracic cavity

pleurisy (ploor'-ih-see): inflammation of pleura

plexus (plek'-sus): a network of spinal nerves

pneumonia (noo-mon'-ya): infection of the lung

poliomyelitis (po"-le-o-mye-lye'-tis): disease of nerve pathways of spinal cord, rarely seen because of polio vaccines

polycythemia (pol"-eh-si-thee'-mee-ah): too many red blood cells

polydipsia (pol'-eh-dip'-see-ah): excessive thirst

polyphagia (pol'-e-fay'-jah): excessive hunger

polypnea (pol"-ip-nee'-uh): very rapid respiration or panting due to increased muscular activity or form emotional trauma

polysaccharide (pol"-ee-sak'-uh-ride): a complex sugar

polyuria (pol'-e-yoor'-ee-ah): excessive urination

pons (ponz): a part of the brainstem

popliteal (pop-lit'-ee-ul): area behind knee

pores (porz): (1) very small openings on a surface, (2) opening ducts of a sweat gland

portal circulation (por'-tul sir-kul-ay'-shun): brings blood from the organs of digestion through the portal vein to the liver

posterior (pos-teer'-ee-ur): located behind or at the back; opposite to anterior

presbyopia (prez"-bee-oh'-pee-uh): farsightedness of advanced age due to loss of elasticity in lens of eye

prime mover (prime muv'-er): muscle which provides movement in a single direction

progesterone (pro-jes'-tur-ohn): steroid hormone secreted by ovary from corpus luteum to help maintain pregnancy

prolapsed uterus (pro-lapst' yoo'-tur-us): normal supportive structures around the uterus weaken and allow the uterus to fall from its normal position

pronation (pro-nay'-shun): (1) condition of being prone, (2) turning of palm of hand downward

prophase (pro'-faze): phase two in the process of mitosis

prostaglandin (pros-tah-glan'-din): hormones secreted by various tissue, their function depends on which tissue they are excreted from

prostate gland (pros'-tate gland): gland located just under the urinary bladder; secretes a thin, milky alkaline fluid that enhances sperm motility

prostatectomy (pros"-tuh-tek'-tuh-mee): surgical removal of all or part of prostate

prostatic urethra (pros'-tat-ik yoo-ree'-thruh): area at the beginning of the urethra, surrounded by the prostate gland

protoplasm (pro'-tuh-plazm): living colloid material of the cell; contains proteins, lipids, inorganic salts and carbohydrates

proximal (prok'-sih-mul): located nearest the center of the body; point of attachment of a structure

pruritus (proo-rye'-tes): itching

psoriasis (so-rye'-ah-sis): chronic inflammatory skin disease with silvery patches

psychic (sigh'-kik): (1) pertaining to psyche, which is the mind or self as a functional unit, helping a person adjust to the changes, demands, or needs of the environment, (2) sensitive to nonphysical forces, (3) mental

puberty (pew'-bur-tee): age when reproductive organs become functional

pubis (pew'-bis): pubic bone, portion of hipbone forming front of pelvis

pupil (pew'-pil): opening in iris of eye for passage of light

pulp cavity (pulp kav'-ih-tee): inside of the tooth contains blood vessels and nerve

pulmonary artery (pool-'ma-ner-ee ar'-ter-ee): structure takes blood from the right ventricle to the lungs

pulmonary veins (pool-'ma-ner-ee vayns): structure which takes blood from the lungs to the right atrium

pulse (puls): measures the number of times the heart beats per minute

Purkinje fibers (per-kin'-jee fye'-burs): conduction fibers which conduct the impulses through the ventricles of the heart

pus (pus): a product of inflammation; a cream-colored liquid that is a combination of dead tissue, dead and living bacteria, dead white blood cells, and blood plasma

pyelonephritis (pye-loh-nef-right'-is): inflammation of the kidneys and the pelvis of the ureter

pylorus (pye-lo'-rus): circular opening of stomach into duodenum

pyrexia (pye-rek'-see-uh): fever

pyrogen (pye'-ra-jen): any fever-producing agent

pyuria (pi-yoor'ee-a): pus in the urine

R

radioactive (ra'dee-oh-ak'tiv): capable of emitting energy in the form of radiation

radius (ra'-dee-us): bone on the thumb side of the forearm

receptor (ree-sep'-tur): sensory nerve that receives a stimulus and transmits it to the CNS

red muscle (red mus'-ul): muscle that appears red in fresh state due to presence of muscle hemoglobin

reflex (ree'-fleks): involuntary action; automatic response

reflex arc (ree'-fleks ahrk): pathway travelled by an impulse during reflex action, going from receptor to effector

reflux (ree'-fluks): return flow

rehabilitation (ree-ha-bil-eh-tay'-shun): the process of restoring function through therapeutic exercise

renal (ree'-nul): pertaining to the kidney

renal pelvis (ree'-nul pel'-vis): funnel shaped structure at the beginning of the ureter

rennin (ren'-in): milk-coagulating enzyme found in gastric juice of ruminating animals, not present in the human stomach

replication (rep"-li-kay'-shun): occurs when an exact copy of each nuclear chromosome is made during the early part of the first stage of mitosis (early interphase)

respiratory distress syndrome (res'-peh-ruh-tor-ee dis-tres' sin'-drome): condition that generally affects premature babies; characterized by the formation of a hyaline-like false membrane within the alveoli which causes the alveoli to collapse

retina (ret'-in-ah): innermost layer of the eye contains the rods and cones

retroperitoneal (ret"-ro-per"-i-toh-nee'-ul): located behind the peritoneum

RH factor (R H fak'-tor): antigen found in red blood cells

rheumatoid arthritis (roo'-mah-toyd arth-ri'-tis) chronic inflammatory disease affects connective tissue and joints

rhinorrhea (rye"-noh-ree'-uh): discharge of thin, watery fluid from the nose

RHOgam: specific preparation of immune globulin given

rhinitis (rih-ni'-tis): inflammation of the lining of the nose

ribonucleic acid (rye'-boh-noo-kley'-ik as'-id): RNA, type of nucleic acid

ribosome (rye'-bo-sohm): submicroscopic particle attached to endoplasmic reticulum, site of protein synthesis in cytoplasm of cell

rickets (rik'-its): bones become soft due to lack of Vitamin D

ringworm (ring'-worm): contagious fungal infection with raised circular patches

rods (rodz): cells in the retina, sensitive to dim light

rotation (roh-tay'-shun): allows a bone to move around a central axis

roughage (raftage) (ruf'-aj): the coarse parts of certain foods that are undigestible and stimulate peristalses

rugae (roo'-jee): wrinkles or folds

rule of nines (rule of nines): measures the percent of the body burned

S

sacroiliac joint (say"-kro-il'-ee-ak joynt): joint between sacrum and ilium

sacrum (sa'-krum): wedge shaped bone below the lumbar vertebra at the end of the spinal column

sagittal (sadj'-ih-tul): longitudinal; shaped like an arrow

sarcoplasm (sahr'-ko-plazm): the hyaline or finely granular interfibrillar material of muscle tissue

salt (salt): compound formed when a negative ion of acid combines with a positive ion of a base

salivary gland (sal'-ah-ver-ee gland): gland located in the mouth that secretes saliva, there are three pairs namely parotid, submandible and sublingual

sarcolemma (sar-koh'-lem-mah): muscle cell membrane

sartorius (sahr-to'-ree-us): thigh muscle

scapula (skap'-yoo-luh): large, flat, triangular bone forming back of shoulder

scar *see* cicatrix

sciatic nerve (siy-at'-ik nurv): largest nerve in the body originates in the sacral plexus, runs through the pelvis and down the leg

sciatica (siy-at'-ik-ah): neuritis of the sciatic nerve

second degree burn *see* burn

sclera (skleer'-uh): tough, white covering, part of external coat of eye

scoliosis (skoh"-lee-oh'-sis): lateral curvature of the spine

scrotum (skro'-tum): pouch that contains the testicles

sebaceous gland (se-bay'-shus gland): gland that secretes sebum, a fatty material

sebum (see'-bum): secretion of sebaceous glands that lubricate the skin

secretin (se-kree'-tin): hormone secreted by the epithelial cells that line the duodenum; stimulated by the acidic gastric juice and the partially digested proteins from the stomach.

sedimentation rate (sed"-e-men-tay'shun rate): time it takes red blood cells to settle to the bottom in an upright tube

selective semipermeable membrane (se-lek'-tiv sem"-ih-per'-mee-ah-bul mem'-brayn): the cell membrane regulates the passage of certain material in and out of the cell

sella turcica (sel'-uh tur'-si-kuh): saddle-shaped depression in sphenoid bone

semen (see'-mun): male reproductive fluid containing sperm

semi-circular canals (sem'-ih-sir'-kuh-lar kan-als'): structures in the inner ear involved with equilibrium

sensory neuron (sen'-soh-ree neur'-on): *see* afferent neuron

semilunar (sem"-ih-lew'-nur): half-moon shaped valve of aorta and pulmonary artery

seminal vesicles (sem'-i-nul ves'-i-kuls): two highly convoluted membranous tubes that produce substances found to help nourish and protect sperm on its journey up the female reproductive system

senescence (se-nes'-unce): old age; senility

septicemia (sep"-tih-see'-mee-a): presence of pathogenic organisms in the blood

septum (sep'-tum): partition; dividing wall between two spaces or cavities, such as the septum between left and right side of heart or nose

serous fluid (seer'-us floo'-id): (1) normal lymph fluid, (2) thin, watery body fluid

serous membrane (seer'-us mem'-brayn): a double walled membrane which produces serous fluid

serum (seer'-um): clear, pale yellow fluid that separates from a clot of blood; plasma that contains no fibrinogen

shaft (shaft): (1) part of the hair which extends from the skin surface; (2) the diaphysis of the long bone

shin splints (shin splintz): injury to muscle tendon in front of the shins

shingles (shing'-elz): herpes zoster, a virus infection of the nerve endings

sickle-cell anemia (sick'-ul sel uh-nee'-mee-uh): blood disorder. The shape of the red blood cell is a sickle shape, which makes the red blood cells clump together.

sigmoid (sig'-moyd): shaped like the letter S; distal, S-shaped part of colon

silicosis (sil'-ah-koh'sis): lung condition caused by breathing dust containing silicon dioxide; lungs become fibrotic

sinoatrial node (sigh"-no-ay'-tree-ul node): dense network of fibers of conduction at junction of superior vena cava and right atrium

sinus (sigh'-nus): recessed cavity or hollow space

skeletal muscle (skel'-e-tul mus'-ul): muscle attached to a bone or bones of skeleton and concerned in body movements; also known as voluntary or striated muscle

slipped disc (slipt disk): a cartilage disc between the vertebra ruptures or protrudes out of place

smooth muscle (smooth mus'-ul): non-striated, involuntary muscle

sneezing (sneez'ing): deep breath followed by exhalation from the nose

solute (sol'-yoot): dissolved substance in a solution

somatic cell (soh-mat'-ik sel): all of the body cells except for sex cells (egg and sperm)

somatotropin (soh'-ma-te-troh'-fin): growth hormone

spastic quadriplegia (spas'-tik kwod'-re-plee'-ja): spastic paralysis of all four limbs

sperm (spurm) the reproductive cell of the male

spermatic cord (spur-mat'-ik kord): the cord that extends from the testis to the deep inguinal ring; contains the ductus deferens, the blood vessels and nerves of the testis and epididymis, and the surrounding connective tissue

spermatogenesis (spur'-mat'-ah-jen'ah-sis): the process of the formation of sperm

sphenoid (sfen'-oid): the key bone of the skull

sphincter (sfink'-tur): circular muscle, such as the anus

spina bifida (spye'-nuh bye'-fi-duh): congenital defect in closure of spinal canal with hernial protrusion of meninges of spinal cord

spinal cord (spye'-nel kord): part of the central nervous system within the spinal column, begins at foramen magnum of occipital bone and continues to the second lumbar vertebra

spinal nerve (spye'-nul nurv): thirty one pairs, originate in the spinal cord

spleen (spleen): lymph organ situated below and behind the stomach

splenomegaly (splen-oh-meg'-ah-lee): enlarged spleen

spondylitis (spon"-di-lye'-tis): inflammation of the vertebrae

spongy bone (spon'-jee bone): when hard bone is broken down it leaves spongy bone

sprain (sprayn): wrenching of a joint, producing a stretching or laceration of ligaments

squamous cell cancer (skwa'-mes sel kan'-ser): cancer of the epidermis

Standard Precautions (stand'-ard pre-caw'-shuns): guidelines to be used during patient care and cleaning

stapes (stay'-peez): stirrup-shaped bone in middle ear

steapsin (stee-ap'-sin): pancreatic lipase

sterile (ster'-el): incapable of reproducing, or free from bacteria or other microorganisms

sternocleidomastoid (stur"-no-klyd-o-mas'-toyd): large muscle extends down side of neck

sternum (stur'-num): flat, narrow bone in median line in front of chest, composed of three parts: manubrium, body, and xiphoid process

steroid (ster'-oyd): lipids or fats which contain cholesterol

stethoscope (steth'-uh-skope): instrument used for detection and study of sounds arising within body

stomach (stum'-ik): a major organ of digestion, a pouch-like structure located in the upper left quadrant of the abdominal cavity, between the esophagus and the duodenum

stomatitis (sto-me-tiy'-tis): inflammation of the mucous membrane of the mouth

stimulus (stim'-ye-lus): any change in environment

strain (strayn): tear in a muscle or stress

stroke *see* CVA

sty (stye): infection of gland along the eyelid

subluxation (sub"-luk-say'-shun): incomplete dislocation

sudoriferous (sue"-dur-if'-ur-us): producing perspiration

sulci (sul'-ce): fissure or grooves separating cerebral convolutions

superior (sue-peer'-ee-ur): in anatomy, higher; denoting upper of two parts, toward vertex

supination (sue-pih-nay'-shun): turning of palm of hand upward, condition of being supine (lying on back)

surfactant (sur-fak'-tunt): surface-active agent

suture (sue'-chur): (1) in osteology, a line of connection or closure between bones, as in a cranial suture. (2) in surgery, a fine thread-like catgut or silk—used to repair or close a wound

sympathetic nervous system (sim-pah-theh'-tik ner'-vus sis'-tem): division of autonomic nervous system

synapse (sin'-aps): space between adjacent neurons through which an impulse is transmitted

synaptic cleft (si-nap'-tik kleft): space between the axon of one neuron and the dendrite of another

synarthroses (sin-ar-thro'-ses): immovable joints connected by fibrous connective tissue

synergist (sin'-er-jist): muscles which help steady a joint

synovia (si-noh'-vee-uh): viscid fluid present in joint cavities

synovial membrane (si-noh'-vee-al mem'-brayn): double layer of connective tissue lines joint cavities and produces synovial fluid

synthesis (sin'-the-sis): in chemistry, processes and operations necessary to build up a compound; in general, a reaction, or series of reactions, in which a complex compound is obtained from elements or simple compounds

syphilis (sif'-eh-lis): infectious disease transmitted by sexual contact

systole (sis'-tuh-lee): contraction of ventricles, forcing blood into aorta and pulmonary artery

T

tachycardia (tak"-i-kahr'-dee-uh): abnormally rapid heartbeat

tachypnea (tack-ip'-nee-uh): abnormally rapid rate of breathing

talus (tay'-lus): ankle bone that articulates with bones of leg

tarsals (tahr'-sals): ankle bones

tarsus (tahr'-sus): instep

Tay-Sachs disease (tay-saks' di-zeez'): genetic mutation caused by lack of a particular enzyme (hexosaminidase) needed for the breakdown of lipid molecules in the brain

taste buds (tayst budz): cells on the papillae of the tongue which can distinguish salt, bitter, sweet and sour qualities of dissolved substances

telephase (tel'-ah-faze): final stage in the mitosis process

temporal (tem'-per-el): side of the head

temporal lobe (tem'-per-el lobe): part of the cerebral hemisphere associated with the perception and interpretation of sound

tendon (ten'-dun): cord of fibrous connective tissue that attaches a muscle to a bone or other structure

tennis elbow (ten'-is el'-boh): inflammation of the tendon which connects the arm muscles to the elbow

testes (tes'-tis): male reproductive organ produces sperm and testosterone

testosterone (tes-tos'-te-rohn): male sex hormone responsible for male secondary sex characteristics

tetanus (tet'-uh-nus): infectious disease, usually fatal, characterized by spasm of voluntary muscles and convulsions caused by toxin from tetanus bacillus (clostridium tetani)

thalamus (thal'-a-mus): part of the diencephalon, relays sensory stimuli to the cerebral cortex

third degree burn see burn

third ventricle see cerebral ventricle

thoracocentesis (thor"-ruh-koh-sen-tee'-sis): aspiration of chest cavity for removal of fluid, usually for empyema

thorax (tho'-raks): chest; portion of trunk above diaphragm and below neck

thrombin (throm'-bin): enzyme found in blood; produced from an inactive precursor, prothrombin, inducing clotting by converting fibrinogen to fibrin

thrombocyte (throm'-bah-site): platelet, part of megakaryocyte cells necessary for blood clotting

thrombocytopenia (throm"-bah-siy-toh-pen'-ee-ah): decrease in the number of platelets

thromboplastin (throm'-boh-plas-tin): substance secreted by platelets when tissue is injured; necessary for blood clotting

thrombosis (throm-boh'-sis): formation of a clot in a blood vessel

thrombus (throm'-bus): blood clot formed in a blood vessel

thymus (thiy'-mus): endocrine located under the sternum, produces T-lymphocytes

thyroid gland (thiy'-royd gland): endocrine gland located on anterior portion of the neck produces thyroxine triiodothyronine and calcitonin

thyroxine (thigh-rok'-seen): hormone secreted by thyroid gland or prepared synthetically

TIA (t-i-a): transient ischemic attacks, temporary interruption of the blood flow in the brain

tibia (tib'-ee-uh): larger, inner bone of the leg, below the knee

tinnitis (tin-i'-tus): ringing sensation in one or both ears

tissue (tish'-yoo): cells grouped according to size, shape and function, epithelial, connective, muscle, and nerve

tonsils (ton'-silz): mass of lymph tissue in the back of the throat which produces lymphocytes

torticollis (tor-ti-kol'-is): a contracted state of the neck muscles producing an unnatural position of the head;also called wryneck

trachea (tray'-kee-ah): a thin walled tube between the larynx and the bronchi, conducts air to the lungs

trait (trate): any characteristic, feature, quality, or property of an organism

transmit (tranz'-mit): to pass on to another person, place, or thing

transverse (trans-vurse'): crosswise; at right angles to longitudinal axis of body

triceps (tri'-seps): three-headed muscle on back of upper arm

tricuspid valve (tri-kus'-pid valv): three part valve located between the right atrium and right ventricle

trigeminal neuralgia (tri-jem'-i-nel noo-ral'-ja): painful condition affecting the fifth cranial nerve also known as "tic douloureux"

true ribs (tru ribz): first seven pairs of ribs which are attached to the sternum by costal cartilage

trypsin (trip'-sin): one of four protein-digesting enzymes found in pancreatic juice

trypsinogen (trip-sin'-uh-jen): the inactive form of trypsin. In the small intestine, trypsinogen is converted to trypsin by the influence of enterokinase, an intestinal enzyme that is secreted by glands lining the small intestine

tuberculosis (too-bur"-kya-loh'-sis): infectious disease caused by tubercule bacillus, mainly affects lung

tumor (too'-mer): abnormal and uncontrolled growth of cell

tunica (too'-ni-kah): layer of tissue found in the blood vessels and specified as tunica adventitia, the outer lining; tunica media, the middle lining and tunica interna, the inner lining

tunica albuginea (tew'-ni-kuh al-bew-jin'-ee-uh): fibrous tissue covering the testes

turbinate (tur'-bin-ut): shaped like a spiral; the three bones situated on the lateral side of the nasal cavity

tympanic membrane (tim-pan'-ik mem'-brayn): membrane that separates the external ear from the middle ear

U

ulcer (ul'-sur): an inflammation that occurs on the mucosal skin surface

ulna (ul'-nuh): bone on inner forearm

umbilicus (um-bil'-i-kus): navel

unicellular (yoo"-nih-sel'-yoo-lur): composed of one cell

unilateral (you"-nih-lat'-ur-ul): pertaining to, or affecting, one side

universal donor (yoo-ih-ver'-sal do'-nur): type O blood; has no A or B antigens; can be donated to all blood types

universal recipient (yoo"-nih-vur'-sul re-sip'-ee-unt): individual belonging to AB blood group

uremia (yoo-ree'-mee-ah): the presence of urea and excess waste products in the blood

ureter (yoor'-ah-ter): the long narrow tube that conveys urine from the kidney to the urinary bladder

urethra (yoo-re'-thra): the tube which takes urine from the bladder to the outside of the body

urinalysis (yoor-i-nal'-ah-sis): the chemical analysis of urine

urinary bladder (yoor'-i-ner-ee blad'-er): a muscular membrane lined sac situated in the anterior part of the pelvic cavity and used to hold urine

urinary meatus (yoor'-i-ner-ee mee'-tus): the opening to the urethra

urtocaria (ur"-ti-kar'-ee-a): skin condition characterized by itching wheals or welts and usually caused by an allergic reaction also known as "hives"

uvula (yoo'-vew-luh): projection hanging from soft palate, in back of throat

V

vacuole (vak'-yoo-ole): (1) clear space in cell, (2) cavity bound by a single membrane; usually a storage area for fat, glycogen, secretions, liquid, or debris

vagina (va-jie'-nuh): sheathlike structure; tube in females, extending from the uterus to the vulva

vaginitis (vadj"-i-nigh'-tis): inflammation of the vagina

valve (valv): structure which permits flow of a fluid in only one direction

varicose veins (var'-i-kose vayns): veins that have become abnormally dilated and tortuous, due to interference with venous drainage or weakness of their walls

vasopressin (vay"-zo-pres'-in): hormone secreted by the posterior pituitary gland; has an antidiuretic effect. Also called antidiuretic hormone (ADH)

vein (vane): vessel which carries blood toward the heart

vena cava (ve'-nah ka'-vah): large blood vessel that returns blood to the right atrium; there are two: superior and inferior

ventral (ven'-trul): front or anterior; opposite of posterior or dorsal

ventricle (ven'-trik-ul): small cavity or chamber, as in heart or brain

venule (ven'-yoo-ul): small vein

vermiform appendix (vur'-mi-form a-pen'-diks): small, blind gut projecting from cecum

vertigo (vur'-ti-go): sensation of dizziness

villi (vil'-eye): hairlike projections, as in intestinal mucous membrane

viscera (vis'-er-ah): internal organs

visceral membrane (vis'-er-al mem'-brayn): the membrane covering each organ in a body cavity

vitamin (vye'-tuh-min): any of a group of organic compounds found in very small amounts in natural food; needed for the normal growth and maintenance of an organism

vitreous humor (vit'-ree-us hew'-mur): transparent, gelatin-like substance filling greater part of eyeball

voluntary (vol'-un-ter"-ee): under control of the will

vomer (vo'-mer): flat thin bone that forms part of the nasal septum

W

whiplash injury (wip'lash in'-jer-ee): trauma to cervical vertebra

white muscle (white mus'-ul): skeletal muscle that appears paler in fresh state than red muscle

whooping cough (hoop'-ing kof): infectious disease characterized by repeated coughing attacks that end in a "whooping" sound. Also called *pertussis*.

wisdom tooth (wiz'-dum tooth): third molar tooth in adult mouth

Z

zona pellucida (so'-nuh pe-lew'-si-duh): thick, solid, elastic envelope of ovum

zygote (zye'-gote): organism produced by union of two gametes

INDEX

License Agreement for Delmar Publishers
an International Thomson Publishing company

Educational Software/Data

You the customer, and Delmar incur certain benefits, rights, and obligations to each other when you open this package and use the software/data it contains. BE SURE YOU READ THE LICENSE AGREEMENT CAREFULLY, SINCE BY USING THE SOFTWARE/DATA YOU INDICATE YOU HAVE READ, UNDERSTOOD, AND ACCEPTED THE TERMS OF THIS AGREEMENT.

Your rights:

1. You enjoy a non-exclusive license to use the enclosed software/data on a single microcomputer that is not part of a network or multi-machine system in consideration for payment of the required license fee, (which may be included in the purchase price of an accompanying print component), or receipt of this software/data, and your acceptance of the terms and conditions of this agreement.

2. You own the media on which the software/data is recorded, but you acknowledge that you do not own the software/data recorded on them. You also acknowledge that the software/data is furnished "as is," and contains copyrighted and/or proprietary and confidential information of Delmar Publishers or its licensors.

3. If you do not accept the terms of this license agreement you may return the media within 30 days. However, you may not use the software during this period.

There are limitations on your rights:

1. You may not copy or print the software/data for any reason whatsoever, except to install it on a hard drive on a single microcomputer and to make one archival copy, unless copying or printing is expressly permitted in writing or statements recorded on the diskette(s).

2. You may not revise, translate, convert, disassemble or otherwise reverse engineer the software/data except that you may add to or rearrange any data recorded on the media as part of the normal use of the software/data.

3. You may not sell, license, lease, rent, loan, or otherwise distribute or network the software/data except that you may give the software/data to a student or and instructor for use at school or, temporarily at home.

Should you fail to abide by the Copyright Law of the United States as it applies to this software/data your license to use it will become invalid. You agree to erase or otherwise destroy the software/data immediately after receiving note of Delmar Publishers' termination of this agreement for violation of its provisions.

Delmar Publishers gives you a LIMITED WARRANTY covering the enclosed software/data. The LIMITED WARRANTY can be found in this product and/or the instructor's manual that accompanies it.

This license is the entire agreement between you and Delmar Publishers interpreted and enforced under New York law.

Limited Warranty

Delmar Publishers warrants to the original licensee/purchaser of this copy of microcomputer software/data and the media on which it is recorded that the media will be free from defects in material and workmanship for ninety (90) days from the date of original purchase. All implied warranties are limited in duration to this ninety (90) day period. THEREAFTER, ANY IMPLIED WARRANTIES, INCLUDING IMPLIED WARRANTIES OF MERCHANTABILITY AND FITNESS FOR A PARTICULAR PURPOSE ARE EXCLUDED. THIS WARRANTY IS IN LIEU OF ALL OTHER WARRANTIES, WHETHER ORAL OR WRITTEN, EXPRESSED OR IMPLIED.

If you believe the media is defective, please return it during the ninety day period to the address shown below. A defective diskette will be replaced without charge provided that it has not been subjected to misuse or damage.

This warranty does not extend to the software or information recorded on the media. The software and information are provided "AS IS." Any statements made about the utility of the software or information are not to be considered as express or implied warranties. Delmar will not be liable for incidental or consequential damages of any kind incurred by you, the consumer, or any other user.

Some states do not allow the exclusion or limitation of incidental or consequential damages, or limitations on the duration of implied warranties, so the above limitation or exclusion may not apply to you. This warranty gives you specific legal rights, and you may also have other rights which vary from state to state. Address all correspondence to:

Delmar Publishers
3 Columbia Circle
P. O. Box 15015
Albany, NY 12212-5015